A GUIDE TO THE CLINICAL CARE OF WOMEN WITH HIV

2000 Preliminary Edition

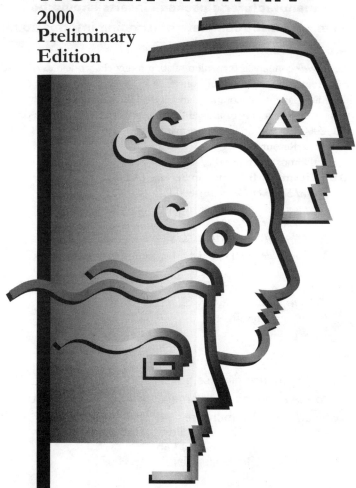

Edited by Jean Anderson, MD

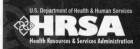

U.S. Department of Health & Human Services
HRSA
Health Resources & Services Administration

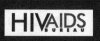

This *Guide* contains information relating to general principles of medical care which should not be construed as specific instructions for individual patients. Recommendations for HIV care change frequently, so the care provider is cautioned that this preliminary edition is dated May, 2000. To find updated information, consult the listings in Chapter XV on Resources.

For the most current HIV/AIDS treatment guidelines, contact the **AIDS Treatment Information Service (ATIS):**

United States & Canada: 1-800-HIV-0440

Fax number: 1-301-519-6616

TTY: 1-888-480-3739

International: 1-301-519-0459

Mailing Address: HIV/AIDS Treatment Information Service
P.O. Box 6303
Rockville, MD 20849-6303

Web site: http://hivatis.org

E-mail: atis@hivatis.org

Send Us Your Comments

E-mail: womencare@hrsa.gov

Fax to the attention of "Womencare": 301-443-0791 (USA)

Postal address: Womencare
Parklawn Building, Room 11A-33
5600 Fishers Lane
Rockville, Maryland 20857
USA

Note that this and subsequent editions of
A Guide to the Clinical Care of Women with HIV
will be available online.

Go to the HIV/AIDS Bureau Web site
and click on the publication *Women's Guide*:
http://www.hrsa.gov/hab

Dedication

A Guide to the Clinical Care of Women with HIV
is dedicated to Donna M. Davis, who died in June 1999.
She worked to improve the lives of women
both in the U.S. and globally.

ACKNOWLEDGEMENTS

A number of people made this *Guide* possible. Joan Holloway's vision provided the framework for the *Guide's* inception and development. Magda Barini-García, MD, the Project Officer, skillfully shepherded and oversaw the project. Helen Schietinger, the Project Manager, coordinated the entire process masterfully and brought it to fruition. Others whose work was essential include staff from HRSA's HIV/AIDS Burearu, Tom Flavin and Brad Read of the Office of Communications, and Carole McGeehan of the DHHS Program Support Center's Media Arts Branch. Carole's work on design, layout, and final production of the *Guide* was artful and invaluable.

For sale by the U.S. Government Printing Office
Superintendent of Documents, Mail Stop: SSOP, Washington, DC 20402-9328

ISBN 0-16-050394-9

ISBN 0-16-050394-9

90000

9 780160 503948

CONTRIBUTING AUTHORS

SILVIA M ABULARACH, MD, MPH
ASSISTANT PROFESSOR
DIVISION OF GYNECOLOGIC ONCOLOGY
JOHNS HOPKINS SCHOOL OF MEDICINE
BALTIMORE, MD

CARLA S. ALEXANDER, MD
ASSISTANT PROFESSOR OF MEDICINE
UNIVERSITY OF MARYLAND SCHOOL OF MEDICINE
BALTIMORE, MD

JEAN ANDERSON, MD
ASSOCIATE PROFESSOR
GYNECOLOGY AND OBSTETRICS
JOHNS HOPKINS SCHOOL OF MEDICINE
BALTIMORE, MD

BARBARA ARANDA-NARANJO, PHD, RN, FAAN
CHIEF, DEMONSTRATION PROJECT DEVELOPMENT AND EVALUATION BRANCH
HIV/AIDS BUREAU, HEALTH RESOURCES AND SERVICES ADMINISTRATION
ROCKVILLE, MD

PATRICIA BARDITCH-CROVO, MD
ASSISTANT PROFESSOR
DIVISION OF INFECTIOUS DISEASES
THE JOHNS HOPKINS SCHOOL OF MEDICINE
BALTIMORE, MD

VICTORIA A CARGILL, MD, MSCE
OFFICE OF AIDS RESEARCH
NATIONAL INSTITUTES OF HEALTH
BETHESDA, MD

LAURA CHEEVER, MD
CHIEF, HIV EDUCATION BRANCH
HIV/AIDS BUREAU, HEALTH RESOURCES AND SERVICES ADMINISTRATION
ROCKVILLE, MD

CONNIE CELUM, MD, MPH
ASSOCIATE PROFESSOR OF MEDICINE
UNIVERSITY OF WASHINGTON
SEATTLE, WA

RACHEL DAVIS, RN
CLINIC COORDINATOR
SOUTH TEXAS FAMILY AIDS NETWORK
UNIVERSITY OF TEXAS HEALTH SCIENCE CENTER
SAN ANTONIO, TX

JUDITH FEINBERG, MD
PROFESSOR OF MEDICINE
UNIVERSITY OF CINCINNATI COLLEGE OF MEDICINE
CINCINNATI, OHIO

HENRY L. FRANCIS, M.D.
DIRECTOR, CENTER ON AIDS AND OTHER MEDICAL CONSEQUENCES OF DRUG ABUSE
(CAMCODA)
NATIONAL INSTITUTE ON DRUG ABUSE
BETHESDA, MD

DONNA FUTTERMAN, MD
ASSOCIATE PROFESSOR OF PEDIATRICS
ALBERT EINSTEIN COLLEGE OF MEDICINE
BRONX, NY

RUTH GREENBLATT, MD
PROFESSOR OF MEDICINE, EPIDEMIOLOGY AND BIOSTATISTICS
UNIVERSITY OF CALIFORNIA AT SAN FRANCISCO
SAN FRANCISCO, CA

NANCY A. HESSOL, MSPH
DEPARTMENT OF MEDICINE
UNIVERSITY OF CALIFORNIA, SAN FRANCISCO
SAN FRANCISCO, CA

JOYCE SEIKO KOBAYASHI, M.D.
ASSOCIATE PROFESSOR
UNIVERSITY OF COLORADO HEALTH SCIENCES CENTER
DENVER, COLORADO

RANI LEWIS, MD
ASSOCIATE PROFESSOR
DEPARTMENT OF OBSTETRICS AND GYNECOLOGY
VANDERBILT UNIVERSITY MEDICAL CENTER
NASHVILLE, TN

JANINE MAENZA, MD
ACTING ASSISTANT PROFESSOR, MEDICINE.
DIVISION OF ALLERGY AND INFECTIOUS DISEASES
UNIVERSITY OF WASHINGTON
SEATTLE, WA

PAUL PHAM, PharmD
RESEARCH ASSOCIATE
DIVISION OF INFECTIOUS DISEASE
JOHNS HOPKINS UNIVERSITY
BALTIMORE, MD

CHIA C WANG, MD, MS
UNIVERSITY OF WASHINGTON
SEATTLE, WA

TABLE OF CONTENTS

FORWARD
Joseph F O'Neill, MD, MPH

Dear Colleagues:

The Ryan White CARE Act program of the Health Resources and Services Administration is pleased to make this *Guide* available to clinicians caring for women living with HIV/AIDS. We believe it is the first comprehensive clinical manual on this topic, and the need for such a guide has never been greater. The World Health Organization estimates that the number of people living with HIV/AIDS is rapidly approaching 50 million, and that women constitute 45%–50% of the total. Already, in several regions of the world, more than half of the people living with HIV/AIDS are women. But these statistics tell only part of the story. In addition to facing unique clinical issues, women living with HIV/AIDS are often challenged by social isolation, poverty, discrimination, and lack of access to quality health care.

Please note that this *Guide* for the care of women has been written almost entirely by women. This is testimony to the enormous contribution that women have made in the battle against HIV/AIDS on every front and in every community across the globe. However, no medical guide can stand alone in assuring that women will receive the best treatment available. In addition to furthering our clinical knowledge, we must commit ourselves to addressing the myriad social and economic issues that hamper effective prevention and access to care for seropositive women.

Regard this preliminary edition as "our" *Guide*. It belongs to the global community of clinicians who struggle daily with HIV/AIDS, caring for people with competence, compassion and equality. Your comments, criticisms and suggestions are needed to shape this manual into a clinical tool that will be of maximum utility to all of us. Throughout the *Guide* you will find requests for your input. Please respond by post, fax, or e-mail. And, if you can, suggest partners who can help have this *Guide* translated into the many languages of "our" community.

We all owe a debt of gratitude to John G. Bartlett, M.D. His guide, *1999 Medical Management of HIV Infection* was the inspiration and template for this volume. He graciously allowed us to adapt many of the charts and algorithms for this book.

Finally, I want offer my personal thanks to the editor, Jean Anderson, M.D., for her tireless dedication and perseverance in creating this *Guide*. Her efforts have made a profound change possible. This *Guide*, I believe, will mark a turning point in significantly improving the care of women living with HIV/AIDS.

Cordially,

Joseph F. O'Neill, MD, MPH
Director, HIV/AIDS Bureau
Health Resources and Services Administration,
U.S. Department of Health and Human Services

Send Us Your Comments

E-mail: womencare@hrsa.gov

Fax to the attention of "Womencare": 301-443-0791 (USA)

Postal address: Womencare
　　　　　　　　Parklawn Building, Room 11A-33
　　　　　　　　5600 Fishers Lane
　　　　　　　　Rockville, Maryland 20857
　　　　　　　　USA

Note that this and subsequent editions of
A Guide to the Clinical Care of Women with HIV
will be available online.

Go to the HIV/AIDS Bureau Web site
and click on the publication *Women's Guide*:
http://www.hrsa.gov/hab

INTRODUCTION
Jean Anderson, MD

Despite the dramatic advances made in understanding the natural history of HIV disease and the development of effective antiretroviral therapies, the AIDS epidemic continues to grow. And that growth has displayed some disturbing trends. HIV/AIDS morbidity and mortality increasingly impact the poor, the disenfranchised, and the young. Women are traditionally over-represented in these groups.

The growing number of women living with HIV/AIDS is a dominant feature of the evolving epidemic. In addition, because they are often diagnosed later and generally have poorer access to care and medications, women tend to have higher viral loads and lower CD4 counts. Women living with HIV/AIDS also must contend with vulnerability related to reproductive issues and domestic violence. Finally, women living with HIV/AIDS are usually relied upon to meet the care needs of children and other family members, many of whom are also HIV-positive.

For these, and other reasons, a manual addressing the primary care needs unique to women with HIV infection is long overdue. This manual represents an attempt to fill this gap. Our target audiences are clinicians who provide primary care to women. This *Guide* might also be of interest to individuals seeking a more in-depth understanding of how to care for women with HIV/AIDS.

The book you have in your hands is a preliminary edition, a work in progress, and we welcome your comments and suggestions. Please send any feedback to the postal, fax, or e-mail addresses found throughout the book and on the inside covers. We are particularly eager for this *Guide* to be translated into other languages. Please let us know if you can help or suggest partners.

This preliminary edition is focused primarily on the problems facing HIV-infected women in the developed nations, primarily the U.S. Our goal is that in future editions of this *Guide* we can take a more global perspective and address the care of women with HIV/AIDS in both developed and developing nations.

I want to offer my personal thanks to Helen Schietinger and Magda Barini-García for their championing this *Guide* throughout its development, displaying enormous tact, tenacity, and attention to detail. Without them, this manual would never have been published.

Finally, we want to acknowledge the women with HIV/AIDS who have been the inspiration for this manual. Their strength is celebrated and their struggle is not forgotten. We offer this *Guide* as a tribute to them, and to the providers who have taken on this struggle and made it their own.

Jean Anderson, MD
Editor

I. EPIDEMIOLOGY AND NATURAL HISTORY OF HIV INFECTION IN WOMEN

Ruth M. Greenblatt, MD and Nancy A. Hessol, MSPH

I. INTRODUCTION

The successful introduction and spread of the human immunodeficiency virus (HIV) into the global human population has occurred for many reasons. The discovery and wide spread use of penicillin and other antibiotics meant that there was treatment and cure for most sexually transmitted diseases. The existence of these new drugs changed how people perceived risks associated with sexual activity. Soldiers in World War II increasingly used prophylactics and the subsequent development of hormonal contraceptives hastened the pace of change in sexual practices, as prevention of pregnancy became a real possibility. Lifestyles also were changing: people were moving into regions that were previously uninhabited by man and long distance travel became easier and was much more common, allowing for more social migration and sexual mixing. Although the virus may have first been introduced to humans earlier in the 20th century (most likely contracted from infected animals), it was in the 1970's that wider dissemination occurred.

For industrialized countries, the first evidence of the AIDS epidemic was among groups of individuals who shared a common exposure risk. In the United States, sexually active homosexual men were among the first to present with manifestations of HIV disease, followed by recipients of blood or blood products, then injection drug users, and ultimately children of mothers at risk. Women have represented an increasing proportion of reported AIDS cases in the United States, accounting for 23% of adult cases from July 1998–June 1999. (CDC, 1999) Eighty percent of AIDS cases in women are in African Americans and Hispanics, as compared to 61% of cases in men.

In developing countries, the AIDS epidemic manifested itself quite differently, both because the signs and symptoms were harder to identify due to other competing causes of morbidity and mortality and because the epidemic did not seem to be limited to "high-risk" groups and, instead, was more generalized. Worldwide, women now represent 43% of all adults living with HIV and AIDS (Table 1-1, next page) and this proportion had been steadily increasing over time. (UNAIDS, 1998)

This chapter reviews the epidemiology of HIV/AIDS: beginning with how HIV is transmitted and the variables involved; the natural history of HIV infection in women, both without treatment and in the era of highly active

TABLE 1-1: REGIONAL HIV/AIDS STATISTICS AND FEATURES, DECEMBER 1998

REGION	EPIDEMIC STARTED	NUMBER OF PERSONS WITH HIV INFECTION	NUMBER OF PERSONS WITH NEW HIV INFECTION	PREVALENCE AMONG ADULTS	PERCENT OF INFECTED ADULTS WHO ARE WOMEN	MAIN MODES OF TRANSMISSION FOR ADULTS
Sub-Saharan Africa	Late 1970s–early 1980s	22.5 million	4 million	8.0%	50%	Heterosexual contact
North Africa and Mid-East	Late 1980s	210,000	19,000	0.13%	20%	Injection drug use, heterosexual contact
South, South-East Asia	Late 1980s	6.7 million	1.2 million	0.69%	25%	Heterosexual contact
East Asia, Pacific	Late 1980s	560,000	200,000	0.068%	15%	Injection drug use, heterosexual contact, male/male sex
Latin America	Late 1970s–early 1980s	1.4 million	160,000	0.57%	20%	Male/male sex, injection drug use, heterosexual contact
Caribbean	Late 1970s–early 1980s	330,000	45,000	1.96%	35%	Heterosexual contact, male/male sex
Eastern Europe, Central Asia	Early 1990s	270,000	80,000	0.14%	20%	Injection drug use, male/male sex
Western Europe	Late 1970s–early 1980s	500,000	30,000	0.25%	20%	Male/male sex, injection drug use
North America	Late 1970s–early 1980s	890,000	44,000	0.56%	20%	Male/male sex, injection drug use, heterosexual contact
Australia, New Zealand	Late 1970s–early 1980s	12,000	600	0.1%	5%	Male/male sex, injection drug use
Total		**33.4 million**	**5.8 million**	**1.1%**	**43%**	

Source: Modified from UNAIDS, 1998.

antiretroviral therapy (HAART); and concludes with future issues regarding the HIV/AIDS epidemic.

II. HIV TRANSMISSION

Epidemiological studies have demonstrated that HIV is transmitted by three primary routes: sexual, parenteral (blood-born), and perinatal. Virtually all cases of HIV transmission can be attributed to these exposure categories. Transmission rates from the infected host to the uninfected recipient vary by both mode of transmission and the specific circumstances. Since HIV is a relatively large virus, has a short half-life in vitro, and can only live in primates, HIV cannot be transmitted from causal (i.e. hugging or shaking hands) or surface (i.e. toilet seats) contact or from insect bites.

A. MODES OF TRANSMISSION

Sexual transmission of HIV from an infected partner to an uninfected partner can occur through male-to-female, female-to-male, male-to-male, and female-to-female sexual contact. Worldwide, sexual transmission of HIV is the predominant mode of transmission. (Quinn, 1996) Among U.S. women with AIDS, sexual transmission constitutes 40% of reported cases as of June 1999. (CDC, 1999) This 40% is probably and underestimate when you take into consideration that a large proportion of the women with AIDS who report no identifiable risk (an additional 15% of AIDS cases in women) are actually also infected via sexual transmission. While receptive rectal and vaginal intercourse appear to present the greatest risk of infection (approximately 0.1–3% and 0.1–0.2%, respectively, per episode), insertive intercourse (both rectal and vaginal) have also been associated with HIV infection (approximately 0.06% and 0.1%, respectively, per episode). (Vittinghoff, 1999; Mastro, 1996) In addition, there have been a few case reports of male-to-male transmission from receptive oral intercourse with an HIV-infected male partner (approximately 0.04% per contact) and female-to-female transmission from oral-vaginal, oral-anal, and digital intercourse. (Marmor, 1986; Monini, 1996; Monzon, 1987; Perry, 1989; Rich, 1993; Sabatini, 1983)

Parenteral transmission of HIV has occurred in recipients of blood and blood products, either through transfusion (estimated 95% risk of infection from transfusion of a single unit of HIV-infected whole blood – (CDC, 1998)) or clotting factors, in intravenous or injection drug users through the sharing of needles (approximately 0.67% risk per exposure (Kaplan, 1992)), and in health care workers through needle sticks (approximately 0.4% risk per exposure, depending on the size and location of the inoculum (Tokar, 1993)) and less commonly mucous membrane exposure. (Hessol, 1989) Among cumulatively reported AIDS cases in U.S. women through June 1999, 42% had injection drug use as their exposure risk and 3% receipt of blood, blood products, or tissue. (CDC, 1999) Parenteral transmission patterns vary by geographic region due to social and economic factors. For instance, in regions where the prevalence of HIV infection is higher, the risk of occupational or nosocomial transmission of HIV is increased over regions where there is lower prevalence. (Consten, 1995) The transmission risk is therefore related to the prevalence of HIV in the population as well as the frequency of exposure to infected body fluids and organs and the method of exposure. (Fraser, 1995) In addition, many developing countries that have a high prevalence of HIV infection also lack the resources to implement universal precautions adequately (Gilks, 1998) and may experience a greater amount of transfusion-associated HIV transmission due to a lack of HIV antibody screening in some areas, a higher residual risk of contamination in blood supplies despite antibody screening (McFarland, 1997), and high rates of transfusion in some groups of patients.

Perinatal transmission can occur in utero, during labor and delivery, or post-partum through breast-feeding. (Gwinn, 1996) Perinatal transmission rates average 25–30% (Blanche, 1989), but vary by maternal stage of disease, use of antiviral therapy, duration of ruptured membranes, practice of breast-feeding, as well as other factors. In the U.S. as of June 1999, 91% of cumulative pediatric AIDS cases were attributed to perinatal transmission. (CDC, 1999) More information on perinatal transmission can be found in Chapter VII on HIV and Reproduction.

B. FACTORS FACILITATING TRANSMISSION

Transmission of HIV infection can be influenced by several factors, including characteristics of the HIV-infected host, the recipient, and the quantity and infectivity of the virus. A summary of factors affecting sexual transmission of HIV is presented in Table 1-2.

INFECTIOUSNESS OF THE HOST

There is an association between the quantity of virus transmitted and the risk of HIV infection. (Roques, 1993) Several studies have found that HIV-infected persons may be more likely to transmit the infection when viral replication is high, both during the initial stage of infection (Palasanthiran, 1993) and at more advanced stages of HIV disease. (Laga, 1989) People with high blood viral load are more likely to transmit HIV to recipients of blood, their sexual partners, and their offspring. (Vernazza, 1999; Quinn, 2000) HIV has been quantified in semen (Coombs, 1998; Speck, 1999; Vernazza, 1997) and detected in female genital secretions (Ghys, 1997; Mostad, 1998), and virus in these locations may facilitate transmission. However, the association between infectivity and disease stage is not absolute; HIV-infected women may transmit virus to a first-born child while not to a second-born child (deNartubim 1991), and temporal studies of semen from HIV-infected men demonstrate waxing and waning viral titers over time. (Krieger, 1991; Tindall, 1992)

TABLE 1-2: BIOLOGIC AND HOST-RELATED FACTORS AFFECTING SEXUAL TRANSMISSION OF HIV

BIOLOGIC FACTOR	HOST-RELATED INFECTIVITY FACTORS		
	HIV CONCENTRATION IN GENITAL SECRETIONS	INFECTIOUSNESS (TRANSMISSION)	SUSCEPTIBILITY (ACQUISITION)
Mutation of chemokine-receptor gene	?	?	▼▼▼
Late stage of HIV infection	▲▲	▲▲▲	Not applicable
Primary HIV infection	▲▲	▲▲	Not applicable
Antiretroviral therapy	▼	▼▼	▼?
Local infection	▲▲	▲	▲▲
Presence of cervical ectopy?	▲▲	▲?	▲▲
Presence of foreskin?	?	▲▲	▲▲
Method of contraception			
Barrier	Not applicable	▼▼▼	▼▼▼
Hormonal contraceptives	▲▲	⬍?	⬍
Spermicidal agents	?	▼?	⬍
Intrauterine devices	?	?	▲▲
Menstration	?	▲▲	▲
Factors that lower cervicovaginal pH?	▼?	▼?	▼?
Immune activation	▲?	▲	▲
Genital tract trauma?	▲?	▲▲	▲▲
Pregnancy	▲▲	▲?	▲?

The degrees of positivity (▲ to ▲▲▲) and negativity (▼ to ▼▼▼) of the associations are indicated with arrows, with three arrows indicating a very strong association. The symbol ⬍ denotes that there is evidence in support of both a positive and negative association. A question mark (?) indicates an unknown or hypothesized association that is not currently supported by data.

Source: Royce, 1997.

Factors that decrease viral titers, including anti-retroviral therapy, may decrease but not eliminate the risk of HIV transmission. (Hamed, 1993) Zidovudine has been shown to reduce vertical transmission from mothers to their fetus even when administered late in pregnancy or during labor. (CDC, 1998) (See Chapter VII on HIV and Reproduction) Individuals receiving anti-retroviral therapy have also shown reduced transmission rates of HIV to their sex partners. (Musicco, 1994) Several studies have suggested that anti-retroviral treatment reduces detection of HIV in female genital secretions (Cu Uvin, 1998) and the concentration of HIV in semen. (Gilliam, 1997; Gupta, 1997) Providers counseling patients on treatment should be clear that precautions to prevent transmission of the virus should be maintained since not all treatment reduce infectiousness and transmissions have been reported among individuals with undetectable HIV RNA levels. (The European Collaborative Study Group, 1999)

Factors which increase the risk of exposure to blood, such as genital ulcer disease (Cameron, 1989; Plummer, 1991), trauma during sexual contact (Marmor, 1986), and menstruation of an HIV-infected woman during sexual contact (The European Collaborative Study Group, 1992; Nair, 1993; St. Louis, 1993) may all increase the risk of transmission.

Method of contraception also affects the likelihood of HIV transmission. (Daly, 1994) There is overwhelming evidence that the correct and consistent use of latex condoms protect both men and women against HIV. However, because of methodologic difficulties in studies of contraceptive use and HIV transmission, it remains unclear whether the use of hormonal contraceptives, IUDs and spermicides alter the risk of HIV transmission.

SUSCEPTIBILITY OF THE RECIPIENT

Similarly, characteristics of the uninfected individual may increase the likelihood of infection for a given exposure to HIV. Specifically, inflammation or disruption of the genital or rectal mucosa (which can occur with sexually transmitted diseases and trauma), and lack of circumcision in heterosexual men may increase the risk of infection. (Cameron, 1989; Moses, 1994; Quinn, 2000) Sex during menstruation may increase women's risk of acquiring HIV infection (Lazzarin, 1991) as may bleeding during sexual intercourse. (Seidlin, 1993) In women, both uclerative and non-uclerative sexually transmitted diseases have been shown to be risk factors for getting infected with HIV. (Laga, 1993; Plummer, 1991) Cervical ectopy has been identified as a risk factor for acquisition of HIV infection in some (Nicolosi, 1994; Plourde, 1994) but not all (Mati, 1994) studies that have evaluated this condition. There is also some evidence that changes in the vaginal flora, as characterized by bacterial vaginosis, may facilitate acquisition of HIV. (Sewankambo, 1997)

Non-barrier contraceptive methods have also been investigated in association with risk of HIV transmission but the results are inconclusive. The most frequently studied methods of contraception have been oral contraceptives, injectable hormones, intrauterine devices, and nonoxynol-9. (Daly, 1994; Plummer, 1998) (See Chapter III on Prevention) Traditional vaginal agents, used in African women for sexual enhancement and self-treatment of vaginal symptoms, has also been investigated as a potential cofactor for HIV transmission. (Dallabetta, 1995) For many of these studies, limitations of the study design preclude any definitive conclusions.

There is increasing evidence that host genetic or immunologic factors may protect against HIV infection. This has been investigated in cohort studies of Nairobi sex workers (Willerford, 1993) and in United States homosexual men (Dean, 1996), both of who remained uninfected despite multiple sexual exposures to HIV. Individuals who are homozygous for a null allele of CCR5 are relatively resistant to sexually transmitted infection with HIV, indicating an important, though not absolute, role for this receptor in viral transmission. However, homozygous CCR5 mutations were not found among 14 hemophiliacs who remained uninfected with HIV after being inoculated repeatedly with HIV contaminated Factor VIII concentrate from plasma during 1980–1985. (Zagury, 1998) In this study, investigators found an over production of beta-chemokines in most of the uninfected individuals.

VIRAL PROPERTIES

Several viral factors have been proposed to play a role in the transmissibility of HIV. These include phenotypic characteristics (e.g., envelope proteins required for transmission), genetic factors that control the replicative capacity and "fitness" of the virus, and resistance to antiviral drugs. (Vernazza, 1999)

Envelope sequences can define viral quasispecies that have been phenotypically arranged according to their ability to induce syncytia formation in infected T-cells. (Paxton, 1998) It appears that the most commonly transmitted phenotype is the non-syncytia-inducing (NSI), M-tropic viral strain, which is frequently found in those who have been recently infected. During the course of HIV infection the development of a more cytopathic, syncytia-inducing (SI), T-tropic viral phenotype can be found and this is often a precursor to the development of AIDS. While some researchers have suggested that NSI isolates of HIV are preferentially transmitted (Roos, 1992), others have not been able to show preferential transmission of this isolate. (Albert, 1995)

Envelope sequences can also be used to define viral subtypes, or clades, and these subtypes may also influence the transmissibility of HIV. The distribution of HIV subtypes differ according to geographic region, with A, C, D, and E predominant in sub-Saharan Africa and Asia and B predominant in the United States, the Caribbean, South America, and Western Europe. (Hu, 1996) In one study, subtype E is reported to have greater tropism for Langerhans' cells than subtype B (Soto-Ramirez, 1996) and may have a greater per contact transmissibility.

Lastly, the transmission characteristics of a viral strain that is resistant to certain antiretroviral agents may differ from transmission of wild type virus. More research is needed in this emerging field of therapy-resistant virus and its characteristics.

III. NATURAL HISTORY AND HIV DISEASE PROGRESSION

The natural history of HIV infection in adults has been extensively documented in the medical literature. The impact of gender on the manifestations and progression of HIV-disease is still being investigated. Concerns about gender-based differences in the course of HIV infection were expressed early in the epidemic. In most industrialized countries, women tended to have lower income, be un- or under-insured for health care, know less about HIV, more likely to be Black or Hispanic, and to have a personal or partner history of injection drug or cocaine use. Women also appeared to have more rapid progression of illness than men and to present with a different constellation of opportunistic conditions than men. When sophisticated statistical methods were applied that controlled for the tendency of women to receive less care, and to present with more advanced disease, gender-based differences in HIV disease course appeared to lessen. More recently, however, with better measures of viral activity and infirmity, the issue of gender-based differences in rate of disease course and virologic parameters has again been raised. These new observations have prompted active research into the impact of gender, hormones and demographic factors on the outcome of HIV infection.

HIV infects and induces cell death in a variety of human cell lines. T-helper lymphocytes (also known as CD4 cells) are a major target of viral infection, and circulating CD4-cells become steadily depleted from peripheral blood in most untreated infected persons. Thus quantification of CD4-cells in blood is a rather simple way of determining cumulative immunologic damage due to HIV. Profound CD4-cell depletion is unusual in persons who do not have HIV infection and are usually iatrogenic or associated with severe illnesses, such as chemotherapy-induced leukopenia. (Aldrich, 2000) Other immunological parameters become altered with HIV-disease progression, and though often used for research purposes, they tend to be more difficult to measure and less reliable or more costly.

Untreated HIV infection is a chronic illness that progresses through characteristic clinical stages; AIDS is an endpoint of HIV infection, resulting from severe immunological damage, loss of an effective immune response to specific opportunistic pathogens and tumors. AIDS is diagnosed by the occurrence of these specific infections and cancers or by CD4-cell depletion to less than $200/mm^3$.

A. STAGING

HIV can cause a wide range of symptoms and clinical conditions that reflect varying level of immunological injury and different predisposing factors. Certain conditions tend to occur in association with each other and at specific CD4 cell counts. Staging systems for HIV-disease facilitate clinical evaluation and planning therapeutic interventions, help determine the individual level of infirmity, and give prognostic information. Untreated HIV infection is a chronic illness that progresses through characteristic clinical stages that can be used to describe infirmity. Several groups have produced organized staging systems to facilitate clinical evaluation and planning therapeutic interventions. In industrialized countries, the most widely used system for classifying HIV infection and AIDS in adults and adolescents was published by the United States Centers for Disease Control in 1993. (CDC, 1992)

TABLE 1-3: 1993 REVISED CLASSIFICATION SYSTEM FOR HIV INFECTION AND EXPANDED SURVEILLANCE CASE DEFINITION FOR AIDS AMONG ADULTS AND ADOLESCENTS

CD4 CELL CATEGORY	CLINICAL CATEGORY A	CLINICAL CATEGORY B	CLINICAL CATEGORY C
1 500 cells/mm³	A1	B1	C1
2. 200–499 cells/mm³	A2	B2	C2
3. < 200 cells/mm³	A3	B3	C3

CATEGORY A CONDITIONS	CATEGORY B CONDITIONS	CATEGORY C CONDITIONS	
■ No symptoms ■ Acute HIV infection (resolves) ■ Generalized lymphadenopathy	■ Bacillary angiomatosis ■ Oropharyngeal candidiasis ■ *Vulvovaginal candidiasis*: persistent, frequent, or poorly responsive to therapy ■ Cervical intraepithelial neoplasia II or III ■ *Constitutional symptoms*: fever, diarrhea > 1month ■ Oral hairy leuko plakia ■ *Herpes zoster*: multiple episodes or involving > 1 dermotome ■ Idiopathic thrombocytopenic purpura ■ Listeriosis ■ *Pelvic inflammatory disease:* particularly if complicated by tubo-ovarian abscess ■ Peripheral neuropathy	■ Candidiasis of bronchi, trachea, lungs or esophagus ■ Invasive cervical cancer ■ *Coccidioidomycosis,* disseminated or extrapulmonary ■ *Cryptococcosis,* extrapulmonary ■ Cryptosporidiosis, (intestinal infection > 1 month duration) ■ *Cytomegalovirus disease* (excluding liver, spleen or lymph nodes) ■ HIV-related encephalopathy ■ *Herpes simplex*: chronic ulcer > 1 month duration, or bronchitis, pneumonitis, or esophagitis ■ *Histoplasmosis*: disseminated or extrapulmonary ■ *Isosporiasis*: > 1 month's duration ■ Kaposi's sarcoma ■ Burkitt's lymphoma ■ Immunoblastic lymphoma ■ Primary lymphoma of the brain ■ *MAC* or M. kansasii:* disseminated or extrapulmonary ■ *M. TB*: any site ■ *Mycobacterium*: other species or unknown species, disseminated or extrapulmonary ■ *Pneumocystis carinii* pneumonia ■ Recurrent pneumonia ■ Progressive multifocal leukoencephalopathy ■ Salmonella septicemia, recurrent ■ Toxoplasmosis of the brain	
Source: CDC, 1992.		■ Wasting syndrome due to HIV	

The case definition (Table 1-3) begins first with confirmation of HIV infection either via serologic testing (combination of a screening method such as enzyme immunoassay and more specific confirmatory test such as Western blot), or direct detection of HIV in patient tissue by viral culture, antigen detection or other test such as polymerase chain reaction (PCR). The definition of each stage of illness is then based on two types of information: peripheral blood CD4 cell counts and clinical manifestations. CD4 cell counts are placed in three strata, ranging from relatively normal (> 500 cells/mm^3) to severe CD4 depletion (< 200 cells/mm^3).

The clinical manifestations of HIV infection are also placed in three strata, generally in accordance with the level of immunologic dysfunction associated with the various conditions. (Table 1-3) Category A includes persons who have minimal clinical findings, clinical findings that do not indicate immune injury (including absence of symptoms), generalized lymphadenopathy or resolved acute HIV infection. Category B includes conditions that indicate the presence of a defect in cell-mediated immunity or conditions that appear to be worsened by HIV infection. Category C includes conditions that are considered AIDS defining, even in the absence of a CD4 cell count less than 200 cell/mm^3. (CDC, 1992) The addition of specific laboratory measures such as plasma HIV RNA level, improves prognostic value even after the occurrence of Category C conditions. (Lyles, 1999)

DEVELOPING WORLD

The CDC criteria require diagnostic testing and case confirmation methods that may not be available in developing countries, so several other sets of criteria have been proposed for these regions. Since lymphocyte subset quantitation is not widely available in many countries, the Global Program on AIDS of the World Health Organization (W.H.O.) proposed a clinically based staging system that is more broadly applicable than the CDC system. (W.H.O., 1993) The system uses clinical historical data, laboratory measures (optional) and indices of physical activity to assess level of infirmity to establish four strata that are summarized in Table 1-4. Laboratory measures include a single assessment absolute CD4 cell count, with the option of replacing this test with total lymphocyte count, each of which are placed in three strata. CD4 cell count is a better prognostic indicator than total lymphocyte count, but the two results correlate well. (Brettle, 1993)

Clinical history and functional measures are placed in four categories that range from asymptomatic to severe disease. In general, when compared with the CDC stages, the W.H.O. system requires less diagnostic test data and fewer direct observations. The definition includes broader categories for conditions that may vary by region (e.g., disseminated infections with endemic mycoses which are common in South East Asian AIDS patients but not in the United States or Europe). The inclusion of performance scale measures permits quantitative clinical assessment that is not dependent on laboratory resources.

TABLE 1-4: THE WORLD HEALTH ORGANIZATION CLINICAL HIV STAGING SYSTEM AND PROPOSED MODIFICATIONS

	LABORATORY COMPONENT		CLINICAL GROUP			
	CD4 CELL COUNT	OR TOTAL LYMPHOCYTE COUNT	1	2	3	4
A	≥500	≥2000	A1	A2	A3	A4
B	200–499	1000–1999	B1	B2	B3	B4
C	< 200	< 1000	C1	C2	C3	C4

CLINICAL STAGE	CLINICAL HISTORY	PERFORMANCE SCALE CRITERIA	PROPOSED MODIFICATIONS
One: Asymptomatic	1. Asymptomatic infection 2. Persistent generalized lymphadenopathy 3. Acute retroviral infection	Normal functional level in performance scales	none
Two: Mild Disease	1. Unintentional weight loss less than 10% of body weight 2. Minor mucocutaneous manifestations 3. Herpes zoster within the previous 5 years 4. Recurrent upper respiratory infections	Performance scale level at which symptoms are present but patients are almost fully ambulatory	1. Substitution of weight loss with BMI of 19–21kg/m²* 2. Specify addition of acute oral or genital ulcers as one of the minor mucocutaneous manifestations* 3. ESR ≤65mm/hr defines Kigali stage II 4. ESR > 65 mm/hr defines Kigali stage III
Three: Moderate Disease	1. Unintentional weight loss greater than 10% of body weight 2. Chronic diarrhea ** 3. Prolonged intermittent or constant fever ** 4. Oral candidiasis 5. Oral hairy leukoplakia 6. Pulmonary tuberculosis developing within the previous year 7. Severe bacterial infections 8. Chronic vulvovaginal candidiasis** or poorly responsive to therapy	Performance scale level at which patients remain in bed < 50% of daytime, but more than normal	1. Suggest exclusion of oral candidiasis and pulmonary tuberculosis* 2. Recommend substitution of weight loss with BMI ≤19 kg/m²* 3. Differentiation of ambulatory vs hospitalized patients improved correlation with laboratory markers (Kassa, 1999) 4. ESR ≤65mm/hr defines Kigali stage II 5. ESR > 65 mm/hr defines Kigali stage III
		Table continues . . .	

TABLE 1-4: THE WORLD HEALTH ORGANIZATION CLINICAL HIV STAGING SYSTEM AND PROPOSED MODIFICATIONS (continued)

CLINICAL STAGE	CLINICAL HISTORY	PERFORMANCE SCALE CRITERIA	PROPOSED MODIFICATIONS
Four: Severe Disease	1. HIV wasting syndrome defined as unexplained weight loss > 10% and either chronic diarrhea** or chronic weakness** and unexplained fever 2. Pneumocystis carinii pneumonia 3. CNS toxoplasmosis 4. Chronic cryptosporidial diarrhea** 5. Chronic isosporiasis with diarrhea ** 6. Extrapulmonary cryptococcosis 7. Cytomegalovirus disease affecting organs other than the liver, spleen or lymph nodes 8. Visceral or chronic** mucocutaneous herpes simplex virus infection 9. Progressive multifocal leukoencephalopathy 10. Any disseminated endemic mycosis 11. Candidiasis of the esophagus, trachea, bronchi or lungs 12. Disseminated atypic Mycobacterium sp. Infection 13. Nontyphoidal Salmonella septicemia 14. Extrapulmonary tuberculosis 15. Lymphoma 16. Kaposi's sarcoma 17. HIV-related encephalopathy	Performance scale at level which patients remain in bed more than 50% of daytime	1. Addition of oral candidiasis 2. Substitution of weight loss with BMI ≤ 19 kg/m^2* 3. Addition of chronic** oral or genital ulcer 4. Addition of pulmonary tuberculosis 5. ESR > 65mm/hr defines Kigali stage III 6. Addition of positive HIV serology*** 7. Addition of invasive cervical cancer***

* Lifson, 1995.

** > 1 month duration

*** De Cock, 1993.

Source: W.H.O., 1993.

The four clinical stages in the W.H.O. system correlated well with CD4 cell counts and HIV RNA levels in a study of 750 Ethiopians (included 336 women) by Kassa and others. (Kassa, 1999) Other studies of patient populations have also demonstrated correlation of W.H.O. clinical stage with CD4 cell count and clinical outcome. (Morgan, 1997; Morgan, 1998; Schechter, 1995) When compared with the CDC staging, the W.H.O. clinical stages demonstrated a high degree of specificity, but a lower level of sensitivity (35–65%) for HIV infection. (Gallant, 1993; Gallant, 1992) In particular all of the systems for disease staging are not perfectly sensitive and specific for HIV infection, but can be improved by the addition of HIV serologies. (Ankrah, 1994; DeCock, 1991) Modifications (Table 1-4) have been proposed that improve the prognostic accuracy of the W.H.O. system. Based on observations made in a study of AIDS mortality among Rwandan women, Lifson and colleagues proposed minor modifications of clinical history definitions, replacement of body mass index (BMI) (weight(in kg) divided by height (in m²)) for weight loss and use of erythrocyte sedimentation rate (ESR) as a laboratory indicator of infirmity. (Lifson, 1995) BMI was significantly better at predicting mortality than percentage of body weight lost over two measurements taken in one year. Both ESR and hematocrit were highly predictive of mortality over a 36 month period of observation. (Lifson, 1995)

Other HIV-disease classifications, such as the Caracas definition proposed by the Pan American Health Organization (Rabeneck, 1996; Weniger, 1992) have been proposed but have not been evaluated as extensively as the CDC and W.H.O. systems.

B. UNTREATED NATURAL HISTORY

PRIMARY OR ACUTE INFECTION

Acute HIV infection is a transient symptomatic illness that can be identified in 40–90% of cases of new HIV infection. It is characterized by a high rate of HIV replication, high titers of virus in blood and lymphoid organs (up to several million copies of HIV RNA per mm³ of plasma), and initiation of an HIV-specific immune response. The amount of virus present in blood and tissues begins to fall after appearance of cytotoxic ("killer") lymphocytes that specifically react with HIV antigens; the vigor of this response varies among individuals and is associated with subsequent rate of disease progression. (Cao, 1995) A pool of persistently infected CD4 cells ("latent reservoirs") emerges early in the course of HIV infection and persists indefinitely. (Chun, 1998)

Symptoms have been identified from 5–30 days after a recognized exposure to HIV. (Schacker, 1998) The signs and symptoms of acute HIV infection are not specific; fever, fatigue, rash, headache, lymphadenopathy, pharyngitis, mild gastrointestinal upset, night sweats, aseptic meningitis and oral ulcerations are most frequently reported. Because the clinical signs of acute HIV infection resemble those of many acute viral illnesses, the correct diagnosis is often missed. Because early treatment at the time of acute infection may be especially beneficial (See Chapter IV on Primary Medical Care), early suspicion of and evaluation for HIV infection should be encouraged. (Kahn, 1998)

ESTABLISHED INFECTION

Regardless of whether the syndrome of acute HIV infection is recognized or not, after the HIV-specific immunological response begins to control the intensity of viremia, a so-called "**viral set-point**" is established, which varies by individual. With exceedingly rare exceptions, the immunological response to HIV does not eliminate infection, but rather establishes a steady state between viral replication and elimination. (Henrad, 1995) A variable level of viremia is attained, which can be measured via quantification of the number of copies of HIV RNA present in blood (viral load). Although the viral load within the first 120 days of HIV infection is not of prognostic value (Schacker, 1998), in most patients a relatively stable viral load is attained after recovery from acute infection, and this viral set point is highly predictive of the rate of future progression of illness, at least as determined in studies that were largely focused on men. In the case of a high viral load set point (i.e. values ranging up from 40,000 copies per mm³) more rapid decline in CD4 cell counts and more rapid occurrence of Clinical Class B and C conditions will occur. Some individuals have viral load set points that are low (below 500 copies per mm³), which indicates a better prognosis; no evidence of progression (CD4 cell depletion or HIV-diseases) is seen for long periods of time in a small subset of patients (see section on long-term progression, below). The viral set point is likely influenced by several factors such as presence of other infections at the time of HIV exposure, genetic characteristics (particularly the type of HIV binding receptors present on lymphocytes), viral characteristics, age and perhaps gender (see below). (Kahn, 1998)

During the period of clinical stability acute illnesses and other events that can stimulate the immune system, such as influenza, herpes simplex outbreaks, and tuberculosis as well as routine vaccinations, have been demonstrated to result in 10–1000 fold increases in viral load; these increases are transient and most often resolve within two months. (Stanley, 1996; Staprans, 1995) Thus, determination of viral load for prognostic purposes should not be done during or shortly after an acute illness.

For most HIV-infected persons, viral quasispecies evolve overtime. Transition for the non-syncytia-inducing macrophage-tropic viral strains, that are commonly present after transmission to syncytia-inducing T-lymphocyte tropic strains occurs in many hosts. While variation of viral quasispecies with time is usual, the mechanism by which this process occurs has not been defined. However, transitions in viral quasispecies and cellular tropism has been observed to coincide with key clinical events such as CD4 cell depletion and development of symptomatic illness. These virologic changes may reflect evolution of a virus that is tailored to an individual's immune response or other genetic characteristics. Interventions that prevent evolution of quasispecies in a host may yield effective therapies in the future.

The HIV RNA level in tissues does not correlate in a linear fashion with blood levels, so even in patients with undetectable plasma HIV RNA, intracellular and tissue HIV RNA can still be detected with more sophisticated techniques. (Hockett, 1999) Thus HIV replication continues at varying pace among infected persons, even those who can control viremia well.

HIV is also frequently present in the genital tract (Fiore, 1999; Iverson, 1998), where expression of inflammatory mediators, and lymphocyte receptors differ from blood and may influence the rate of viral replication and numbers of virions present. (Anderson, 1998; Hladik, 1999) While the quantities of HIV present in cervicovaginal fluid are generally similar to blood (Hart, 1999; Shaheen, 1999), they differ in some individuals. The finding that HIV isolates from the lower genital tract can have different genotypic markers than blood isolates from a single host (DiStefano, 1999; Shaheen, 1999), supports the concept that the lower genital tract sometimes functions as a separate virologic compartment.

TIME COURSE

In most studies of seroconverters, (persons for whom the date of the HIV infection can be estimated), 50–60% of adults will be diagnosed with an AIDS-defining condition within 10 years of infection (for the pre-HAART treatment era). Forty-eight percent of seroconverters die (due to any cause) after 10 years of infection. Increasing age is the factor most consistently associated with rate of progression and death in most groups of patients studied to date. (Alioum, 1998; UK Register of HIV Seroconverters Steering Committee, 1998; Pezzott, 1999; Prins, 1999) Date of infection also influences time from infection to an AIDS diagnosis, at least in some locations, demonstrating that even in the pre-HAART era, improvements in treatment resulted in tangible benefits. (Webber, 1998)

LABORATORY INDICATORS AND PREDICTORS

A large number of laboratory tests have been evaluated as prognostic indicators in HIV infection. For the most part, the tests can be divided into three groups: A. measures of HIV replication, B. measures of immune function and C. measures of inflammation. Group A is specific to HIV infection, Group B, when indicating severe CD4 cell depletion is relatively specific to HIV infection and Group C are generally not specific to HIV infection. Table 1-5, on the following page, summarizes these laboratory measures, outcomes, their advantages and disadvantages. HIV RNA quantitation, performed on fresh or fresh-frozen plasma or serum, is a powerful and accurate prognostic indicator in HIV infection, and is uniquely useful in determining response to antiretroviral therapy. (Saag, 1996) In general the best measures of prognosis and staging include combinations of HIV RNA level, CD4 cell count and perhaps

TABLE 1-5: LABORATORY INDICATORS OF PROGNOSIS AND/OR STAGE OF ILLNESS IN HIV INFECTION (BLOOD SPECIMEN).

Group	Test	Interpretation in HIV	Advantages	Disadvantages
A	HIV RNA level	Higher level, greater rate of viral replication, poorer prognosis	Direct measure of current viral activity, excellent prognostic indicator. Useful as indicator of treatment response.	Requires freshly frozen and separated sample, expensive and technically demanding (O'Brien, 1996; Saag, 1996)
A	P24 antigen level	Higher level indicates greater level of viremia, poorer prognosis	Simple and relatively inexpensive	Of less prognostic value than most other assay (Coombs, 1989; Fahey, 1990)
A	Syncytium-inducing (SI) HIV phenotype	Emergence of SI strains is an independent predictor of progression to AIDS	An indicator of viral virulence for CD4 cells, adds to prognostic information provided by CD4 and HIV RNA level	Requires viral culture or DNA assay, which is cumbersome and costly (Koot, 1993)
B	Lymphocyte count	Lymphopenia suggests greater immune injury	Indicates current status, cumulative over variable time	Nonspecific, can be influenced by large number of concurrent conditions and treatments
B	CD4 subset (absolute count, % or CD8 ratio	Depletion of CD4 cells suggests immune injury and poorer prognosis, excellent prognostic indicator	Indicates current status, cumulative over variable time, severe depletion relatively specific for HIV	Large range of variation some introduced by differences among labs, expensive, must be performed on fresh (not frozen specimen)
B	Lymphocyte markers of immunologic activation	Presence of specific sets of activation markers on lymphocytes, depending on type, indicates favorable or unfavorable prognosis. Excellent prognostic indicators	Highly specific marker of long term stability or decline	Methods not standardized, costly and has limited availability (Giorgi, 1994)
B	HIV-specific cytotoxic lymphocytes	Strong cytotoxic responses to HIV indicate favorable prognosis	Highly specific marker of long term stability	Methods not standardized, costly and has limited availability (Harrer, 1996)

Table continues . . .

TABLE 1-5: LABORATORY INDICATORS OF PROGNOSIS AND/OR STAGE OF ILLNESS IN HIV INFECTION (BLOOD SPECIMEN) *(continued)*			
Group	**Test**	**Interpretation in HIV**	**Advantages**	**Disadvantages**
C	C-reactive protein			
C	ESR		Simple to perform	General marker of inflammation, nonspecific (Planella, 1998)
C	B-2 microglobulin	Higher B-2 microglobulin levels associated with risk of progression		
C	Neopterin	Higher neopterin levels associated with risk of progression	Perhaps best prognostic indicator among group C. Simple to perform assay.	Not as good a prognostic indicator as CD4 cell count. (Fahey, 1990)

lymphocyte function (cytotoxic lymphocyte response to HIV). (Spijkerman, 1997; Vlahov, 1998)

LONG TERM NON-PROGRESSORS

In untreated adults the median time from HIV infection to AIDS in developed countries is 8–10 years. However, approximately 8–15% of HIV infected persons (most studies focus on men) remain symptom free for much longer periods of time , a phenomenon that has been named long-term survival (LTS). Among these individuals who remain clinically stable without treatment for 5–8 years, two groups can be discerned, those who have stable CD4 cell counts and those who have low CD4 cell counts, but no AIDS defining conditions. (Schrager, 1994) Several factors have been found to be associated with long-term survival including host characteristics such as the presence of specific anti-HIV cytotoxic lymphocyte responses, and viral characteristics such as defective genes and gene products. (Kirchhoff, 1995) LTS patients tend to have consistently lower levels of HIV RNA after the period of acute infection suggesting better control of viral replication. (Vesanen, 1996) For example viral growth in peripheral mononuclear cells taken from LTS was markedly less than in PBMCs taken from healthy HIV-uninfected donors. (Cao, 1995)

GENDER EFFECTS

In general the predictors of the rate of HIV-disease progression and survival among women are the same as in men. CD4 cell count depletion and higher HIV RNA level are strong pre-

TABLE 1-6: FACTORS THAT INFLUENCE RATE OF HIV-DISEASE PROGRESSION

HOST FACTORS	Effect	Notes	Reference
Age	Increasing age associated with more rapid progression	Increasing age at the time of infection is consistently associated with rate of progression to AIDS and survival after AIDS diagnosis	Committee, 1998; Del Amo, 1998; van Benthem, 1998
Gender	? lower HIV RNA level among women, without progression benefit		
Race	No consistent effect in various studies		Del Amo, 1998
Chemokine receptor and ligand mutations: CCR5, CCR2, SDF-1	Homozygous mutation protective versus primary infection, hetero-zygotes appear to have slower progression	These mutations are much more common among Caucasians	Winkler, 1998; Zimmerman, 1997; Martin, 1998
HLA type	HLA differences associated with differing HIV RNA levels and rate of progression	Not currently of clinical utility, may provide clues to immunopathogenesis	Saah, 1998
HIV risk behavior	Higher CD4 cell counts in persons with a history of IDU	This effect seen in several studies	Brettle, 1995
VIRAL FACTORS	Effect	Notes	Reference
Clade/Location	Mixed evidence, possible impact of viral subtype (or clade) on rate of progression	No clinical application currently	Prins, 1999; Kanki, 1999

Table continues . . .

TABLE 1-6: FACTORS THAT INFLUENCE RATE OF HIV-DISEASE PROGRESSION *(continued)*

VIRAL FACTORS *(continued)*	Effect	Notes	Reference
Mutations	Mutation of viral genes can produce attenuated viral strains that are associated with slowed disease progression	Mutation resulting in attenuation appears relatively rare.	Deacon, 1995; Learmont, 1999
ACQUIRED FACTORS	**Effect**	**Notes**	**Reference**
Immunologic activation			
Concurrent viral infection			
Concurrent bacterial infection			
CLINICAL INDICATORS	**Effect**	**Notes**	**Reference**
Wasting			
Oral candidiasis and hairy leukoplakia	The presence of oral candidiasis or hairy leukoplakia suggests HIV infection and progression to impaired immunological function. Oral candidiasis adds to the predictive value of HIV RNA in persons with low CD4 cell counts	Accuracy of diagnosis varies with clinician experience, but oral manifestations are particularly useful prognostic indicators in resource-poor environments and important points of HIV recognition world-wide	Carre, 1998; Greenspan, 1996
Constitutional symptoms			

dictors of progression and survival in women. (Anastos, 1996b) Several recent reports, however, describe gender-based differences in HIV RNA level and in rate of CD4 cell depletion; women had HIV RNA levels that were 30–50% lower than men who had comparable CD4 cell counts. (Bush, 1996; Evans, 1997; Farzadegan, 1998) Similar results occurred when analysis was restricted to seroconverters or when HIV culture was used to quantify viremia rather than RNA assays. ()Lyles, 1998; Sterling, 1999) Intuitively, lower levels of circulating HIV RNA, which suggest lower steady state level of viremia, should be associated with better outcome. However, the findings of several recent studies suggest that the lower HIV RNA level does not provide benefit to women. Women experienced more rapid CD4 cell depletion and faster progression to AIDS and death than men at similar HIV-RNA levels, even when race and age were taken into consideration. (Anastos, 1999a; Farzadegan, 1998)

Determination of the effect of gender on the rate of progression, time until occurrence of an AIDS defining condition and death is a complicated process. Unless the date of HIV infection can be established, duration of infection becomes a significant unknown factor in studies. In addition, particularly in developed countries, HIV-infected women and men differ by more than just their gender. Women tend to have lower income, be members of minority ethnic groups, have been born in Africa, have used injection drugs or cocaine, or to have a sexual partner who has done so, all of which are risk factors for poor health in general. In most studies women have shorter duration of infection prior to AIDS and death than men, but these differences tend to disappear when CD4 cell count and drug use are taken into consideration. (Alioum, 1998; UK Register of HIV Seroconverters Steering COmmittee, 1998; Pezzotti, 1999; Santoro-Lopes, 1998) Several studies have reported an excess proportion of infections or deaths due to bacterial infection, often pneumonia (Feldman, 1999), among women compared with men. (Melnich, 1994; Weisser, 1998)

A summary of factors that influence disease progression is shown in Table 1-6.

C. NATURAL HISTORY IN HAART ERA

INDUSTRIALIZED COUNTRIES

In countries that are able to provide highly affective antiretroviral treatments (HAART), HIV-associated morbidity and mortality have declined significantly. (Michales, 1998; Miller, 1999a; Miller 1999b; Palella, 1998; Pezotti, 1999) (See Primary Medical Care in Chapter IV for more information). These population findings, based on regional surveillance systems, were preceded by a multitude of clinical trials that demonstrated clinical and virologic benefits of HAART. (Bartlett, 1996; Collier, 1996; Deeks, 1997; Hammer, 1997) Despite the promise and documented benefits of HAART, clinical progression continues to occur among recipients, particularly among persons who received antiretroviral treatment prior to initiation of HAART. (Ledergerber, 1999) Viral resistance to HAART components can occur via several mechanisms, which for the most part involve mutation of viral target proteins. (Richman, 1996; Schapiro, 1999) The emergence of antiretroviral resistance is a function of several factors: prior treatment, pre-treatment level of viremia, drug levels (adherence to medication regimens, bioavailability of medications, adequate dosing) and specifics of the regimen. (Guilick, 1998; Ledergerber, 1999; Shafer, 1998) Multiple daily doses, side effects and in some cases, dietary restrictions aggravate the problem of achieving optimal drug levels since protease inhibitor agents are relatively poorly bioavailable. Suppression of viral replication and prevention of resistance are directly related to level of antiretroviral drug. Persistent viral replication provides opportunity of occurrence of resistance mutations, and selective pressure to support continued presence of such mutants. (Condra, 1998; Feinberg, 1997; Wong, 1997) Besides clinical treatment failure, emergence of antiretroviral resistance is now associated with transmission of resistant virus to previously uninfected persons, a finding that could portend significant limits to the effectiveness of these treatments in populations over long periods of time. (Boden, 1999; Brodine, 1999; Yerly, 1999)

DEVELOPING COUNTRIES

The high cost of antiretroviral drugs and the need for clinical and laboratory services for monitoring response to and efficacy of these treatments has greatly restricted provision of HAART in the developing world. Thus the reductions in morbidity and gains in survival in HIV patients that have been demonstrated in many industrialized countries do not extend to developing countries in which the majority of HIV cases worldwide occur. A consensus statement regarding provision of these therapies has been released based on meetings held in Dakar and Abidjan during 1997. The key recommendations of conference participants include: efforts must be made to expand provision of ART, ART only makes sense in the setting of effective AIDS control programs, funding must be sustained to provide uninterrupted treatment and continuity of care, care providers must be trained in use of the treatments and basic patient rights, resources for assessment of efficacy and tolerance must be available, sentinel monitoring for resistance pattern determination should be available, 3-drug combination regimens should be used when possible, treatment of pregnant women to prevent perinatal transmission must be a priority, and new drug development should focus on less costly medications. (International AIDS Society, 1999)

V. FUTURE ISSUES

A. GLOBAL IMPACT

The HIV/AIDS epidemic continues to spread without full control in any country. Over forty million people have been infected worldwide. By the end of 1998, the United Nations Program on AIDS (UNAIDS) estimated that 33.4 million people were living with HIV, a figure which includes 13.8 million adult women (UNAIDS, 1998) (Table 1-1, page 2). In 1998 it is estimated that 5.8 million new HIV infections occurred of with 2.1 million of these occurring in women. After steady increases of the prevalence of disease among women during the 1990s, currently 43% of all persons over the age of 15 years living with HIV are women. Globally, AIDS is now the fourth leading cause of mortality; 2.5 million deaths have been attributable to AIDS, of which 900,000 occurred in women. The notable improvements in AIDS mortality reported in North America and Europe, in association with the introduction of highly active combination antiretroviral therapies, do not extend to most of the world's cases which occur in regions in which this expensive type of treatment is not available.

More than 95% of HIV-infected people live in the developing world, most in Sub-Saharan Africa. Seventy percent of infections that occurred during 1998 took place in this epicenter. The region has also experienced 83% of all AIDS deaths. Unfortunately prior projections of the epidemic course in Southern Africa underestimated the incidence of infection by half. (Balter, 1998) Improved data have revealed that the prevalence rates in southern Africa are staggering: 20–26% of adults (aged 15–49 years) are infected; in some regions 20–50% of pregnant women are infected and are likely to transmit infection to 1/3 of their offspring. The declining mortality rate, and population growth taking place in other regions cannot be extended to Sub-Saharan Africa, due to the extent of AIDS mortality. (Bongaarts, 1998) AIDS has now surpassed malaria as the leading cause of death in this region. (Balter, 1999) Life expectancy will fall from 64 to 47 years by 2015. AIDS will cost, on an average, 17 years of life expectancy in the 9 Sub-Saharan countries with a > 10% prevalence of HIV infection among adults. The child mortality rates in this region are also elevated by AIDS; rates are approximately double that expected without the HIV epidemic. (UNAIDS, 1998) Within one year 2,400 Zimbabweans will succumb to AIDS per week, many in the prime of life, many leaving dependent children as orphans (up to 1 in 5 children are likely to become orphans). The United States Surgeon General, David Satcher, notes that "the progress of decades of work immunizing children, controlling diseases, and improving nutrition is being negated by HIV." (Satcher, 1999)

In Asia, the epidemic has a mixed pattern that includes countries with slow growth in HIV prevalence, countries with some success in control efforts and regions that appear to be experiencing explosive epidemics. Currently 7 million Asians are infected with HIV. Rapidly accelerating epidemics are possible in China, Cambodia, Vietnam and India. While urban areas were initially of greatest concern in many countries, recent information has revealed very active epidemics in specific rural areas (up to 2% of the general population), which are hosts to large proportions of the region's population.

While the outlook for AIDS in Asia is bleak, there is also cause for hope. Growth of the epidemic in the Philippines is notably slow. (Jacobs, 1999) Thailand has been successful in reducing the incidence of infection in sentinel population groups (such as members of the military and pregnant women) using a combination of good surveillance, effective policy response, implementation of educational and condom promotion programs. The incidence of HIV infection among pregnant women in Thailand has dropped from a peak of 2.4% in 1995 to 1.7% in 1997. (Phoolchareon, 1998) However ongoing political upheaval and cuts to the national HIV prevention budget may modify this pattern of success in the near future.

In the Americas the epidemic continues to grow in specific subgroups. In the United States, as summarized earlier in this chapter, the highest incidence of infection is occurring among poor women, particularly among women of color. In Mexico the incidence of infection among men who have sex with men continues high, while in Brazil and the Caribbean heterosexual transmission is increasing. At surveillance sites in the Dominican Republic and Haiti the prevalence of HIV infection among pregnant women has reached 8%. (UNAIDS, 1998)

Rapid spread of infection among injection drug users in Eastern Europe and Central Asia likely to foreshadow a large number of cases among women and increasing prevalence of perinatal transmission. The introduction of HIV into these high-risk populations has been paralleled by tremendous increases in the incidence of syphilis and other sexually transmitted diseases. (Gollub, 1999)

B. CONTAINING THE EPIDEMIC

Control of the HIV epidemic should be a worldwide health priority. Complex interactions of social, economic and cultural factors have preceded AIDS with epidemics of other sexually transmitted diseases, and now hinder control of HIV itself. Global disparities in economic status have limited efforts to control sexually transmitted diseases that are much simpler to diagnose and treat than HIV. The effect of limited monetary resources are compounded by stigmatization of HIV and sexually transmitted diseases that effect willingness to seek care, social support of afflicted individuals and health policy decision making. Traditional cultural values regarding the role of women also tends to intensify the problems. Lack of acceptance of the right of women to make decisions about child bearing and work outside the home limit options for individuals who wish to reduce risk of infection via sexual exposures. Economic independence is a crucial factor enabling women to make some decisions themselves. The options for employment outside of sex work, for divorced or widowed women, in many societies are quite restricted. These fundamental values may directly conflict with efforts to empower women to avoid risk of HIV and other sexually transmitted diseases.

To control the HIV epidemic, societies need to make deep commitments that may require an uncomfortable loss of highly valued cultural norms. Without social acceptance and encouragement, behaviorally mediated risk reduction strategies may not assume full efficacy. Vaccination is, at present, an optimal but unavailable solution. The prospects for development of an effective vaccine in the near future are not promising. Thus we have good cause to fear for the effects of HIV on women worldwide, and to increase our attention to this enormous problem as we enter the twenty-first century and the third decade of the HIV pandemic.

REFERENCES

Albert, J, Fiore, J, Fenyo, EM, et al. Biological phenotype of HIV-1 and transmission [letter]. *AIDS, 9*(7): 822–3, 1995.

Aldrich, J, Gross, R, Adler, M, et al. The effect of acute severe illness on CD4+ lymphocyte counts in nonimmunocompromised patients. *Arch Int Med, 160*:715–6, 2000.

Alioum, A, Leroy, V, Commenges, D, Dabis, F, and Salamon, R. Effect of gender, age, transmission category, and antiretroviral therapy on the progression of human immunodeficiency virus infection using multistate Markov models. *Epidemiol, 9*: 605–612, 1998.

Alliegro, MB, Dorrucci, M, Phillips, AN, et al. Incidence and consequences of pregnancy in women with known duration of HIV infection. Italian seroconversion study group. *Arch Int Med, 157*: 2585–2590, 1997.

Anastos, K, Gange, SJ, Lau, B, et al. The Women's Interagency HIV Study (WIHS) and the Multicenter AIDS Cohort Study (MACS). Gender Specific Differences in QuantitativeHIV-1 RNA levels. Paper presented at the 6th Conference on Retroviruses and Opportunistic Infections, Chicago, IL, 1999a.

Anastos, K, Kalish, LA, Hessol, N, et al. The relative value of CD4 cell count and quantitative HIV-1 RNA in predicting survival in HIV-1-infected women: results of the women's interagency HIV study. *AIDS*(13), 1999b.

Anderson, DJ, Politch, JA, Tucker, LD, et al. Quantitation of mediators of inflammation and immunity in genital tract secretions and their relevance to HIV type 1 transmission. *AIDS Res Hum Retroviruses, 14S*: S43–S49, 1998.

Ankrah, TC, Roberts, MA, Antwi, P, et al. The African AIDS case definition and HIV serology in medical in-patients at Komfo Anoyke Teaching Hospital, Kumasi, Ghana. *W African J Med, 13*(2): 98–101, 1994.

Balter, M. HIV incidence: 'more serious than we imagined'. *Science, 280*: 1864, 1998.

Balter, M. AIDS now World's fourth biggest killer. *Science, 284*: 1101, 1999.

Bartlett, JG. Protease inhibitors for HIV infection. *Ann Intern Med, 124*(12): 1086, 1996.

Bessinger, R, Clark, R, Kissinger, P, Rice, J, and Coughlin, S. Pregnancy is not associated with the progression of HIV disease in women attending an HIV oupatient program. *Am J Epidemiol, 147*(5): 434–40, 1998.

Blanche, S, Rouzioux, C, Moscato, ML, et al. A prospective study of infants born to women seropositive for human immunodeficiency virus type 1. HIV Infection in Newborns French Collaborative Study Group. *N Engl J Med, 320(25):*1643–8, 1989.

Boden, D, Hurley, A, Zhang, L, et al. HIV-1 drug resistance in newly infected individuals. *J Am Med Assoc, 282*: 1135–1141, 1999.

Bongaarts, J. Global population growth: demographic consequences of declining fertility. *Science, 282*: 419–420, 1998.

Brettle, RP, Gore, SM, Bird, AG, and McNeil, AJ. Clinical and epidemiological implications of the Centers for Disease Control/World Health Organization reclassification of AIDS cases. *AIDS, 7*: 531–539, 1993.

Brettle, RP, Raab, GM, Ross, A, et al. HIV infection in women: immunological markers and the influence of pregnancy. *AIDS, 9*: 1177–1184, 1995.

Brodine, SK, Shaffer, RA, Starkey, MJ, et al. Drug resistance patterns, genetic subtypes, clinical features, and risk factors in military personnel with HIV-1 seroconversion. *Ann Intern Med, 131*: 502–506, 1999.

Buchbinder, SP, Katz, MH, Hessol, NA, O'Malley, PM, and Holmberg, SD. Long-term HIV-1 infection with immunologic progression. *AIDS, 8*: 1123–1128, 1994.

Bush, CE, Donovan, RM, Markowitz, N, et al. Gender is not a factor in serum human immunodeficiency virus type 1 RNA levels in patients with viremia. *J Clin Microbiol, 34*(4): 970–972, 1996.

Buskin, SE, Diamond, C, and Hopkins, SG. HIV-infected pregnant women and progression of HIV disease. *Arch Int Med, 158*: 1277–1278, 1998.

Cameron, D. W., Simonsen, J. N., LJ, D. Costa, et al. Female to male transmission of human immunodeficiency virus type 1: risk factors for seroconversion in men. *Lancet, 2*(8660): 403–7, 1989.

Cao, Y, Qin, L, Zhang, L, Safrit, J, and Ho, DD. Virologic and immunologic characterization of long-term survivors of human immunodeficiency virus type 1 infection. *N Engl J Med, 332*(4): 201–208, 1995.

Carre, N, Boufassa, F, Hubert, JB, et al. Predictive value of viral load and other markers for progression to clinical AIDS after CD4+ cell count falls below 200/ml. *Int J Epidemiol, 27*: 897–903, 1998.

CDC. 1993 revised classification system for HIV infection and expanded surveillance case definition for AIDS among adolescents and adults. *Morbid Mortal Wkly Rep, RR-17*, 1992.

CDC. Management of possible sexual, injecting-drug-use, or other nonoccupational exposure to HIV, including considerations related to antiretroviral therapy. *Morbid Mortal Wkly Rep, 47:* (RR-17);1–14, 1998.

CDC. Administration of zidovudine during late pregnancy and delivery to prevent perinatal HIV transmission — Thailand, 1996–1998. *Morbid Mortal Wkly Rep, 47*: 151–4, 1998.

CDC. *HIV/AIDS Surveillance Report* . Atlanta, Georgia: U.S. Department of Health and Human Services, 1999.

Chun, T-W, Engel, D, Berrey, MM, et al. Early establishment of a pool of latently infected, resting CD4+ T cells during primary HIV-1 infection. *Proc Natl Acad Sci, 95*: 8869–8873, 1998.

Collier, AC, Coombs, RW, Schoenfeld, DA, et al. Treatment of human immunodeficiency virus infection with saquinavir, zidovudine, and zalcitabine. AIDS Clinical Trials Group. *N Engl J Med, 334 (16)*: 1011–7, 1996.

Condra, JH. Resisting resistance: maximizing the durability of antiretroviral therapy. *Ann Intern Med, 128*(11): 951–953, 1998.

Consten, EC, van Lanschot, JJ, Henny, PC, Tinnemans, JG, and van der Meer, JT. A prospective study on the risk of exposure to HIV during surgery in Zambia. *AIDS, 9*(6): 585–8, 1995.

Coombs, RW, Collier, AC, Allain, J-P, et al. Plasma viremia in human immunodeficiency infection. *N Engl J Med, 321*: 1626–1631, 1989.

Coombs, RW, Speck, CE, Hughes, JP, et al. Association between culturable human immunodeficiency virus type 1 (HIV-1) in semen and HIV-1 RNA levels in semen and blood: evidence for compartmentalization of HIV-1 between semen and blood. *J Infect Dis, 177*(2): 320–30, 1998.

Cu Uvin, S, Caliendo, AM, Reinert, SE, et al. HIV-1 in the female genital tract and the effect of antiretroviral therapy. *AIDS, 12*(7): 826–7, 1998.

Dallabetta, GA, Miotti, PG, Chiphangwi, JD, et al. Traditional vaginal agents: use and association with HIV infection in Malawian women. *AIDS, 9*(3): 293–7, 1995.

Daly, CC, Helling-Giese, GE, Mati, JK, and Hunter, DJ. Contraceptive methods and the transmission of HIV: implications for family planning. *Genitourin Med, 70*(2): 110–7, 1994.

De Cock, KM, Lucas, S, Coulibaly, D, Coulibaly, I-M, and Soro, B. Expansion of surveillance case definition for AIDS in resource-poor countries. *Lancet, 342*: 437–438, 1993.

De Cock, KM, Selick, R, Soro, B, Gayle, H, and Colebunders, RL. AIDS surveillance in Africa: a reappraisal of case definitions. *Br Med J, 303*: 1185–1188, 1991.

de Martino, M., Tovo, P. A., Galli, L., et al. HIV-I infection in perinatally exposed siblings and twins. The Italian Register for HIV Infection in Children. *Arch Dis Child, 66*(10): 1235–8, 1991.

Deacon, NJ, Tsykin, A, Solomon, A, et al. Genomic structure of an attenuated quasi species of HIV-1 from a blood transfusion donor and recipients. *Science, 270*: 988–991, 1995.

Dean, M., Carrington, M., Winkler, C., et al. Genetic restriction of HIV-1 infection and progression to AIDS by a deletion allele of the CKR5 structural gene. Hemophilia Growth and Development Study, Multicenter AIDS Cohort Study, Multicenter Hemophilia Cohort Study, San Francisco City Cohort, ALIVE Study. *Science, 273*(5283): 1856–62, 1996.

Deeks, SG, Smith, M, Holodniy, M, and Kahn, JO. HIV-1 protease inhibitors: a review for clinicians. *J Am Med Assoc, 277*: 145–153, 1997.

Del Amo, J, Petruckevitch, A, Phillips, A, et al. Disease progression and survival in HIV-1 infected Africans in London. *AIDS, 12*: 1203–1209, 1998.

Di Stefano, M, Fiore, JR, Monno, L, et al. Detection of multiple drug-resistance-associated pol mutations in cervicovaginal secretions. *AIDS, 13*: 992–994, 1999.

European Collaborative Study Group. Maternal viral load and vertical transmission of HIV-1: an important factor but not the only one. *AIDS*, 13: 1377–85, 1999.

European Study Group. Comparision of female to male and male to female transmission of HIV in 563 stable couples. European Study Group on Heterosexual Transmission of HIV. *BMJ, 304*(6830): 809–13, 1992.

Evans, JS, Nims, T, Cooley, J, et al. Serum levels of virus burden in early-stage human immunodeficiency virus type 1 disease in women. *J Infect Dis, 175*(4): 795–800, 1997.

Fahey, JL, Taylor, JMG, Detels, R, et al. The prognostic value of cellular and serologic markers in infection with human immunodeficiency virus type 1. *N Engl J Med, 322*: 166–172, 1990.

Farzadegan, H, Hoover, DR, Astemborski, J, et al. Sex differences in HIV-1 viral load and progression to AIDS. *Lancet, 352*: 1510–1514, 1998.

Feinberg, M. Hidden dangers of incompletely suppressive antiretroviral therapy. *Lancet, 349*: 1408–1409, 1997.

Feldman, C, Glatthaar, M, Morar, R, et al. Bacteremic pneumococcal pneumonia in HIV-seropositive and HIV-seronegative adults. *Chest, 116*: 107–114, 1999.

Fraser, VJ, and Powderly, WG. Risks of HIV infection in the health care setting. *Annu Rev Med, 46*: 203–11, 1995.

French, R, and Brocklehurst, P. The effect of pregnancy on survival in women infected with HIV: a systematic review of the literature and meta-analysis. *Br J Obstet Gynecol, 105*: 827–835, 1998.

Gallant, JE, Eldred, LJ, Leslie, JM, Chaisson, RE, and Quinn, TC. Impact of the 1993 revision of the CDC case definition on the performance of the W.H.O. and PAHO clinical case definitions for AIDS. *AIDS, 7*(10): 1396–1397, 1993.

Gallant, JE, Somani, J, Chaisson, RE, et al. Diagnostic accuracy of three clinical case definitions for advanced HIV diseases. *AIDS, 6*(3): 295–299, 1992.

Ghys, P. D., Fransen, K., Diallo, M. O., et al. The associations between cervicovaginal HIV shedding, sexually transmitted diseases and immunosuppression in female sex workers in Abidjan, Cote d'Ivoire. *AIDS, 11*(12): F85–93, 1997.

Gilks, C. F., and Wilkinson, D. Reducing the risk of nosocomial HIV infection in British health workers working overseas: role of post-exposure prophylaxis. *BMJ, 316*(7138): 1158–60, 1998.

Gilliam, B. L., Dyer, J. R., Fiscus, S. A., et al. Effects of reverse transcriptase inhibitor therapy on the HIV-1 viral burden in semen. *J Acquir Immune Defic Syndr Hum Retrovirol, 15*(1): 54–60, 1997.

Giorgi, JV, Ho, HN, Hirji, K, and al, et. CD8+ lymphocyte activation at human immunodeficiency virus type 1 seroconversion: development of HLA-DR+ CD38-CD8+ cells is associated with subsequent stable CD4+ cell levels. *J Infect Dis, 170*: 775–781, 1994.

Gollub, EL, and Metzger, D. Community-level HIV intervention work for women means restructing society and culture. *Am J Public Health, 89*(11): 1762, 1999.

Greenspan, D, and Greenspan, JS. HIV-related oral disease. *Lancet, 348*: 729–733, 1996.

Gulick, RM, Mellors, JW, Havlir, D, et al. Similtaneous vs sequential initiation of therapy with indinavir, zidovudine, and lamivudine for HIV-1 infection: 100-week follow-up. *J Am Med Assoc, 280*: 35–41, 1998.

Gupta, P, Mellors, J, Kingsley, L, et al. High viral load in semen of human immunodeficiency virus type 1-infected men at all stages of disease and its reduction by therapy with protease and nonnucleoside reverse transcriptase inhibitors. *J Virol, 71*(8): 6271–5, 1997.

Gwinn, M, and Wortley, PM. Epidemiology of HIV infection in women and newborns. *Clin Obstet Gynecol, 39*(2): 292–304, 1996.

Hamed, KA, Winters, MA, Holodniy, M, Katzenstein, DA, and Merigan, TC. Detection of human immunodeficiency virus type 1 in semen: effects of disease stage and nucleoside therapy. *J Infect Dis, 167*(4): 798–802, 1993.

Hammer, SM, Squires, KE, Hughes, MD, et al. A controlled tiral of two nucleoside analogues plus indinavir in persons with human immunodeficiency virus infection and CD4 cell counts of 200 per cubic millimeter or less. *N Engl J Med, 337*(11): 725–33, 1997.

Harrer, T, Harrer, E, Kalams, SA, et al. Cytotoxic T lymphocytes in asymptomatic long-term nonprogressing HIV-1 infection: breadth and specificity of the response and relation to *in vivo* viral quasispecies in a person with prolonged infection and low viral load. *J Immunol, 156*: 2616–2623, 1996.

Hart, CE, Lennox, JL, Pratt-Palmore, M, et al. Correlation of human immunodeficiency virus type 1 RNA levels in blood and the female genital tract. *J Infect Dis, 179*: 871–882, 1999.

Henrad, DR, Phillips, JF, Muenz, LR, et al. Natural history of HIV-1 cell-free viremia. *J Am Med Assoc, 274*(7): 554–558, 1995.

Hessol, NA, Lifson, AR, and Rutherford, GW. Natural history of human immunodeficiency virus infection and key predictors of HIV disease progression. *AIDS Clin Rev*: 69–93, 1989.

Hladik, F, Lentz, G, Delpit, E, McElroy, A, and McElrath, MJ. Coexpression of CCR5 and IL-2 in human genital but not blood T cells: implications for the ontogeny of the CCR5+ Th1 phenotype. *J Immunol, 163*: 2306–2313, 1999.

Hocke, C, Morlat, P, Chene, G, Dequae, L, and Dabis, F. Prospective cohort study of the effect of pregnancy on the progression of human immunodeficiency virus infection. The Groupe d'Epidaemiologie Clinique Du SIDA en Aquitaine. *Obstet Gynecol, 86*: 886–891, 1995.

Hockett, RD, Kilby, JM, Derdeyn, CA, et al. Constant mean viral copy number per infected cell in tissues regardless of high, low, or undetectable plasma HIV RNA. *J Exp Med, 189*(10): 1545–1554, 1999.

Hu, DJ, Dondero, TJ, Rayfield, MA, et al. The emerging genetic diversity of HIV. The importance of global surveillance for diagnostics, research, and prevention. *JAMA, 275*(3): 210–6, 1996.

International AIDS Society. Place of antiretroviral drugs in the treatment of HIV-infected people in Africa. *AIDS, 13*(2): IAS 1–3, 1999.

Jacobs, L. *UNAIDS chief warns against complacency in battle against AIDS in Asia.* Paper presented at the 5th International Congress on AIDS in Asia and the Pacific, Kuala Lumpur, 1999.

Kahn, JO, and Walker, BD. Acute human immunodeficiency virus type 1 infection. *N Engl J Med, 339*(1): 33–39, 1998.

Kanki, PJ, Hamel, DJ, Sankale, J-L, et al. Human immunodeficiency virus type 1 sub-types differ in disease progression. *J Infect Dis, 179*: 68–73, 1999.

Kaplan EH, Heimer R. A model-based estimate of HIV infectivity via needle sharing. *JAIDS, 5*:1116–8, 1992.

Kassa, E, de Wit, R, Hailu, E, et al. Evaluation of the World Health Organization staging system for HIV infection and disease in Ethiopia: association between clinical stages and laboratory markers. *AIDS, 13*: 381–389, 1999.

Kirchhoff, F, Greenough, TC, Brettler, DB, Sullivan, JL, and Desrosiers, RC. Brief report: absence of intact *nef* sequences in a long-term survivor with nonprogressive HIV-1 infection. *N Engl J Med, 332*(4): 228–232, 1995.

Koot, M, and et al. Prognostic value of HIV-1 syncytium-inducing phenotype for rate of CD4+ cell depletion and progression to AIDS. *Annals of Internal Medicine, 118*: 681–688, 1993.

Krieger, JN, Coombs, RW, Collier, AC, et al. Recovery of human immunodeficiency virus type 1 from semen: minimal impact of stage of infection and current antiviral chemotherapy. *J Infect Dis, 163*(2): 386–8, 1991.

Laga, M, Manoka, A, Kivuvu, M, et al. Non-ulcerative sexually transmitted diseases as risk factors for HIV-1 transmission in women: results from a cohort study. *AIDS, 7*: 95–102, 1993.

Laga, M, Taelman, H, Van der Stuyft, P, et al. Advanced immunodeficiency as a risk factor for heterosexual transmission of HIV. *AIDS, 3*(6): 361–6, 1989.

Lazzarin, A, Saracco, A, Musicco, M, and Nicolosi, A. Man-to-woman sexual transmission of the human immunodeficiency virus. Risk factors related to sexual behavior, man's infectiousness, and woman's susceptibility. Italian Study Group on HIV Heterosexual Transmission. *Arch Intern Med, 151*(12): 2411–6, 1991.

Learmont, JC, Gecy, AF, Mills, J, et al. Immunologic and virologic status after 14 to 18 years of infection with an attenuated strain of HIV-1: a report from the Sydney blood bank cohort. *N Engl J Med, 340*: 1715–1722, 1999.

Ledergerber, B, Egger, M, Oprovil, M, et al. Clinical progression and virologic failure on highly active antiretroviral therapy in HIV-1 patients: a prospective cohort study. *Lancet, 353*: 863–868, 1999.

Lifson, AR, Allen, S, Wolf, W, et al. Classification of HIV infection and disease in women from Rwanda: evaluation of the World Health Organization HIV staging system and recommended modifications. *Ann Intern Med, 122*: 262–270, 1995.

Lifson, AR, O'Malley, PM, Hessol, NA, et al. HIV seroconversion in two homosexual men after receptive oral intercourse with ejaculation: implications for counseling concerning safe sexual practices. *Am J Public Health, 80*(12): 1509–11, 1990.

Lyles, CM, Vlahov, D, Farzadegan, H, et al. Comparisons of two measures of human immunodeficiency virus (HIV) type 1 load in HIV risk groups. *J Clin Microbiol, 36*(12): 3647–3652, 1998.

Lyles, RH, Chu, C, Mellors, JW, et al. Prognostic value of plasma HIV RNA in the natural history of Pneumocystis carinii pneumonia, cytomegalovirus and Mycobacterium avium complex. *AIDS, 13*: 341–349, 1999.

Marmor, M, Weiss, LR, Lyden, M, et al. Possible female-to-female transmission of human immunodeficiency virus. *Ann Intern Med, 105*(6): 969, 1986.

Martin, MP, Dean, M, Smith, MW, et al. Genetic acceleration of AIDS progression by a promoter variant of CCR5. *Science, 282*: 1907–1911, 1998.

Mastro TD, de Vincenzi I. Probabilities of sexual HIV-1 transmission. *AIDS 10 (suppl A):* S75–82, 1996.

Mati, JK, Mbugua, S, and Wanderi, P. Cervical cancer in Kenya: prospects for early detection at primary level. *Int J Gynaecol Obstet, 47*(3): 261–7, 1994.

McFarland, W, Mvere, D, Shandera, W, and Reingold, A. Epidemiology and prevention of transfusion-associated human immunodeficiency virus transmission in sub-Saharan Africa. *Vox Sang, 72*(2): 85–92, 1997.

Melnick, SL, Sherer, R, Louis, TA, and al, et. Survival and disease progression according to gener of patients with HIV infection: the Terry Beirn Community Programs for Clinical Research on AIDS. *J Am Med Assoc, 272*: 1915–1921, 1994.

Michaels, SH, Clark, R, and Kissinger, P. Declining morbidity and mortality among patients with advanced human immunodeficiency virus infection. *N Engl J Med, 339*(6): 405–406, 1998.

Miller, V, Mocroft, A, Reiss, P, et al. Relations among CD4 lymphocyte count nadir, antiretroviral therapy, and HIV-1 disease progression: results from the EuroSIDA Study. *Ann Intern Med, 130*: 570–577, 1999a.

Miller, V, Staszewski, S, Nisius, G, et al. Risk of new AIDS diseases in people on triple therapy. *Lancet, 353*: 463, 1999b.

Monini, P, Rotola, A, DeLellis, L, et al. Latent BK virus infection and Kaposi's sarcoma pathogenesis. *Int J Cancer, 66*: 717–722, 1996.

Monzon, OT, and Capellan, JM. Female-to-female transmission of HIV. *Lancet, 2*(8549): 40–1, 1987.

Morgan, D, Maude, GH, Malamba, SS, et al. HIV-1 disease progression and AIDS-defining disorders in rural Uganda. *Lancet, 350*: 245–250, 1997.

Morgan, D, Ross, A, Mayanja, B, Malamba, S, and Whitworth, J. Early manifestations (pre-AIDS) of HIV-1 infection in Uganda. *AIDS, 12*: 591–596, 1998.

Moses, S, Plummer, FA, Bradley, JE, et al. The association between lack of male circumcision and risk for HIV infection: a review of the epidemiological data. *Sex Trans Dis, 21*(4): 201–10, 1994.

Mostad, SB, Jackson, S, Overbaugh, J, et al. Cervical and vaginal shedding of human immunodeficiency virus type 1-infected cells throughout the menstrual cycle. *J Infect Dis, 178*(4): 983–991, 1998.

Munoz, A, Kirby, AJ, He, YD, et al. Long-term survivors with HIV-1 infection: incubation period and longitudinal patterns of CD4+ lymphocytes. *Journal of Acquired Immune Deficiency Syndromes and Human Retrovirology, 8*: 496–505, 1995.

Musicco, M, Lazzarin, A, Nicolosi, A, et al. Antiretroviral treatment of men infected with human immunodeficiency virus type 1 reduces the incidence of heterosexual transmission. Italian Study Group on HIV Heterosexual Transmission. *Arch Intern Med, 154*(17): 1971–6, 1994.

Nair, P, Alger, L, Hines, S, et al. Maternal and neonatal characteristics associated with HIV infection in infants of seropositive women. *J Acquir Immune Defic Syndr, 6*(3): 298–302, 1993.

Nicolosi, A, Correa Leite, ML, Musicco, M, et al. The efficiency of male-to-female and female-to-male sexual transmission of the human immunodeficiency virus: a study of 730 stable couples. Italian Study Group on HIV Heterosexual Transmission. *Epidemiology, 5*(6): 570–5, 1994.

O'Brien, WA, Hartigan, PM, Martin, D, et al. Changes in plasma HIV-1 RNA and CD4+ lymphocyte counts and the risk of progression to AIDS. *N Engl J Med, 334*: 426–431, 1996.

Palasanthiran, P., Ziegler, J. B., Stewart, G. J., et al. Breast-feeding during primary maternal human immunodeficiency virus infection and risk of transmission from mother to infant. *J Infect Dis, 167*(2): 441–4, 1993.

Palella, FJ, Delaney, KM, Moorman, AC, et al. Declining morbidity and mortality among patients with advanced human immunodeficiency virus infection. *N Engl J Med, 338*(13): 853–860, 1998.

Paxton, WA, and Kang, S. Chemokine receptor allelic polymorphisms: relationships to HIV resistance and disease progression. *Semin Immunol, 10*(3): 187–94, 1998.

Perry, S, Jacobsberg, L, and Fogel, K. Orogenital transmission of human immunodeficiency virus (HIV). *Ann Intern Med, 111*(11): 951–2, 1989.

Pezotti, P, Napoli, PA, Acciai, S, et al. Increasing survival time after AIDS in Italy: the role of new combination antiretroviral therapies. *AIDS, 13*: 249–255, 1999.

Pezzotti, P, Galai, N, Vlahov, D, et al. Direct comparison of time to AIDS and infectious disease death between HIV seroconverter injection drug users in Italy and the United States: results from the ALIVE and ISS studies. *J Acquired Immune Defi Syndr Hum Retrovirol, 20*: 275–282, 1999.

Phoolchareon, W. HIV/AIDS prevention in Thailand: success and challenges. *Science, 280*: 1873–1874, 1998.

Planella, T, Cortes, M, Martinez-Bru, C, et al. The predictive value of several markers in the progression to acquired immunodeficiency syndrome. *Clin Chem Lab Med, 36*: 169–173, 1998.

Plourde, PJ, Pepin, J, Agoki, E, et al. Human immunodeficiency virus type 1 seroconversion in women with genital ulcers. *J Infect Dis, 170*(2): 313–7, 1994.

Plummer, FA, Simonsen, JN, Cameron, DW, et al. Cofactors in male-female sexual transmission of human immunodeficiency virus type 1. *J Infect Dis, 163*(2): 233–9, 1991.

Plummer, FA. Heterosexual transmission of human immunodeficiency virus type 1 (HIV): interactions of conventional sexually transmitted diseases, hormonal contraception and HIV-1. *AIDS Res Human Retroviruses*, Suppl: S5–10, 1998.

Prins, M, Brettle, RP, Robertson, JR, et al. Geographical variation in disease progression in HIV-1 seroconverted injecting drug users in Europe? *Int J Epidemiol, 28*: 541–549, 1999.

Quinn, TC. Global burden of the HIV pandemic. *Lancet, 348*(9020): 99–106, 1996.

Quinn, TC, Wawer, MJ, Sewankambo, N, et al. Viral load and risk of heterosexual transmission of HIV-1 among sexual partners. 7th Conference on Retroviruses and Opportunistic Infections, San Francisco, January 30-February 2, 2000.

Rabeneck, L, Hartigan, PM, Huang, IW, Souchek, J, and Wray, N. Predicting progression to AIDS: an evaluation of two approaches. *J Gen Intern Med, 11*: 622–624, 1996.

Rich, JD, Buck, A, Tuomala, RE, and Kazanjian, PH. Transmission of human immunodeficiency virus infection presumed to have occurred via female homosexual contact. *Clin Infect Dis, 17*(6): 1003–5, 1993.

Richman, DD. Antiretroviral drug resistance: mechanisms, pathogenesis, clinical significance. *Antiviral Chemother, 4*: 383–395, 1996.

Roos, MT, Lange, JM, de Goede, RE, et al. Viral phenotype and immune response in primary human immunodeficiency virus type 1 infection. *J Infect Dis, 165*(3): 427–32, 1992.

Roques, P, Marce, D, Courpotin, C, et al. Correlation between HIV provirus burden and in utero transmission. *AIDS, 7 Suppl 2*: S39–43, 1993.

Royce, RA, Sena, A, Cates, W, Jr, and Cohen, MS. Sexual transmission of HIV. *N Engl J Med, 336*(15): 1072–8, 1997.

Saag, MS, Holodniy, M, Kurtizkes, DR, et al. HIV viral load markers in clinical practice. *Nature Med, 2*(6): 625–629, 1996.

Saah, AJ, Hoover, DR, Weng, S, et al. Association of HLA profiles with early plasma viral load, CD4+ cell counts and rate of progression to AIDS following acute HIV-1 infection. *AIDS, 12*: 2107–2113, 1998.

Sabatini, MT, Patel, K, and Hirschman, R. Kaposi's sarcoma and T-cell lymphoma in an immunodeficient woman: a case report. *AIDS Res, 1*(2): 135–7, 1983.

Samuel, MC, Hessol, N, Shiboski, S, et al. Factors associated with human immunodeficiency virus seroconversion in homosexual men in three San Francisco cohort studies, 1984–1989. *J Acquir Immune Defic Syndr, 6*(3): 303–12, 1993.

Santoro-Lopes, G, Harrison, LH, Moulton, LH, et al. Gender and survival after AIDS in Rio de Janeiro, Brazil. *J Acquired Immune Defi Syndr Hum Retrovirol, 19*: 403–407, 1998.

Satcher, D. The global HIV/AIDS epidemic. *J Am Med Assoc, 281*: 1479, 1999.

Schacker, TW, Hughes, JP, Shea, T, Coombs, RW, and Corey, L. Biological and virologic characteristics of primary HIV infection. *Ann Intern Med, 128*(8): 613–620, 1998.

Schapiro, JM, Lawrence, J, Speck, R, et al. Resistance mutations to zidovudine and saquinavir in patients receiving zidovudine plus saquinavir or zidovudine and zalcitabine plus saquinavir in AIDS clincial trials group 229. *J Infect Dis, 179*: 249–253, 1999.

Schechter, MT, Le, N, Craib, KJP, et al. Use of the Markov model to estimate the waiting times in a modified W.H.O. staging system for HIV infection. *J Acquired Immun Defi Synd Hum Retrovirol, 8*: 474–479, 1995.

Schrager, LK, Young, JM, Fowler, MG, Mathieson, BJ, and Vermund, SH. Long-term survivors of HIV-1 infection: definitions and research challenges. *AIDS, 8*(suppl 1): S95–S108, 1994.

Seidlin, M, Vogler, M, Lee, E, Lee, YS, and Dubin, N. Heterosexual transmission of HIV in a cohort of couples in New York City. *AIDS, 7*(9): 1247–54, 1993.

Sewankambo, N, Gray, RH, Wawer, MJ, et al. HIV-1 infection associated with abnormal vaginal flora morphology and bacterial vaginosis. *Lancet, 350*: 546–550, 1997.

Shafer, RW, Winters, MA, Palmer, S, and Merigan, TC. Multiple concurrent reverse transcriptase and protease mutations and multidrug resistance of HIV-1 isolates from heavily treated patients. *Ann Intern Med, 128*(11): 906–911, 1998.

Shaheen, F, Sison, AV, McIntosh, L, Mukhtar, M, and Pomerantz, RJ. Analysis of HIV-1 in the cervicovaginal secretions and blood of pregnant and nonpregnant women. *J Hum Virol, 2*: 154–166, 1999.

Soto-Ramirez, LE, Renjifo, B, McLane, MF, et al. HIV-1 Langerhans' cell tropism associated with heterosexual transmission of HIV. *Science, 271*(5253): 1291–3, 1996.

Speck, C. E., Coombs, R. W., Koutsky, L. A., et al. Risk factors for HIV-1 shedding in semen. *Am J Epidemiol, 150*(6): 622–31, 1999.

Spijkerman, IJB, Prins, M, Goudsmit, J, et al. Early and late HIV-1 RNA level and its association with other markers and disease progression in long-term AIDS-free homosexual men. *AIDS, 11*: 1383–1388, 1997.

St Louis, ME, Kamenga, M, Brown, C, et al. Risk for perinatal HIV-1 transmission according to maternal immunologic, virologic, and placental factors. *JAMA, 269*(22): 2853–9, 1993.

Stanley, SK, Ostrowski, MA, Justement, JS, et al. Effect of immunization with a common recall antigen on viral expression in patients infected with human immunodeficiency virus type 1. *N Engl J Med, 334*: 1222–1230, 1996.

Staprans, SI, Hamilton, BL, Follansbee, SE, et al. Activation of virual replication after vaccination of HIV-1-infected individuals. *J Exp Med, 182*(6): 1727–37, 1995.

Sterling, TR, Lyles, CM, Vlahov, D, et al. Sex differences in longitudinal human immunodeficiency virus type 1 RNA levels among seroconverters. *J Infect Dis, 180*: 666–72, 1999.

Taha, TE, Gray, RH, Kumwenda, NI, et al. HIV infection and disturbances in vaginal flora during pregnancy. *JAIDS, 20*(1): 52–9, 1999.

Tindall, B, Evans, L, Cunningham, P, et al. Identification of HIV-1 in semen following primary HIV-1 infection. *AIDS, 6*(9): 949–52, 1992.

Tokars JI, Marcus R, Culver DH , et al, for the CDC Cooperative Needlestick Surveillance Group. Surveillance of HIV infection and zidovudine use among health care workers after occupational exposure to HIV-infected blood. *Ann Intern Med 118*: 913–9, 1993.

UK register of HIV seroconverters steering committee. The AIDS incubation period in the UK estimated from a national register of HIV seroconverters. *AIDS, 12*: 659–667, 1998.

UNAIDS. *AIDS epidemic update: December 1998* . Geneva: United Nations, 1998.

van Benthem, BHB, Veuglers, PJ, Cornelisse, PGA, et al. Is AIDS a floating point between HIV seroconversion and death? Insights from the tricontinental seroconverter study. *AIDS, 12*: 1039–1045, 1998.

Vernazza, PL, Eron, JJ, Fiscus, SA, and Cohen, MS. Sexual transmission of HIV: infectiousness and prevention. *AIDS, 13*(2): 155–66, 1999.

Vernazza, PL, Gilliam, BL, Dyer, J, et al. Quantification of HIV in semen: correlation with antiviral treatment and immune status. *AIDS, 11*(8): 987–93, 1997.

Vesanen, M, Stevens, CE, Taylor, PE, Rubinstein, P, and Saksela, K. Stability in controlling viral replication identifies long-term nonprogressors as a distinct subgroup among human immunodeficiency virus type 1-infected persons. *J Virol, 70*(12): 9035–9040, 1996.

Vittinghoff, E, Douglas, J, Judson, F, et al. Per-contact risk of human immunodeficiency virus transmission between male sexual partners. *Am J Epidemiol, 150*(3): 306–11, 1999.

Vlahov, D, Graham, N, Hoover, D, et al. Prognostic indicators for AIDS and infectious disease death in HIV-infected injection drug users: plasma viral load and CD4+ cell count. *J Am Med Assoc, 279*(1): 35–40, 1998.

Webber, MP, Schoenbaum, EE, Gourevitch, MN, et al. Temporal trends in the progression of human immunodeficiency virus disease in a cohort of drug users. *Epidemiol, 9*: 613–617, 1998.

Weisser, M, Rudin, C, Battegay, M, et al. Does pregnancy influence the course of HIV infection? Evidence from two large Swiss cohort studies. *J Acquired Immune Defi Syndr Hum Retrovirol, 17*: 404–410, 1998.

Weniger, BG, Quinhaoes, EP, Sereno, AB, et al. A simplified surveillance case definition of AIDS derived from empirical clinical data. The Clinical AIDS Study Group, and the Working Group on AIDS case definition. *J Acquired Immun Defi Synd Hum Retrovirol, 5*(12): 1212–1223, 1992.

W.H.O. International Collaborating Group for the Study of the W.H.O. Staging. Proposed 'World Health Organization Staging System for HIV-Infection and Disease': preliminary testing by an international collaborative cross-sectional study. *AIDS, 7*: 711–718, 1993.

Willerford, DM, Bwayo, JJ, Hensel, M, et al. Human immunodeficiency virus infection among high-risk seronegative prostitutes in Nairobi. *J Infect Dis, 167*(6): 1414–7, 1993.

Winkler, C, Modi, W, Smith, MW, et al. Genetic restriction of AIDS pathogenesis by an SDF-1 chemokine gene variant. *Science, 279*: 389–393, 1998.

Wong, JK, Gunthard, HF, Havlir, DV, et al. Reduction of HIV-1 in blood and lymph nodes following potent antiretroviral therapy and the virologic correlates of treatment failure. *Proc Natl Acad Sci, USA, 94*: 12574–12579, 1997.

Yerly, S, Kaiser, L, Race, E, et al. Transmission of antiretroviral-drug-resistant HIV-1 variants. *Lancet, 354*: 729–733, 1999.

Zagury, D, Lachgar, A, Chams, V, et al. C-C chemokines, pivotal in protection against HIV type 1 infection. *Proc Natl Acad Sci U S A, 95*(7): 3857–61, 1998.

Zimmerman, PA, Buckler-White, A, Alkhatib, G, et al. Inherited resistance to HIV-1 conferred by an inactivating mutation in CC chemokine receptor 5: studies in populations with contrasting clinical phenotypes, defined racial background, and quantified risk. *Molecular Med, 3*(1): 23–36, 1997.

This *Guide* is a PRELIMINARY EDITION.

We need YOUR HELP to make the NEXT EDITION as useful as possible!

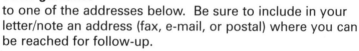

Please send your
comments
criticisms
corrections
suggested changes, and
other guidance
to one of the addresses below. Be sure to include in your letter/note an address (fax, e-mail, or postal) where you can be reached for follow-up.

Translation Partners Needed

Write to us if you can help us find partners to help us have this *Guide* translated into your native language. For instance, provide us with a contact who works with translation in your country's Ministry of Health, or tell us about a group at a medical school that translates medical texts.

Send Us Your Comments

E-mail: womencare@hrsa.gov

Fax to the attention of "Womencare": 301-443-0791 (USA)

Postal address: Womencare
Parklawn Building, Room 11A-33
5600 Fishers Lane
Rockville, Maryland 20857
USA

Note that this and subsequent editions of
A Guide to the Clinical Care of Women with HIV
will be available online.

Go to the HIV/AIDS Bureau Web site
and click on the publication *Women's Guide*:
http://www.hrsa.gov/hab

II. Approach to the Patient
Jean Anderson, MD

The woman with HIV infection is indistinguishable from most women seen in primary care today. Women with HIV cover the spectrum of age, color, geography, education, cultural background, and income level, and have all of the health and lifestyle concerns any other woman has, in addition to those related to HIV. She is often asymptomatic, and may not know she is infected. She is frequently a mother and a caretaker for other family members. The issues most important to her will be those shaped by her personal circumstances — HIV is part of these circumstances, but her own perception of how big a part will vary from woman to woman and from time to time. The health care provider-patient relationship begins with where the individual woman is. To be most effective, it must become a partnership, based on mutual trust and respect.

This chapter reviews general guidelines for interaction with all patients, highlighting points that are particularly relevant to women with HIV infection, and provides an overview of the initial and ongoing medical and psychosocial evaluation.

I. GENERAL GUIDELINES

A. COMMUNICATION

The initial interaction of patient and provider should begin with introductions and from there, it should be highlighted with communication that is clear and nonjudgmental. Language and terminology used should be sensitive, inoffensive, and easily understandable to the individual patient. This will vary depending on the patient's age, cultural background and level of education. Translation will be needed for women unable to adequately understand or express themselves in the language of the medical provider.

Whenever possible, questions should be asked in an open-ended manner, including questions about behavior and treatment adherence, and the woman should be given permission to be honest and to acknowledge failure in terms of relapse or nonadherence. She should be given adequate time and opportunity to ask questions and express concerns.

Women undergoing gynecologic exams often feel special anxiety, vulnerability, embarrassment, or simply fear of discomfort or the discovery of pathology. It is important to adequately prepare her verbally for the exam and visually as well, if possible, showing her charts, models, or equipment (such as specula), which may demystify the whole process. Explain what will be done and why, as well as the degree of discomfort to be expected. During the exam tell her what you are going to do before doing it, describe what is seen or felt, reassure when findings are normal.

Do not underestimate the importance of nonverbal communication. Facial expression and body posture are often far more articulate than words, and the most effective providers are sensitive to these cues and use their own body language with care. Maintaining frequent eye contact encourages the patient's candor, builds rapport and trust, helps allay embarrassment and fear, and conveys your interest and attention.

Patients should be given written instructions on how to reach their providers when there are problems or questions and to make appointments. Whenever possible, written information about HIV and its treatment, as well as other health issues, should be available to supplement face-to-face discussions.

B. RESPECT

Every person deserves respect. Do not be condescending or patronizing. Under no circumstances should a patient ever be treated as a sexual object, particularly when assessing risk behaviors or performing the pelvic exam. Although different circumstances may dictate different levels of formality, addressing the patient by her first name (without her express consent) or, especially, by terms of familiarity (e.g. honey, dear) is usually inappropriate and often offensive.

Respect for the individual includes respect for her beliefs and values. Use of complimentary therapies among HIV-infected individuals is common and should be respected, not ridiculed, even while discouraging potentially harmful remedies and emphasizing the proven effectiveness of currently recommended regimens.

C. SENSITIVITY

Sensitivity is essential to gather and impart important information, to foster trust, and to insure ongoing follow-up. It requires attention to how words are used, questions are asked, and to a great deal that is unspoken. Responding to a patient's fear, anxiety, denial, or anger is inevitably part of the health provider's role and requires consideration of more than a disease process, but of a whole person and the entire context of her life. Any chronic and life-threatening disease carries with it an enormous burden of vulnerability and loss of control. Anything the provider can do to give back some control to the woman will help ease that burden. The importance of adherence to antiretroviral regimens for optimal effectiveness and to reduce the development of drug resistance has been well established. Allowing the patient to be involved in choosing her treatment regimen will allow her values and lifestyle (job schedule, etc) to be considered and is believed to enhance adherence. Understanding her cultural background enhances your sensitivity. For example, involvement of the patient's spouse or mother during visits may be particularly important and reassuring for Hispanic women.

D. CONFIDENTIALITY

Confidentiality is a major cornerstone of the therapeutic relationship. It carries special meaning for HIV-infected individuals who have experienced discrimination in the workplace and other settings; stigmatization; and occasional abandonment by friends or family. HIV-positive women may be particularly vulnerable to these effects because of lower economic status, cultural traditions and general societal beliefs about the role of women, minority status, and child-care or other caretaking responsibilities. Information about a patient's HIV status or details about her medical condition should be kept strictly confidential by providers and shared only with the express permission of the woman herself. At the same time she should be encouraged and assisted in disclosing her status to others who need to know, i.e. sexual partners and health care providers.

II. THE EVALUATION OF THE HIV-INFECTED WOMAN

A. TEAM APPROACH

Because of the medical and social complexity of HIV disease, a team approach to the care of women with HIV is essential. Expertise needed includes HIV medical expertise (including management of antiretroviral regimens), gynecology, nursing, counseling, and social service assistance/case management. Throughout the course of HIV infection, multidisciplinary medical collaborations should be available for evaluation and management of the varied medical problems associated with HIV. The use of peer counselors may be especially helpful as women deal with negotiating safer sexual practices, contraception and other reproductive concerns, medication adherence, and other issues where similar cultural background and personal experience with HIV may facilitate education and candid discussion.

B. HIV EXPERIENCE

Care by a medical provider with HIV experience is one of the few specific factors that has been shown to prolong the life of HIV-infected individuals (Laine, 1998; Kitahata, 1996). This is increasingly important as antiretroviral treatment becomes steadily more complicated and recommendations change on an almost monthly basis. Awareness of drug interactions and strategies to avoid the development of antiretroviral resistance are but two issues that have a significant impact on both the short- and long-term health of the

HIV-positive individual. Primary providers with little or no HIV experience should link with providers with HIV expertise to provide optimal care by referral or regular consultation. Current USPHS treatment guidelines, several as living documents with regular online updating, can be accessed at **http://www.hivatis.org**. The Health Resources and Services Administration also supports the AIDS Education and Training Centers warmline (1-800-933-3413), which is a resource for clinical providers needing expert consultation.

C. CULTURAL SETTING/BACKGROUND

The ability to give optimal patient care depends on an understanding of where the patient "begins," her traditions and beliefs. These affect her understanding of health and disease and her acceptance of conventional medical treatment, as well as possible reliance on alternative or complementary therapies. These also affect her view of herself as a woman, her role and responsibilities in society, and issues related to childbearing and contraception. The role of cultural sensitivity in the care of HIV-positive women will be more fully addressed in Chapter VIII on Psychosocial and Cultural Considerations.

D. SPIRITUALITY

The spiritual dimension of a person's life encompasses their beliefs and values and what gives their life meaning and a sense of wholeness. (Puchalski, 1999) Spirituality is important throughout life, during both health and illness, and an individual's beliefs and values can have a profound effect on the way they view illness and its treatment. Some women may view HIV as a punishment and this belief may lessen her acceptance of treatment or may put her at risk of nonadherence. Major spiritual questions which often arise during illness are:

- What gives my life meaning?
- Why is this thing happening to me?
- How will I survive this loss?
- What will happen to me when life ends?

    It is important that the health care provider consider spirituality as an important component of physical, emotional, and mental health and assess the woman's beliefs and learn what is important to her. The spiritual history should include specific questions about the patient's faith or beliefs; the importance and influence of these in her life; her involvement in a spiritual or religious community and its importance to her; and how the health care provider can help address these issues as part of her health care. Spirituality should be addressed as an ongoing issue, and referrals to ministers, priests, rabbis, other spiritual guides or similar community resources can be an important component of care. The provider's own spiritual beliefs can be a source of strength personally and can enhance the patient-provider relationship, but should not be imposed on the patient-her own beliefs should be respected.

E. IDENTIFYING SUPPORT SYSTEMS/DISCLOSURE

During the initial evaluation, the HIV-infected woman's social and emotional support system should be identified and reinforced and updated information about this support system should be obtained at each visit. To whom has she disclosed her HIV status and what was the response? Many HIV-positive women experience feelings of guilt and shame, or are fearful of violence or abandonment, and so are reluctant to trust anyone with knowledge of their infection or their feelings about it. Their sense of isolation is harmful to both their physical and emotional well-being, and may result in avoiding clinic visits and nonadherence with drug therapy. The use of peer advocates or support groups may offer additional support for many women with HIV.

Special issues involve disclosure to sexual partners, children, and other health care providers. Disclosure to those individuals who may be at risk for transmission of HIV from the patient should be encouraged and barriers to disclosure, such as fear of violence, should be identified and addressed. The provider should offer assistance with disclosure when appropriate. Disclosure of a mother's HIV status to her children, who may or may not be infected themselves, is a personal decision and should be honored. The provider should discuss the various considerations in this decision and offer assistance, if needed.

F. MEDICAL EVALUATION

INITIAL EVALUATION

The initial evaluation of an HIV-infected woman should include a comprehensive medical assessment, including a detailed HIV history: date of diagnosis, possible routes of exposure, HIV-related symptoms or opportunistic infections, previous antiretroviral or prophylactic therapies, disclosure history and support systems (see above). Prior antiretroviral treatments should be documented in as much depth as possible, including specific medications, length of treatment, side effects or complications, response, and adherence. Current employment, relationship status and childcare responsibilities, insurance status, and drug and alcohol abuse must all be considered in decision-making about further therapeutic regimens. A comprehensive gynecologic history should be obtained, including menstrual history, sexual practices, contraception and condom use history, previous sexually transmitted and other genital tract infections, prior abnormal pap smears, and other gynecologic illnesses or symptoms. The initial physical examination should include a baseline pelvic exam with pap smear and other studies as needed based on history and physical findings. Various studies (Anderson, 1989; Frankel, 1997; Minkoff, 1999) have found that both prevalence and incidence of gynecologic problems are high in HIV-infected women throughout their disease course.

This initial assessment should take place over several closely-spaced visits. This will allow the woman and her clinical care team to become familiar with one another and to begin to develop the trust and partnership that will form the foundation of her ongoing care. This is particularly important for the woman with newly diagnosed HIV, who is often struggling with the shock, fear, denial and despair that accompany the discovery of a life-threatening illness; she should be given the opportunity to assimilate information about HIV and her own clinical status in small bites.

FOLLOW-UP VISITS

Follow-up visits should be scheduled at intervals based on the woman's HIV clinical, immunologic, and virologic status; other medical or comorbid conditions, including substance abuse or mental illness; and other individual needs for counseling or psychosocial support. CD4 cell counts and HIV-RNA levels should be monitored at 3–4 month intervals and more often if results suggest inadequate or failing therapeutic response, or with development of clinical signs or symptoms. At each interval visit the woman should be questioned about new symptoms, side effects/adherence with medications, and psychosocial issues and concerns. Last menstrual period should be documented, as well as current sexual activity, and interval use of condoms and contraception. Risk behaviors should be reassessed at regular intervals, since sexual and drug use patterns may vary, and safe practices should be reinforced. Pelvic examination should be repeated at least annually, and more frequently with history of abnormal pap smears, unsafe sexual practices, exposure to STDs, or development of gyn signs or symptoms. STD screening should be performed when the patient reports recent or ongoing high-risk sexual activity. Pelvic examination every six months may be considered in women with clinically advanced disease, low CD4 cell counts, and/or high viral loads since their incidence of certain HIV-related gynecologic problems may be increased. The medical and gynecologic evaluation of the HIV-infected woman is described in more detail in Chapter IV on Primary Medical Care and Chapter VI on Gynecologic Problems.

G. FAMILY-CENTERED CARE

HIV is a disease of families. Not only may the woman be infected, but her husband or partner and children may also be living with HIV. Even when other family members are not infected, they are deeply affected by the presence of chronic and life-threatening illness within the family, possible fears of transmission of infection, and often stigma. The HIV-positive woman may neglect her own care while providing care to sick family members or to her children. The provider should encourage all HIV-positive family members to receive appropriate care and should help enlist family support for the infected woman, by providing information and education about HIV and updates on the woman's condition (with her permission), and by assistance in identifying support systems for the entire family.

H. EDUCATION AND COUNSELING

Despite the dramatic advances in therapy, decreases in mortality and hospital-izations, and overall improvement in quality of life, HIV remains a life-threat-ening and often life-ending disease with no cure on the horizon. For women it is often enveloped by poverty; isolation; person, partner, or community drug use; and the competing priorities of children and family. Not dissimilar to dia-betes, modern management of HIV disease requires a basic understanding of HIV infection and an intense personal involvement in one's own care — tak-ing multiple medications on fairly strict schedules, food requirements, recog-nizing and managing side effects, etc. Unlike most other chronic medical conditions, HIV-positive individuals remain infectious for the rest of their lives and must learn about and become empowered to change behaviors that put themselves or others at risk. This learning process is ongoing and life-long and requires continuous reinforcement. It should aim to correct misconcep-tions and myths and should recognize that relapses in unsafe sexual or drug-using behaviors and at least episodic problems with adherence are the norm rather than the exception. Peer advocates (HIV-affected women from similar cultural backgrounds) can be effective members of the clinical team to help educate patients, advocate for them, and provide counseling as needed.

I. ACCESS TO CARE

A recent report from the HIV Cost and Services Utilization Study (HCSUS), using a national sample representative of the adult US population infected with HIV and in ongoing care, found significant variations in service utiliza-tion and receipt of medication. Women were more likely than men to use the Emergency Department and to be hospitalized and were less likely to have received antiretroviral therapy including a protease inhibitor or nonnucleoside reverse transcriptase inhibitor by early 1998. Other predictors for poor access to care included racial or ethnic minority status and lack of insurance (Shapiro, 1999). If women with HIV are to benefit equally from the advances in under-standing and management of this infection, attention must be paid at the indi-vidual, community, and societal level to the factors hindering equal access to care: stigma and isolation; lack of empowerment; competing concerns (e.g. food, housing, care for other family members); childcare; transportation; insur-ance; violence against women, and many more.

REFERENCES

Anderson J, Horn J, King R, et al. Selected gynecologic issues in women with HIV infection. Int Conf AIDS 1989 June 4–9; 5: 760 (abst # Th.D.P.10).

Frankel R, Selwyn P, Mezger J, Andrews S. High prevalence of gynecologic disease among hospitalized women with human immunodeficiency virus infection. *Clin Infect Dis* 25 (3):706–712, 1997.

Kitahata M, Koepsell T, Deyo R, et al. Physicians' experience with the acquired immunodeficiency syndrome as a factor in patients' survival. *N Engl J Med* 334 (11):701–706, 1996.

Laine C, Markson L, McKee L. The relationship of clinic experience with advanced HIV and survival of women with AIDS. *AIDS* 12: 417–424, 1998.

Minkoff HL, Eisenberger-Matityahu D, Feldman J, Burk R, Clarke L. Prevalence and incidence of gynecologic disorders among women infected with human immunodeficency virus. *Am J Obstet Gynecol* 180 (4):824–836,1999.

Puchalski CM et al. FICA. A spiritual assessment. *J Palliative Care* 1999 (in press).

Shapiro MF, Morton SC, McCaffrey DF, et al. Variations in the care of HIV-infected adults in the United States: Results for the HIV Cost and Services Utilization Study. *JAMA* 281(24):2305–2315, 1999.

III. PREVENTION OF HIV

Chia Wang, MD, MS and Connie Celum, MD, MPH

I. INTRODUCTION

Two decades into the human immunodeficiency virus (HIV) epidemic, scientists and clinicians on both the biomedical and behavioral fronts continue to be faced with daunting challenges. While scientists have made progress in vaccine development and in understanding the complexities of the viral-host immune response, the prospect of highly effective, widely available biomedical preventative measures are still in developmental stages. Thus, there remains a critical need to identify and implement effective behavioral strategies and to more effectively address the complex forces that fuel the heterosexual HIV epidemic, including poverty, migration of populations, social and cultural disruption, gender discrimination, and stigma about STDs and HIV.

Many of the measures that women can take to prevent acquisition of STDs and HIV have been known for the past decade: abstaining from intercourse, selecting low-risk partners, negotiating partner monogamy and male condom use. However, the high rates of incident HIV infections among women in many parts of the world and the rising incidence among women in the United States is a testament to prevention barriers facing women in heterosexual relationships. Women often are unaware of their partners' infection status or level of risk, and in many cases, are unable to negotiate sexual safety. Importantly, in many parts of the world, prevalence figures suggest that girls are exposed to HIV earlier than boys (UNAIDS, 1999). Young girls are often emotionally immature, economically disadvantaged, and socially inexperienced, making them vulnerable to sexual relationships that may expose them to HIV and to other sexually transmitted infections that can potentiate HIV transmission. Women in economically disadvantaged nations and in socially marginalized groups in the industrialized world may have less access to medical care for treatment of STDs and contraception, and may also not feel empowered to negotiate for condom use, abstinence, or monogamy within their sexual relationships. Thus, culturally-sensitive interventions that target both behavioral and biologic risk factors for HIV are necessary to reduce transmission to women and girls.

This chapter discusses issues regarding HIV testing, including risk assessment and pre- and post-test counseling, and then goes on to review models of behavioral intervention strategies for HIV prevention, published behavioral intervention trials, and some practical aspects of counseling women on how to reduce sexual risk behavior. Biologic cofactors that may increase risk and thus may be targets for intervention are briefly examined. Finally, new approaches to HIV and STD prevention, including microbicides, vaccines, and post-exposure antiviral medication are reviewed. The important issues of substance abuse and strategies for changing drug use behavior are not addressed in this chapter, but are reviewed extensively in Chapter X.

II. RISK ASSESSMENT FOR STD/HIV INFECTIONS

■ **Unprotected sex increases a woman's risk of HIV infection, based in large part on her partner(s)' risk behaviors.**

Just as most people would find celibacy an impractical means of reducing sexual risk, many individuals may find changing other specific sex behaviors difficult or unacceptable. While some sexual behaviors may be less "mainstream" than others, it is important to remember that participation in such behaviors does not necessarily reflect a lack of morals or willpower, but rather different perceptions of enjoyable and common sex behavior. Furthermore, sexually active women may not realize that they are practicing behaviors that put them at risk for HIV infection. Because of the heterogeneous nature of sexual practices, individual risk assessment is crucial in any attempt to reduce risk of HIV by changing sex behavior. In pre-and post-test HIV counseling, individual risk assessment provides a framework in which to conduct further behavioral intervention and identifies patients appropriate for HIV and STD screening. Guidelines for physicians and other care practitioners recommend that HIV and STD risk assessment be conducted for every patient; however, most primary care physicians do not routinely incorporate questions about sexual behavior into routine patient care.

■ **Clinician discomfort and fear of embarrassing or offending the patient when discussing sex are impediments to conducting effective risk assessment.**

In such circumstances, the clinician may find it more acceptable to "frame" the discussion by explaining the routine nature of such questions, thus demonstrating that the patient is not singled out because of mannerisms, appearance, or ethnicity. One approach may be to emphasize the importance role of this information for patient care: "To be able to provide the best care for you today, we need to understand your risk for certain infections by talking about your sexual practices." Another may be to allude to the universality of many concerns: "Many women find it difficult to get their men to wear condoms; has this been a problem for you?" (Curtis, 1999)

■ **As with any type of medical history taking, open-ended questions probably serve as the most effective means of eliciting information when taking a sexual history.**

Language should be clear, easy to understand, nonoffensive, and nonjudgemental. Many clinicians prefer closed-ended questions when they are functioning under time pressures. In such cases, a questionnaire that the patient completes in the waiting room may be a preferred tool. Whenever possible, however, clinician-patient interaction serves as the ideal forum for sexual risk assessment.

■ **Many clinicians are not familiar with risk factors for HIV infection specifically relevant to women.**

Risk factors for HIV infection in male homosexuals and intravenous drug users have been well described. In contrast, factors that may increase risk in women, such as a history of unwanted pregnancy, or an incarcerated sex partner, are less specific, and less well recognized. While some risk factors for women can be derived from epidemiologic studies, such as history of "high-risk STDs" (i.e. gonorrhea or syphilis), crack cocaine use, and intravenous drug use, some women are at risk through monogamous partner relationships with their HIV-infected husbands. Therefore, identifying risk behaviors in women requires a careful and skilled clinician. In many cases, a low threshold for recommending HIV testing is necessary. Important risk topic areas to cover are listed in Table 3-1.

TABLE 3-1: RISK ASSESSMENT FOR STD/HIV FOR WOMEN
Number of sex partners in the previous year_____, and lifetime: _____
Sex with: ❑men, ❑women, or ❑both
History of abnormal pap smear: ❑yes, or ❑no
History of sexually transmitted disease: ❑yes, or ❑no
History of using: ❑intravenous drugs, ❑sharing needles, ❑use of crystal methamphetamines, or ❑crack cocaine
History of a sex partner who was incarcerated: ❑yes, or ❑no
History of alcohol abuse: ❑yes, or ❑no
History of feeling that the sex partner puts the patient at risk: ❑yes, or ❑no
How does the woman protect herself from AIDS?
How does the woman protect herself from unplanned pregnancy?
Is there anything else that she feels she should mention to ensure good medical care?

III. HIV COUNSELING AND TESTING

■ **There are clear benefits to HIV testing.**

For a woman, knowledge of her serostatus is essential to prevent vertical transmission to her infant and horizontal transmission to her partners, and to seek medical care for herself. With the proven efficacy of several peripartum antiviral regimens to reduce vertical transmission rates and medical therapy to improve survival among HIV-infected individuals, there are even stronger reasons to urge sexually active women to seek HIV testing for themselves and their partners.

■ **Screening strategies range from mandatory screening of pregnant women to selective screening of high-risk women.**

Selective screening strategies have targeted intravenous drug users, STD clinic attendees, and economically-disadvantaged individuals (Ades, 1999). The advantage of selective screening is cost-savings, particularly in low-prevalence parts of the world. Many experts favor a universal recommendation for HIV screening, at least for pregnant women. The advantage of universal screening is not only increased detection rates, but perhaps also increased test acceptance. Universal screening removes the stigma of HIV testing by eliminating any targeted testing based on sexual orientation, socioeconomic status, or race. When HIV testing is stigmatized, women in high-risk groups may be reluctant to identify themselves. On the other hand, the cost of universal HIV testing is significantly higher than voluntary, selective screening strategies, and there are both practical and ethical issues in implementing universal screening, even in perinatal care.

A. PRE- AND POSTTEST HIV COUNSELING

■ **The counseling that occurs before and after HIV testing has three principal goals (Celum, 1999):**

1. to provide counseling about risk reduction for HIV-negative persons;

2. to identify HIV-infected persons for clinical interventions; and

3. to provide counseling to HIV-positive persons about potential transmission.

■ **The components of HIV pre-test and post-test counseling are outlined in Table 3-2**

Pre-test counseling should include discussion about the basic facts of HIV infection, the acquired immunodeficiency syndrome (AIDS), and HIV testing. However, in most situations, emphasis should be placed less on didactic material than on individualized discussion of risk and risk-reduction unless the patient has very limited understanding of HIV/AIDS. Post-test counseling should reinforce these concepts in the context of the test result. Regardless of the test result, resources and referrals for the patient and/or their partner, should be provided. For patients at risk for domestic violence, the potential domestic turmoil that a positive test result can elicit should be

Table 3-2: Components of HIV Pre- and Post-test Counseling

Pre-test Counseling

- Assess understanding of HIV transmission and natural history; psychological stability; social support; impact of a positive result
- Discuss likelihood and meaning of positive, negative, and indeterminate test results*
- Discuss provisions made at the site for confidentiality. (In the United States, some states have name-based reporting of HIV, and clients should be informed about the availability of anonymous testing)
- Ensure that follow-up is available
- Emphasize the importance of obtaining test results
- Discuss risk reduction plan and referral to other services
- Obtain informed consent for HIV antibody testing

* For patients who identify a high-risk exposure, the clinician should explain that tests are generally positive within 3 months of exposure. Therefore, repeat testing should be recommended 3 months after exposure, if the initial test is negative.

Post-test Counseling

- Ensure that the client is ready to receive results
- Disclose and interpret results:
  - *For HIV seronegative persons:*
    - ► Readdress and reinforce risk reduction plan
    - ► Discuss the need for repeat testing for those with recent (< 3 months) exposure or ongoing risk behavior
  - *For persons with indeterminate HIV-1 Western blots:*
    - ► Discuss prevalence of and risk factors for indeterminate
    - ► *For persons with p24 bands and persons with high risk behavior:*
      - ♦ Discuss the possibility of acute HIV infection and need for repeat testing in 1, 3, and 6 months
      - ♦ Perform HIV polymerase chain reaction, if available, to confirm infection status and determine viral load
  - *For HIV seropositive persons:*
    - ► Differentiate between being HIV-infected and having AIDS
    - ► Emphasize the importance of early clinical intervention, if available, and make medical referral, if necessary
    - ► Counsel patient that he/she is HIV positive and discuss ways to avoid transmitting HIV to others
    - ► Assess need for psychological support and provide referral, if necessary and if available
    - ► Assess possibility of domestic violence and provide referral, if necessary and if available
    - ► Ensure that the patient has follow-up

emphasized. This issue will be further addressed in the section on ethnic and gender considerations.

■ Make use of an opportunity to provide client-centered counseling

Any time spent with the patient, however short, provides an opportunity for the clinician to conduct individualized counseling about recognizing and reducing high-risk sexual behaviors. Patients who present with concerns or symptoms of sexually transmitted diseases (STDs) are usually also at risk or concerned about risk for STD, including HIV. In the context of a negative HIV test, the post-test counseling session provides a valuable opportunity to develop a risk reduction plan in a woman who has identified herself as someone who concerned about risk and may be at high risk. Many clinicians may find it effective to deliver the negative test result in the context of a "second chance," thus emphasizing that current behaviors are unsafe and can be changed.

B. RAPID TESTS

■ **Rapid tests are a good alternative in certain circumstances.**

After all, HIV testing is only of value if patients return for their test results and post-test counseling. Many testing programs in the United States use an initial enzyme-linked immunosorbent assay (ELISA) with confirmation through Western blot (WB). In less developed areas, two ELISAs run in sequence are often used. With both protocols, the patient is required to return to clinic one to two weeks after testing for results. In 1995, 25% of persons testing HIV-positive and 33% of persons testing HIV negative at publicly funded HIV testing sites in the U.S. failed to return for test results (CDC, 1998d). Similar low return rates have been described in Nairobi, Kenya, and in other parts of the world.

Rapid testing for HIV would result in substantial cost savings and circumvent patient no-show rates. At least 10 rapid tests, defined as tests requiring less than two hours, are currently available internationally, although only one test (Single Use Diagnostic System HIV-1 Test) is approved for use in the United States (See Chapter IV on Primary Care) (Kassler, 1997; Spielberg, 1996). The W.H.O. has developed alternative testing strategies using sequential rapid tests, thus obviating the need for expensive and delayed confirmatory testing. Some tests require as little as five minutes and are easy to perform in the field. Most tests are 95% to 100% sensitive and specific. In the United States, the CDC has published recommendations that clients receive the results of rapid HIV tests on the day of testing. Patients who test negative can be given a definitive negative result without a return visit. For patients who test positive, it is recommended that they be informed that their screening test was positive, and that they should return to receive a confirmed test result.

In the United States, rapid testing is most appropriate in areas of high prevalence where clinic return rates are low (STD clinics, Emergency departments) or an HIV diagnosis will influence immediate management decisions (post-exposure prophylaxis, unknown HIV status in a pregnant woman presenting to Labor & Delivery). In many ways, rapid testing is most appropriate in economically disadvantaged countries where HIV seroprevalence is high, laboratory resources are limited, and patient travel to and from clinic may be very inconvenient.

■ **Rapid tests may result in unwanted test results**

Critics of rapid testing for HIV are concerned about the ability to provide appropriate counseling outside the framework of two visits for pre- and post-test counseling. Importantly, the prompt sequence of events associated with rapid testing may not give the patient enough time to digest counseling information. However, for many women in areas where rapid tests are likely to be used, rapid testing presents several difficulties. Women may find it difficult to decline an unwanted test, sometimes related to a cultural injunction against refusing a test offered by a health care worker perceived as an authority figure. Furthermore, women may fear that refusing HIV testing may result in not receiving other health care services offered by the clinic. Therefore, availability of rapid tests may result in subtle coercion of a woman to consent to HIV testing. Informal surveys in the context of HIV research in Kenya have revealed that many women feel that an interval of one week between testing and results is ideal. In some cases, failure to return to clinic for HIV test results may reflect a desire not to have had the test in the first place.

C. IMPACT OF HIV COUNSELING AND TESTING ON PREVENTION

What is the evidence that HIV testing may change risk behavior? The literature in this area is difficult to synthesize, largely because of evolving counseling practices, varying lengths of follow-up, and lack of a well-defined endpoint. In one large prospective study the incidence of STDs was determined for patients who received HIV testing and counseling at a public STD clinic in Baltimore. Both HIV positive and negative patients demonstrated high rates of STDs 6 to 23 months after receiving HIV test results and posttest counseling (Zenilman, 1992). In another study, the incidence of gonorrhea was measured after receipt of HIV result and post-test counseling. HIV testing and counseling was associated with a moderate decreased in gonorrhea infection among patients who tested positive for the virus, but with a slight increase in incidence in patients who tested negative (Otten, 1993). These findings suggest that learning of a positive HIV test result may have a modest effect on sexual risk-taking. The studies also raise important concerns about the effectiveness of HIV testing and counseling in impacting sexual risk-taking, and about potential disinhibition after receiving a negative test result.

Results from a study of discordant couples in Zaire were more promising; among 149 discordant couples who voluntarily attended an HIV counseling center, HIV testing and post-test counseling resulted in a increase in consistent condom use from less than 5% to more than 70% (Kamenga, 1991). During 100 person years of follow-up, incidence of new HIV infections was only 3%. The difference between these results and the results obtained in Baltimore and Miami may reflect varying levels of baseline HIV knowledge, the differences between individuals in long-term relationships versus casual relationships, and cultural and geographic influences.

IV. BEHAVIORAL INTERVENTION MODELS

■ **The Health Belief Model, the Social Cognitive Theory, the Theory of Reasoned Action, and the Stages of Change Theory** (Bandura, 1996; Fishbein 1999) have been developed to explain determinants of human behavior change. These models all have in common the theory that perceived risks and benefits of behavioral change predict the likelihood of behavior change as well as can guide the approach to behavioral interventions. These models are described and contrasted in Table 3-3.

■ **The AIDS Risk Reduction Model (ARRM)** integrates the concepts of the above-mentioned theoretical models into a framework providing information, motivation, and behavioral skills specific to AIDS risk reduction (Catania, 1990) (Fisher, 1992). With this model, counselors help patients to identify sexual behaviors that put them at risk for acquiring HIV, formulate plans to change these behaviors, and take action to realize these plans.

■ **The Stage of Change (SOC) behavioral theory** proposes that the process of behavioral change occurs along a continuum of five fundamental stages (Table 3-3) (Coury-Doniger, 1999). The stages can be used to tailor the counselor's approach to an individual by assessing where an individual is on that continuum for a specific behavior. For example, an individual with multiple partners who sees no need to use condoms consis-

---

TABLE 3-3: BEHAVIORAL THEORIES RELEVANT TO SEXUAL RISK REDUCTION COUNSELING

HEALTH BELIEF MODEL

Adopting health-protective behavior depends on a person feeling personally threatened by a disease with serious negative consequences, and must feel that the benefits of making the behavior change will be outweigh the costs of not changing.

SOCIAL COGNITIVE THEORY

Adopting health-protective behavior depends on a person believing that he or she has the ability to change (self-efficacy) and that the benefits of making the behavior change will outweigh the costs of not changing.

THEORY OF REASONED ACTION

Adopting health-protective behavior depends on a person's strength of intention to perform that behavior. The strength of the intention is based on the person's overall positive or negative attitude towards performing the behavior, based on perceived outcomes, as well as whether the person believes that important family members and friends believe that he or she should alter behavior.

STAGES OF CHANGE

Adoption of new behavior involves five distinct stages:

1. *Precontemplative*	Does not see need to do target behavior
2. *Contemplative*	Sees a need to do target behavior, but is ambivalent
3. *Ready for Action*	Ready to do target behavior soon, or has already started
4. *Action*	Doing target behavior consistently 3–6 months
5. *Maintenance*	Doing target behavior consistently > 6 months

---

tently would be in the Precontemplative stage. In contrast, a woman in a mutually monogamous relationship who sees the need to know her partner's HIV status, but fears angering her partner by this request, would be in the Action stage. A counselor's approach to these two patients would be different. For the first individual, counseling directed at recognition of risk would be most appropriate, while for the second woman, communication and goal-setting skills should be emphasized. Importantly, individuals do not always move forwards linearly along this continuum, but may "relapse" and move forwards and backwards between the stages. At the Rochester STD clinic, clinicians who have formally incorporated the SOC in their risk assessment and counseling of STD clients report a high degree of satisfaction with the SOC model as a diagnostic tool that guides their specific counseling interventions with a client.

V. PUBLISHED BEHAVIORAL INTERVENTION TRIALS

Several well-designed randomized controlled trials have been conducted to assess the efficacy of various behavioral intervention strategies, and most conclude that such interventions result in decreased sexual risk-taking, primarily unprotected sex, and in some studies, STD and HIV incidence. In contrast to didactic education sessions, behavioral interventions focus on recognizing risk and formulating effective risk reduction strategies. Knowledge alone does not motivate change. To translate this concept into an issue many of us have experienced, consider the issue of weight reduction and diet modification. Despite widespread knowledge about the adverse health effects of eating fatty foods, adhering to a diet is notoriously difficult. Similarly, knowledge about STDs and HIV is not enough to implement change in sexual behavior.

Randomized controlled studies using STD incidence as an outcome provide objective evidence of health-related endpoints, thus representing the most valid measurement of an intervention's efficacy. Five such trials have been published in the past few years examining the efficacy of behavioral intervention strategies using STD incidence as an outcome measure. (Table 3-4) All five studies used similar intervention approaches incorporating education, motivation, and development of a concrete plan for behavioral change. Sessions were structured as individual or group counseling.

■ **Behavioral interventions can lead to lower rates of STD acquisition**

As shown in Table 3-4, results of these studies varied. The discrepancy in reported outcomes may be related to several factors. The sample sizes of the NIMH study (NIMH, 1998) and CDC-funded Project RESPECT (Kamb, 1998) study were large, providing excellent ability to detect even a modest effect of the intervention. In the San Francisco study (Boyer, 1997), for example, the sample size provided only 45% power to detect the approximate 20% change in STD incidence detected in the RESPECT study. However, an appreciable effect of the intervention was detected in

TABLE 3-4: RESULTS OF LARGE RANDOMIZED TRIALS OF BEHAVIORAL INTERVENTIONS

	NATIONAL INSTITUTE OF MENTAL HEALTH (MULTICENTER)	PROJECT RESPECT STUDY GROUP (MULTICENTER)	UNIVERSITY OF TEXAS (SAN ANTONIO)	CENTERS FOR DISEASE CONTROL (HOUSTON)	UNIVERSITY OF CALIFORNIA (SAN FRANCISCO)
Population	Inner city clinics in multiple cities/men and women screened with questionnaire (74% African American, 25% Hispanic, 58% female)	Inner city clinics in multiple cities/men and women screened with questionnaire (59% African American, 19% Hispanic, 43% female)	Public health clinics/women with non-viral STD (69% Mexican American, 30% African American, 100% female)	Medical Center STD Clinic (90% African American, 44% female)	STD clinic/men and women (46% African American, 16% Hispanic, 37% female)
Sample size	3706	5758	617	964	399
Intervention type	Small group	Individual	Small group	Small group	Individual
Number of sessions	7 bi-weekly sessions of 90–120 minutes each	2 or 4 weekly sessions of 60 minutes each	3 weekly sessions of 3–4 hours each	4 bi-weekly sessions and a booster group session at 2 months	4 weekly sessions of 60 minutes each
Control group	1 hour didactic AIDS* education	2 didactic 5 minute AIDS education sessions	1 standard 15 minute session	2 standard 20 minute sessions	1 standard 15 minute session
Adherence rates	63% attended ≥6 sessions	82% attended all sessions	75% attended all sessions	47% attended ≥4 sessions	48% attended all sessions
Number of STD exams	1 (at 12 months)	2–4 (at 3, 6, 9, 12 months, 3 and 9 months optional)	2 (at 6 and 12 months)	4 (at 2, 6, 9, and 12 months)	2 (at 3 and 5 months)
Follow-up rates	82%	81% at least 1, 51% all 4	90%	72% at least 1 visit, 47% all 4	72% at least 1visit, 52% both

Table continues . . .

Table 3-4: Results of Large Randomized Trials of Behavioral Interventions *(continued)*			
Findings in intervention group compared to control group	■ Improved self-reported prevention efforts ■ Fewer STD symptoms ■ No difference in STD incidence 12 months after intervention, determined by chart review, STD exam	■ 30% lower STD incidence after 6 months ■ 20% lower STD incidence after 12 months ■ 2 session and 4 session interventions had equivalent results	■ 34% lower STD incidence after 6 months ■ 49% lower STD incidence after 12 months	■ Self-reported risky sexual behavior and incidence of STDs were similar between intervention and control groups	■ No change in STD incidence ■ Improved self-reported prevention efforts in men ■ No improvement in self-reported prevention efforts in women
Cited behavioral intervention models	■ Risk reduction counseling, model not specified	■ Theory of Reasoned Action ■ Social Cognitive Theory	■ AIDS Risk-Reduction Model	■ AIDS Risk-Reduction Model	■ AIDS Risk-Reduction Model

the San Antonio study (Shain, 1999) despite a sample size of only 617. In this study, ethnic-specific tools and counselors were used, thus perhaps enhancing the effect of the intervention. Indeed, in this study, a 49% decreased STD incidence was detected after 12 months, compared to a 20% decrease reported in the RESPECT study. Finally, adherence to behavioral session schedule and follow-up with STD exam are crucial elements affecting study validity. The NIMH, RESPECT, and San Antonio studies all reported higher adherence rates and follow-up rates compared to the Houston (Branson, 1998) and San Antonio studies, thus providing increased ability to measure the effectiveness of the intervention.

■ **Even brief (two 20 minute) counseling sessions can result in lower STD rates and can be incorporated into clinical settings**

The 20 minute Project RESPECT counseling sessions may be most applicable to busy practitioners interested in conducting effective behavioral counseling. This study demonstrated that individual "brief" counseling, involving two sessions of 20 minutes each, was as effective in reducing STD incidence as "enhanced" four one hour sessions. Both intervention arms, the two 20 minute and four one hour counseling sessions, were superior to a didactic message. The first of the two brief 20-minute sessions focused on recognizing HIV risk and barriers to risk reduction. After working with the client to agree on an achievable risk reduction plan, the counselors concluded the sessions by identifying a small risk-reduction step which could be achieved before the second session. At the second session, counselors reviewed progress and barriers in achieving the behavioral goal, and helped to clients to arrive at a long-term risk reduction plan. Although the four one-hour "enhanced" sessions also included recognizing risk and formulating risk reduction plans, more energy was focused on key theoretical behavioral elements such as self-efficacy, attitudes, and social norms underlying risk behavior. The fact that the brief two 20 minute counseling sessions demonstrated equivalent efficacy to four hours of counseling is encouraging to practitioners who would like to integrate effective HIV counseling into busy clinical settings.

VI. PRACTICAL ASPECTS OF COUNSELING PATIENTS ABOUT SEXUAL RISK REDUCTION

All of this information may seem overwhelming to the health care provider who has no special training in behavioral theory. However, the underlying principle is one that can be applied by any practitioner in any setting: counseling should be individualized to the person receiving the counseling. Any attempt to accomplish individualization of approach would be superior to simply providing a didactic message. Some practical aspects of counseling are listed in Table 3-5 and discussed below.

■ **Focus the counseling session**

The cornerstone of the counseling session is to focus the session on the patient's recent sexual activities, their perception of their risk, and motivation to reduce their risk of HIV/STD exposure, redirecting the patient to this topic whenever necessary. Clinicians and counselors may become distracted by providing excessive information about scientific data and principles in response to patient questioning. Such information is probably more effectively dispensed in pamphlet form or by referral to other patient information sources. In addition, women at risk for STDs including HIV frequently come to clinic with multiple complicating issues, including poverty, domestic violence, substance abuse, and child care problems. Often the counselor begins to feel responsible for addressing all of these issues and

TABLE 3-5: PRACTICAL ASPECTS OF COUNSELING
■ Focus the counseling session on risk reduction topics
■ Listen and react to the patient
■ Don't stick to a practiced script
■ Avoid over-ambitious risk reduction plans; focus on realistic goals
■ Give the patient a written documentation of the risk reduction plan
■ Use culturally sensitive and ethnic-specific language and terminology, when available and appropriate
■ Consider issues specifically relevant to women

TABLE 3-6: APPROPRIATE RISK REDUCTION TOPICS

■ Enhance self-perception of risk
  - Identify risk behavior
  - Assess level of concern
  - Identify ambivalent feelings about risk

■ Explore specifics of most recent risk
  - Identify specific risk details
  - Assess patient acceptable risk level
  - Address ability to communicate with partner
  - Identify situations that make the patient vulnerable to risk
  - Identify triggers of high-risk behavior
  - Assess patterns of risk behavior

■ Review previous risk reduction experience
  - Identify successful attempts at risk reduction
  - Identify obstacles to risk reduction

■ Synthesize risk patterns
  - Summarize and reflect patient risk
  - Address rish in context of patient's life
  - Convey concerns and urgency regarding risk
  - Support and encourage the patient to action

Source: Adapted from Kamb ML, Fishbein M, Douglas JM, et. al. Efficacy of risk-reduction counseling to prevent human immunodeficiency virus and sexually transmitted disease: a randomized controlled trial. *JAMA* 280:1161–1167, 1998.

---

discouraged by the fact that many of them seem so insurmountable. Furthermore, the patient may be uncomfortable discussing her own risk, and may therefore be emotionally invested in distracting the counselor from that subject. For these reasons, it is important for the counselor to remember that the goal during the limited interaction period with the woman is to directly address, and hopefully impact, risky sexual behavior. Some appropriate topics are listed in Table 3-6. Other longstanding issues may not be easily solvable, and may be more appropriately referred to a social worker, substance abuse counselor, or mental health counselor.

■ **Listen and react**

At the same time, it is important to listen and react to the patient. It is a human quality that we enjoy talking and thinking about ourselves. A counseling technique of summarizing patient's descriptions and viewpoints about her risk is an extremely effective communication tool. In an effort to be non-judgmental, counselors may find themselves nodding supportively to just about any statement that the patient may make. Instead, sometimes direct and clear feedback from the counselor about self-destructive behavior may communicate more effectively the importance of reducing risk (Figure 3-1). For example, if a patient is describing an evening during which she had sex with multiple men while using crack cocaine, it may be more appropriate for the counselor to respond with emphasis that such behavior is dangerous. It would also be important to explore the

---

emotional or physical needs leading to such risky sexual behavior and to identify potential alternatives to fulfilling such needs.

■ Don't stick to a practiced script

In an effort to focus, some counselors may restrict themselves to a practiced script and thus squander opportunities to effectively impact risk behavior. Specific counseling scenarios a provider might encounter are described below:

- references to suicide: "I could have killed myself"
- self-deprecating comments: "I was so stupid"
- over-acceptance of risk: "Even if I would have known he was HIV-positive, I wouldn't have used a condom"
- inappropriate behavior: giggling, putting feet up on the table

Such statements are usually pleas from patients for a direct and honest response, and taking such opportunities to acknowledge and problem-solve risky behavior is important in establishing the objectives of the session. Inappropriate patient behavior such as excessive giggling, angry postures, or demonstrations of boredom, should also elicit comment and questions from the counselor. Overlooking such behavior in an effort to be professional, polite, or focused detracts from the ability to communicate.

■ Avoid over-ambitious risk reduction plans

The most common error made by counselors is to develop an over-ambitious risk reduction goal, particularly during sessions in which good rapport has been developed. In many cases, counselors may convince themselves that the woman has acknowledged her risk to such a degree that she is now ready to eliminate any subsequent episodes of unprotected sex. Such goals are likely unrealistic. Behavioral specialists favor extremely concrete goals, such as "On Friday night I am going to ask my partner to wear a condom." Even modest goals, such as stopping at a drug store and purchasing condoms on the way home from the session, may be suggested. Other possible goals are listed in Table 3-7 on the following page.

■ Put it in writing

Furnishing written documentation of patient goals reinforces verbal instructions and provides additional motivation.

■ Use time wisely

The question then remains: what amount of time is necessary to effect a behavioral intervention? The Project RESPECT study demonstrated successful intervention with two 20 minute sessions within 10 days of each other. An ongoing follow-up study, RESPECT 2, compares a single 1 hour visit with rapid HIV testing to the two 20 minute sessions. In busy clinics, where care for genital tract infections and other medical problems may be occurring simultaneously with patient counseling, clinicians may not feel that they have sufficient time to counsel effectively. However, in many

FIGURE 3-1: LISTEN AND REACT TO THE PATIENT

React to what a woman tells you. Use words and body language to express yourself.

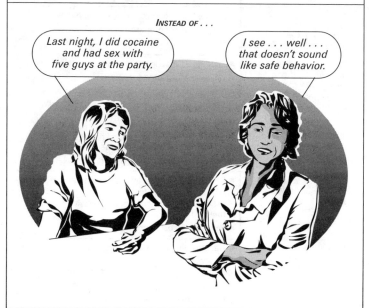

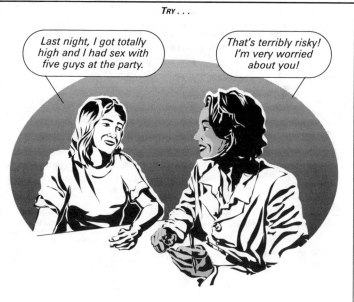

TABLE 3-7: EXAMPLES OF CONCRETE INDIVIDUALIZED RISK REDUCTION PLANS

TYPE OF PLAN	DESCRIPTION
1. Patient will talk about HIV/STD concern/risk to partner/friends	■ Disclosure or communication with partner ■ Disclosure or communication with peers ■ Disclosure or communication with others
2. Patient plans to get herself tested or have partners tested for HIV/STDs prior to having sex	■ Patient will test herself again to ensure uninfected ■ Have partner tested for HIV/STD ■ Use condoms until partner tested for HIV/STD ■ Abstain from sex until partner tested for HIV/STD
3. Patient plans to reduce, change, or eliminate at-risk partner(s)	■ Break up with high risk partner(s) ■ Eliminate a particular type of high risk partner (prostitute, anonymous partner) ■ Patient will have fewer partners
4. Patient will change the type of partners she has	■ Patient will get to know partners better before having sex ■ Patient will remain monogamous with one partner (3 months) ■ Patient will abstain from sex (3 months)
5. Patient plans to change use of alcohol and drugs	■ Decrease/eliminate alcohol/drug use when having sex ■ Generally decrease/eliminate a specific drug/alcohol ■ Change venue where use needles/drugs/alcohol ■ Do not share needles (exchange or obtain new) ■ Clean needles or only share with known negative partner
6. Patient plans to increase condom use or increase situations that she uses condoms	■ Talk to partner(s) about using condoms ■ Buy condoms or have them more available ■ Sex with condoms more often ■ Use condoms with all partners (vaginal/anal sex) ■ Use with all non-main partner (vaginal/anal sex) ■ Use condoms with main partner (vaginal/anal sex)
7. Patient plans to change the kind of sex she will have	■ Have oral sex instead of vaginal or anal sex ■ Have mutual masturbation or petting (no penetrative sex)
8. Patient plans to make changes in the situation she is in that are associated with risk behavior	■ Eliminate going to particularly risky place (bar-park) ■ Reduce number of times going to particularly risky place ■ Substitute behavior — go to . . . gym, movies, etc

Source: Adapted from Kamb ML, Fishbein M, Douglas JM, et. al. Efficacy of risk-reduction counseling to prevent human immunodeficiency virus and sexually transmitted disease: A randomized controlled trial. JAMA 280:1161–1167, 1998 and from Beth Dillon, Project RESPECT training materials.

cases, patients spend much more time waiting in the reception area or in the exam room than they actually do with the clinician. Optimizing use of patient time by providing educational materials during waiting periods may allow the clinician to limit the amount of didactic information dispensed in clinic and to spend more time in interactive behavioral modification. A self-assessment of the counseling session will allow clinicians to measure their counseling skills. Goals for the counseling session include exploring behaviors most associated with risk, identifying a reasonable risk reduction plan, and assessing the patient support system. A reasonable checklist for a behavioral intervention session is listed in Table 3-8.

TABLE 3-8: A CHECKLIST FOR THE BEHAVIORAL INTERVENTION COUNSELING SESSION

❏ Explored behaviors most associated with risk
❏ Identified behaviors most amenable to change
❏ Identified reasonable change step
❏ Developed the change step into a plan for action
❏ Problem-solved obstacles to the plan
❏ Confirmed with patient that the plan is reasonable
❏ Assessed patient's support system
❏ Identified referral resource, if necessary and available
❏ Reviewed date, time, and goals for next visit
❏ Recognized behavior change as a challenge

Source: Adapted from Kamb ML, Fishbein M, Douglas JM, et. al. Efficacy of risk-reduction counseling to prevent human immunodeficiency virus and sexually transmitted disease: a randomized controlled trial. *JAMA* 280:1161–1167, 1998 and from Beth Dillon, *Project RESPECT training materials.*

VII. ETHNIC AND GENDER CONSIDERATIONS IN RISK REDUCTION COUNSELING

■ **Language, visual materials, and descriptive terms sensitive to specific cultures and ethnicities may be important in improving communication techniques.**

Ethnographic data from the San Antonio study found that African-American women in their study population displayed an emphasis on infectious disease prevention, referring to sharing eating utensils as "eating behind" and sharing needles as "fixing behind." The authors suggested that use of terms such as having sex "behind" someone might be an effective means of communicating the concept of unsafe sexual practices in their study population. In contrast, people of Asian background often conceptualize the human body of being made up of "hot" and "cold" components and may think of disease processes such as STDs as "hot". Referring to a condom as "cold" may emphasize the effectiveness of such preventative measures. Finally, some studies have shown that the use of visual tools enhances verbal communication in Spanish. It is important to recognize, however, that such colloquialisms or cultural preferences may vary between regions, socio-economic strata, and religions. If used in the wrong setting, approaches designed for one ethic group may offend another, and detract from the counselor's ability to communicate. In the absence of a validated communication tool, the counselor should take their cues from the patient.

■ **Some counseling concerns are particularly relevant to women.**

In many economically-disadvantaged areas of the world, poverty engenders oppression of women. When education and jobs are scarce, many economies preferentially educate and employ men, thus leaving women financially dependent on their husbands, vulnerable to "sugar daddies," and bartering sex for food and clothing either in informal relationships or in a structured brothel setting. Many cultures sanction a family structure in which the mother of the husband lives in the home and is responsible for directing household activities and ensuring the well-being of her son. Many cultures also may place more value on men than on women, and may mythologize male prowess and discourage condom use. Finally, many societies do not recognize the legal rights of women in custody battles, thus leaving women tied to their husbands if they wish to remain with their children. In conditions in which women are economically and emotionally dependent on men, women often neglect their basic human rights. Such barriers may be extremely daunting to counselors, and the temptation may be to attempt to debunk societal inequalities or to degenerate into a "male-bashing" session. In such cases, the basic tenets of behavioral counseling should be recalled; focus on risk and tailor the session to the readiness of the woman for behavioral change. Clear, feasible risk reduction plans should be formulated, usually involving self-education about risk and recognition of responsibility to reduce risk.

■ **Unfortunately, the issue of domestic violence may also need to be addressed.**

Domestic violence continues to be a prevalent problem, affecting 20–30% of households in the United States and possibly even higher numbers in other parts of the world. A study of HIV testing of women in Nairobi, Kenya, has produced some disturbing results. Out of 243 women informed that they were HIV positive, only 66 (27%) informed their partner of their result. Of these 66, 11 (17%) were chased from the home, 7 (11%) were beaten, and 1 (1%) committed suicide. When the testing protocol was changed to informing women that returning for HIV test results was optional, only one-third of women returned for their results (Temmerman, 1995).

Fear of domestic violence may also impede a woman's ability to assert her rights in a relationship to reduce her risk of HIV infection. Counselors must realize that such fear may be entirely reasonable, and that counseling patients about domestic violence may be beyond their area of expertise. Whenever possible, appropriate patients should be referred to domestic violence centers. At the same time, counselors can help patients formulate risk reduction plans in the setting of domestic violence. The counselor must approach the issue of HIV testing while mentioning and indeed when appropriate, emphasizing, the possibility of domestic violence and social stigma. While counselors must encourage disclosure in order to avoid the potential of infecting an uninfected partner, they must remember that the safety of the patient is their first priority. Unfortunately, only initiation of widespread testing and recognition of seroprevalence will succeed in destigmatizing HIV infection. Meanwhile, on the individual level, care must be taken to help the woman identify ways to reduce her risk of physical harm and excessive emotional stress while at the same time initiating the process of recognizing and reducing risk behavior.

VIII. SEXUALLY TRANSMITTED DISEASES AND THE RISK OF HIV INFECTION

■ **Genital tract infections increase susceptibility to HIV infection**

The fact that STDs are important cofactors for HIV infection has been well-established by prospective studies examining risk factors for seroconversion in high-risk populations. In such studies, the increased risk for HIV-1 acquisition in women with genital ulcer diseases and gonococcal and chlamydial cervicitis has been estimated at two to four above baseline. Women with candida and trichomonal vaginitis have been estimated to have an approximately two to three times increased risk above baseline (Laga, 1993).

■ **Bacterial vaginosis may also increase susceptibility to HIV infection**

In an important recent study in Malawi, bacterial vaginosis was shown to be a significant risk factor for HIV seroconversion in pregnant women attending an antenatal clinic. In this study, bacterial vaginosis (defined by vaginal pH > 4.5, homogeneous vaginal discharge, absence of other etiologic agents of cervicitis or vaginitis, presence of clue cells, and positive amine odor) was a prevalent condition, affecting 30% of women. Presence of BV at the enrollment exam was associated with a three- to four-fold increased risk of HIV seroconversion over the median 2.5 years of follow-up (Taha, 1998). An association between bacterial vaginosis and HIV-1 seroconversion has also been reported in a study of nonpregnant women; women with bacterial vaginosis in the 60 days before HIV testing were 1.4 times more likely to have incident HIV infection than women without genital infections (multivariate p=.07) (Martin, 1998).

■ **Syndromic management of STDs decreased HIV acquisition rates, but mass treatment of STDS did not in two different community randomized trials**

From these studies, one can conclude that a healthy genital tract reduces a woman's susceptibility to HIV infection. This conclusion was further solidified by the results of a community-based randomized trial conducted in Mwanza, Tanzania demonstrating that syndromic management of STDs resulted in a 40 percent reduction in HIV-1 seroconversion in the intervention communities (Hayes, 1995; Mayaud, 1997). In contrast, a randomized controlled trial of mass antibiotic treatment conducted during almost the same time period in Rakai, Uganda, failed to demonstrate a reduction in HIV seroincidence (Wawer, 1999). The reason for the difference in findings in these two trials testing a STD intervention is likely related to the stage of the epidemic in the two locations. In Mwanza, the baseline prevalence of HIV was only 4%, indicating an early phase of the epidemic. In comparison, the Rakai study was conducted in a population with a baseline prevalence of 16%, indicating a more mature epidemic. Experts feel that the core group of high-risk individuals crucial to epidemic transmission was already saturated in Rakai, thus minimizing the impact of the intervention. The Rakai intervention also did not address genital herpes which was the most common cause of genital ulcer disease in the Rakai communities. The disparate findings of these studies emphasize the complexities of the association between HIV and cofactors affecting transmission.

■ **How should we counsel women at risk for STDs and HIV?**

Important issues in counseling women at risk for STDs and HIV are presented in Table 3-9. Reducing the prevalence and incidence of STDs should reduce the susceptibility to HIV transmission. Measures to reduce STDs include female and male condom use, seeking early diagnosis and treatment of genital tract symptoms, and frequent STD screening and should be a part of HIV prevention in the U.S. as well as in developing countries (CDC, 1998b). Infections such as yeast vaginitis and bacterial vaginosis are not sexually transmitted, but arise from disruption of a woman's genital tract flora. For this reason, these infections are often under-emphasized in programs to diagnose and treat genital tract infections. However, these are prevalent conditions, and studies have shown that both yeast vaginitis and bacterial vaginosis may increase risk of HIV acquisition. Clinicians should diagnose and have a low threshold to treat both bacterial vaginosis and candida vaginitis in women with high-risk sexual behavior. Douching may increase the risk of developing bacterial vaginosis or pelvic inflammatory disease.

TABLE 3-9: MEASURES TO REDUCE SEXUALLY TRANSMITTED DISEASES (STDs)

■ Encourage male and female condom use
■ Encourage seeking medical care early for diagnosis and treatment of genital tract symptoms
■ Routine screening for genital tract infections, including chlamydia cervicitis, yeast vaginitis, and bacterial vaginosis among sexually active women
■ Discourage douching
■ Educate women about risk factors for yeast vaginitis
■ Teach how to recognize genital herpes recurrences and prodromes and offer antiviral treatment to shorten or suppress recurrences

---

Douching has no therapeutic benefit and should be strongly discouraged. Preventable risk factors for candida vaginitis include uncontrolled diabetes mellitus, antibiotics, and high-estrogen oral contraceptives. Other possible risk factors that are less well-documented include wearing poorly ventilated clothing, use of low-estrogen oral contraceptives, frequent swimming, feminine hygiene sprays, and use of spermicidal jelly.

Finally, many studies have shown that genital ulcer diseases (i.e., syphilis, chancroid, and genital herpes) are important co-factors for HIV transmission. Women with a history of genital herpes or with serologic evidence of HSV-2 infection should be taught how to recognize prodromes and recurrences. Suppressive herpes antiviral therapy should be considered in women with frequent recurrences who report high-risk sexual behavior (CDC, 1998a).

IX. CONDOMS AND PREVENTION OF HIV INFECTION

Readers of history may know that decorative penile covers have been mentioned in Egyptian writings as far back as 1350 BC. In 1564, the Italian anatomist, Fallopius, described the concept of a penile barrier for the prevention of venereal disease. The famous romancer, Casanova, is said to have protected himself with sheets of sheep intestine. Since that time, technology has allowed the production of latex male condoms, and more recently, polyurethane male condoms and female condoms. Important issues to discuss while counseling women on use of male and female condoms are listed in Table 3-10, on the following page, and discussed below.

A. MALE CONDOMS

■ **Male condoms prevent transmission of many STDs**

The literature on the role of barrier contraception as protection against STDs is vast and the reported degree of protection against specific STDs varies from paper to paper. A distillation of available data produces the conclusion that, of available barrier methods that have been adequately tested, latex male condoms provide substantial protection against infection with HIV and most other STDs, and are currently the most reliable protective measure. Most studies describe a seven- to eight-fold decrease in risk of HIV-1 seroconversion for people who use condoms consistently. Some have reported no seroconversions at all among consistent despite repeated coital exposure (Carlin, 1995). In terms of other STDs, male condoms may be less reliably protective against transmission of herpes and human papilloma viruses.

■ **Latex male condoms must be stored and used properly**

Male condom failures are more likely caused by post-manufacture defects secondary to latex deterioration than to manufacturing defects. Latex male

TABLE 3-10: IMPORTANT ISSUES FOR PATIENTS BEING COUNSELED ON CONDOM USE
■ *Store in a cool, dry place, such as a bedroom drawer*
● Avoid excessive humidity, such as in a bathroom
● Avoid excessive heat, such as in a wallet carried in a trouser pocket
● Avoid exposure to direct sunlight
■ *Use appropriate spermicide or lubricating jelly*
● Mineral-oil containing compounds, such as petroleum jelly, cooking oils, shortening, or lotions, can weaken latex
■ *Use male condom properly*
● Use male condom at the onset of male arousal, even before penetration
● Make sure that the male condom is unrolled to extend completely to the penis base
● Use enough lubrication to prevent excessive friction that might lead to breakage
● Hold the male condom at the base during withdrawal to prevent slippage
■ *Use female condom properly*
● The inner ring must be placed completely onto the cervix or the condom may twist
● Additional lubrication may be needed to prevent the condom from twisting
● Care must be taken not to insert the penis between the condom and vaginal wall
● The outer ring may need to be held in place to keep the condom from slipping into the vagina or anus
● During anal intercourse, the insertive partner may have to keep thrusts shallow, because the condom is not as long as the rectum. It also might be advisable to remove the inner ring for anal sex to reduce likelihood of rectal bleeding.

condoms have proved impermeable to HIV in vitro. In contrast, natural membrane ("skin") condoms have been shown to be permeable to small amounts of HIV and other infectious agents, and are not recommended for disease prevention. Transmission of HIV that occurs with use of latex male condoms is likely due to technical failures or improper usage rather than to manufacturing defects. Since 1987, the Food and Drug Administration (FDA) in the United States has maintained a high level of quality by limiting the number of defective condoms to four per 1000 count batch. Patients should be counseled that stored male condoms should be replaced often, as temperature, light, and animal pests all can contribute to latex deterioration and decreased effectiveness. In clinical studies, breakage rates range from 0.5% to 7% (Stratton, 1993). Studies reporting higher breakage rates tended to include populations from under-developed areas or those who participated in anal intercourse.

■ **Male condoms must also be used properly in order to be effective.**

Using oil-based lubricating materials such as petroleum jelly, cooking oils, shortening, or lotions during intercourse weakens latex and promotes breakage. Common errors that patients should be cautioned about include delaying condom use until just prior to full penetration, failure to extend the condom all the way to the penis base, insufficient application of a water-based lubricant, and failure to hold the condom at the base during withdrawal.

■ **Polyurethane male condoms may be a future alternative**

Acceptability of male condom use is limited by complaints of decreased male sensitivity and limitation of sexual enjoyment by both men and women. Polyurethane has been hailed as an attractive alternative to latex because of increased tensile strength that should, theoretically, allow for a thinner condom wall translating into increased penile sensation. A male polyurethane condom, Avanti, has been popular since its introduction in late 1994, but after increasing numbers of complaints of condom breakage, the manufacturers have changed specifications to produce a thicker condom labeled "Intended for Latex Sensitive Condom Users Only." Breakage rates, patient acceptability, and the ability of this product to protect against STD and HIV infection are yet to be demonstrated.

B. FEMALE CONDOMS

Also made of polyurethane, the female condom has been available for use in the United States since 1993 (Bounds, 1997) and offers women more control over use than with the male condom. The female condom is a sheath, closed at one end, with flexible rings at both ends (Figure 3-2 on the following page). The device is inserted into the vagina by compressing the closed-end ring and pushing against the cervix, while the outer ring covers the labia (Figure 3-3 on the following page). Only one female condom is currently available, marketed under the name "Reality" in the United States and Canada and "Femidom" in other parts of the world. Limited data are available on the efficacy of the female condom in preventing HIV and STDs, although most experts have extrapolated from the data on male latex and polyurethane condoms to conclude that, if used properly, female condoms would be impermeable to most viruses and other micro-organisms. In a study sponsored by the United Nations Programme on HIV/AIDS (UNAIDS), female commercial sex workers in Thailand were randomized into a group instructed to consistently use male condoms, and a group given the option to use female condoms if the male refused to wear a condom (Fontanet, 1998). Both groups reported universal male or female condom use rates of approximately 97%, although 9% of the women in the "option group" used the female condom. Before introduction of the female condom, women in the study population were experiencing an average of two STDs per year (trichomoniasis, chlamydial infection, gonococcal infection, genital ulcer disease). This rate was surprisingly high, particularly given the high rate of reported condom use, and may be due to overreporting of condom use (given the Thai 100% condom use policy) or STDs acquired from their husbands or nonpaying partners. Nevertheless, the group randomized to the option to use either type of condom demonstrated a 24% decrease in the incidence of STD compared to the male condom only

FIGURE 3-2: THE FEMALE CONDOM

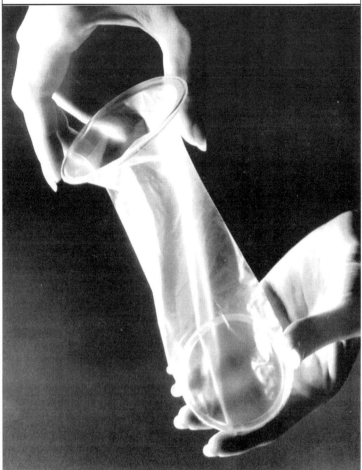

group. Importantly, female condoms were reportedly well accepted both by the women and their clients. Condom tears occurred less frequently with the female condom than the male condom.

C. ACCEPTABILITY OF MALE AND FEMALE CONDOMS

Factors influencing condom use are presented in Table 3-11. These factors are complex, and often differ between men and women. Surveys have shown that both men and women are influenced by perceived social norms and attitudes about condom use, and by the recognition that condoms may prevent STDs. Ability to obtain condoms without excessive cost or embarrassment, ease of using the condom, and preservation of pleasurable sexual sensation are clearly

FIGURE 3-3: FEMALE CONDOM INSERTION AND POSITIONING

STEP 1

Inner ring is squeezed for insertion.

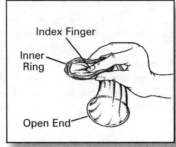

STEP 2

Sheath is inserted, similarly to a tampon.

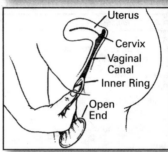

STEP 3

Inner ring is pushed up as far as it can go with index finger.

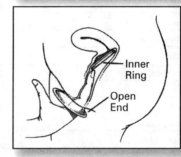

STEP 4

Female condom is in place

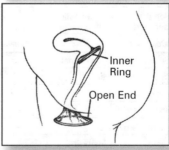

Source: Adapted from Reality brand female condom literature.

concerns for both men and women. Acceptability of the male condom for both men and women is increased by normal appearance and feel, lack of odor, lack of slippage, the presence of a reservoir tip, and spermicidal lubrication. Men may be more likely to use the male condom if they feel that the woman may perceive them as being more sensitive and caring if they do so. Women, on the other hand, have complained that the interruption of foreplay negatively affects the acceptability of the male condom. For the female condom, both men and women have complained about the aesthetic appearance of the external ring, and the noise during intercourse. The fact that the female condom is made of polyurethane and not latex may increase its acceptability, particularly

TABLE 3-11: Factors Associated with Condom Use and Non-use

CONDOMS IN GENERAL	IMPORTANT TO MEN	IMPORTANT TO WOMEN
Negative image of condom use associated with disease, promiscuity, and distrust of sex partner	■	■
Actual and perceived social norms governing condom use	■	■
Perceived ability to protect against sexually transmitted diseases	■	■
Ease of obtaining or purchase	■	■
Ease of putting on or in	■	■
Slippage during intercourse	■	■
Adequate lubrication	■	■
Sensation during intercourse	■	■
MALE CONDOMS	**IMPORTANT TO MEN**	**IMPORTANT TO WOMEN**
Normal appearance and feel	■	■
Lack of odor	■	■
Reservoir tip	■	■
Spermicide coating	■	■
Interruption of foreplay		■
Inferior contraceptive method		■
Perception that partner may believe user is sensitive and caring	■	
FEMALE CONDOMS	**IMPORTANT TO MEN**	**IMPORTANT TO WOMEN**
Aesthetic appearance of external ring	■	■
Noise during intercourse	■	■
Polyurethane material	■	■
Interruption of foreplay		■
Female controlled device		■
Inferior contraceptive method		■

Source: Adapted from Grady WR, Klepinger DH, Nelson-Wally A. Contraceptive characteristics: the perceptions and priorities of men and women. *Fam Plann Perspect* 1999;31:168–75.

among latex-allergic users. Women have reported that inserting the female condom interrupts foreplay. Interestingly, in several surveys, more women have said that they would be likely to use the female condom again than have said that they liked using it, suggesting that women may be willing to sacrifice comfort and pleasure during sex for protection against STDs and pregnancy. Many women have also strongly expressed a preference for a female-controlled device to prevent STDs. Finally, in surveys, pregnancy prevention is more important to women than to men, and most women feel that both the male and female condom may be inferior to other contraceptive methods. (Grady, 1999)

X. OTHER FORMS OF CONTRACEPTION AND THE RISK OF HIV INFECTION

■ **The role of hormonal contraceptives in HIV transmission is controversial**

The association between hormonal contraception and HIV infection has been the subject of controversy. Because of the unique considerations that contribute to contraceptive choice, a clinical trial randomizing a woman to contraception or placebo is probably not feasible. Thus, although many studies presenting data on the association have been published, all are population surveys or observational studies. The reported effects of oral contraceptives on HIV susceptibility are widely divergent, ranging from protective, to no effect, to an increased risk. A meta-analysis on the subject reported that the use of oral contraceptives may be associated with a small increased risk of HIV infection (Wang, 1999). When the results of all 28 published studies were combined, a pooled odds ratio of 1.2 (95% CI 0.99-1.42) was found. This pooled risk estimate increased with increasing study quality, suggesting that a true association, albeit small, does exist. In addition, two cross-sectional studies and two prospective studies have reported that women using depo medroxyprogesterone acetate (Depo-Provera) are at increased risk of HIV infection. In a study conducted in Mombasa, Kenya, commercial sex workers (n=779) were followed for a median of 224 days; in multivariate analysis, women using Depo-Provera demonstrated two times increased risk of HIV seroconversion (Martin, 1998). Insufficient data exist on other hormonal contraceptive methods to reach a conclusion about the effect on a woman's susceptibility to HIV.

■ **Barrier contraceptives other than condoms**

Other forms of barrier contraception, such as the diaphragm and the cervical cap, do not cover the vagina, and therefore would not be expected to provide substantial protection against HIV infection, although the diaphragm with nonoxynol-9 containing spermicide has been associated with a modest decrease in bacterial STDs. N-9 spermicides alone provide modest protection against bacterial STDs but no apparent effect on HIV in randomized clinical trials despite evidence of in vitro activity against HIV.

Furthermore, N-9 spermicides have been associated with chemical irritation or epithelial disruption in the lower genital tract at higher doses of N-9 or with frequent use, raising concerns that these women may be at increased risk for HIV transmission if they use spermicides only. The use of spermicides alone should be discouraged in at-risk women and the potential benefits (lubrication, possible increase in protection if the condom breaks) and risks of spermicide use with condoms should be discussed. Intrauterine devices (IUDs) have been associated with an increased risk of pelvic inflammatory disease, especially around the time of insertion. A two- to threefold increased risk of HIV infection in women who use IUDs has been reported (Kappa, 1994). The foreign body reaction induced in the endometrium by an IUD, with accompanying inflammation, ulceration, and thinning, as well as generally longer and heavier menses (which may increase risk bidirectionally), provide a easily-conceived biologic basis for increased susceptibility to HIV infection.

■ **Sterilization and prevention of HIV infection**

Female sterilization by tubal ligation has no effect on male-to-female HIV transmission. Early penile withdrawal, while theoretically reducing the innoculum size, has not been studied and should not be recommended. While the exact effect of vasectomy on the ability to transmit HIV from male to female is unknown, HIV has been cultured from the ejaculate of vasectomized men (Anderson, 1991).

■ **Contraception and prevention of infection are separate issues**

The issue of contraception for sexually active, reproductive age women, is obviously complex. The importance of preventing unwanted pregnancies is clear. Any counselor working with women is familiar with the issue of controlling and planning family size while taking into account economic factors, maternal health, and social pressures. Hormonal contraception is one of the most effective means to prevent pregnancy. The message conveyed to

TABLE 3-12: CONTRACEPTION AND PREVENTION OF HIV-1 INFECTION			
METHOD	**MAY INCREASE RISK***	**NO EFFECT OR CONFLICTING DATA***	**PROTECTIVE — STRONG EVIDENCE**
Male condom			■
Female condom			■
Intrauterine device	■		
Diaphragm		■	
Cervical cap		■	
Tubal ligation		■	
Vasectomy		■	
Early penile withdrawal		■	
Oral contraceptives		■	
Depo-Provera		■	
* Counsel that condoms should be used to prevent HIV-1 infection			

women must be that contraception and protection against STDs, including HIV, are separate considerations. For women who choose to use hormonal contraception, counselors must emphasize that male and female condoms are the only means to prevent STD transmission

The effectiveness of various contraceptive methods in reducing risk of HIV infection is summarized in Table 3-12.

XI. NEW APPROACHES TO HIV AND STD PREVENTION: MICROBICIDES, VACCINES, AND POST-EXPOSURE PROPHYLAXIS

Given the difficulties that many women encounter in negotiating condom use, other prevention strategies under the control of women have been sought, such as topical microbicides. While microbicides have generated considerable enthusiasm, progress in this area has been relatively slow. Most of the research in microbicides over the past 10 years has focused on safety and efficacy of nonoxynol 9 (N-9). The findings have not been consistent across all studies, complicated by different concentrations and formulations of N-9 used, insufficient sample size, and differing frequency of condom use by the women studied. Data on N-9 are well-summarized in a recent meta-analysis (Roddy, 1998a).

■ **In general, the data available from randomized trials do not support significant efficacy of N-9 against HIV (Roddy, 1998a).**

Current efficacy trials of N-9 by UNAIDS and HIVNET will hopefully answer remaining questions about whether the lack of efficacy of N-9 in vivo was due to high condom use or too low a dose of N-9.

■ **While the concept of topical microbicides is promising, the process to developing and testing new microbicidal products for safety, and ultimately efficacy in preventing HIV, in clinical trials will take a number of years**

New topical microbicidal products in early clinical trials include broad-spectrum microbicides (such as natural lactobacilli, buffering products such as BufferGel, and surfactants such as C31G), inhibitors of viral entry and cell fusion (such as PC503 which has activity against HIV, HSV, and C. trachomatis; and PRO2000) and inhibitors of HIV replication (such as nucleotide reverse transcriptase inhibitors such as PMPA). Many challenges face the study of topical microbicides, including the standardization of in vitro exposure assays for meaningful and consistent comparisons of activities of different compounds against HIV and other STDs and identification of placebos that have similar viscosity and pH to the active ingredient.

■ **Vaccines hold the most promise for protecting the largest number of HIV infections transmitted sexually, perinatally, or through drug use.**

However, no HIV-1 vaccine with proven efficacy currently exists, and the necessary components of an immunogen that can induce protection against

HIV-1 infection are poorly understood. Clues have emerged from dissecting the properties of immunity that correspond to protection against other pathogens, and more particularly in vaccine studies in the related SIV/HIV primate models. In addition, persons demonstrating unusual control of HIV-1 infection, e.g., those repeatedly exposed to HIV-1 without overt infection, HIV-1 long-term non-progressors, and HIV-2-infected persons, may have acquired a unique host defense against HIV that merits induction by vaccination.

Our understanding of the mechanism of action of other effective viral vaccines and HIV pathogenesis is guiding HIV vaccine development. Most licensed vaccines prime host immunity to control initial infection more efficiently, rather than to provide sterilizing immunity. Protection is commonly mediated by induction of antibodies that block infection, which allows time for antigen-specific T cells to mature and overtake any cells that do become infected. HIV-1 preferentially targets T helper cells, and either destroys them or establishes latent infection; a vaccine must restrict HIV-1 "seeding" and reemergence over time. HIV-1 is not easily neutralized by antibody, so that mimicking the largely safe recombinant protein strategy for Hepatitis B virus vaccines is less apt to be successful with HIV-1. HIV-1 transmission occurs predominantly by sexual contact; thus, protection may require both mucosal as well as systemic immunity.

■ **Most experts believe that regimens priming both the cellular and humoral immune arms are the best candidates for protection, based on strong evidence in both experimental and human viral infections.**

HIV vaccines that can stimulate a cellular immune response include poorly replicating viral or bacterial vectors expressing HIV gene products, such as poxviruses, vaccinia and avipox. These products (e.g., the canarypox vector with gag, nef, and env genes) can elicit CD8+ cytotoxic T cell responses in approximately one-third of volunteers. Macaque studies suggest that the less virulent, modified vaccinia Ankara (MVA) recombinant may induce even stronger T cell responses, and its safety profile from previous use internationally looks quite good. Other recombinant vectors containing HIV-1 gene inserts that hold promise for clinical testing include Venezuelan equine encephalitis virus, adenovirus, poliovirus, and bacterial vectors (e.g., salmonella or listeria), but these as yet have not reached phase I testing. DNA vaccines may have promise, based on studies in the macaque model for SIV in which CD4+ and CD8+ T cell immunity and low-level antibodies were elicited. DNA vaccines are stable and will not require continuous cold storage, and may be more readily altered as the pool of viruses in the infected transmitting populations evolve, but immunogenicity has not been optimal at up to 3 mg doses.

Building upon these insights, vaccine development has ensued and several strategies have been tested in the phase I/II setting. Of the vaccine regimens tested thus far in HIV-1 high-risk populations, no single approach is devoid of "breakthrough" infections. Clinical trials to test vaccine efficacy are expensive and large scale and have not as yet been endorsed except by private industry (VaxGen) which is testing the efficacy of a bivalent gp120 vaccination approach in North America and Thailand. At present, among the agents available and demonstrating acceptable safety in phase II trials, the next vaccine candidates to move to efficacy trials are likely to be a multivalent vaccine regimen with a canarypox vector prime and subunit gp120 boost, which induce neutralizing and non-neutralizing antibodies primarily recognizing the variable envelope regions of strains closely similar to that of the immunogen and cytotoxic T cells. An intermediate-sized efficacy trial in the next several years may answer whether the potency of antibodies and frequency of antigen-specific T cells elicited by the canarypox prime-gp120 boost is adequate for protection.

■ **Post-exposure prophylaxis (PEP) is a method which may reduce the likelihood of HIV infection** after a high-risk exposure.

Theoretically, PEP may either prevent establishment of infection or prevent new infection while allowing clearance of already infected cells. The rationale for PEP with sexual exposure is that the probability of infection after a single exposure was similar to needlestick exposures (i.e., 0.1–3% for unprotected receptive anal intercourse or 0.1–0.2% for vaginal intercourse) (USPHS, 1998; Katz 1997, 1998). Animal models indicate that PEP may be effective, particularly when used within 24–48 hours of exposure with potent antiretroviral agents. The data for efficacy of antiretrovirals for occupational exposure primarily is derived from a case-control study, in which health care workers who took zidovudine after needlesticks had an 80% lower likelihood of being infected, but which may suffer biases due to the case-control design. This study has been criticized because of its retrospective nature, small number of cases, and other potential sources of bias. There are also reported cases in which ZDV failed to prevent HIV infection in health care workers. However, no prospective studies have assessed the efficacy of PEP for either occupational or sexual exposures due to ethical and pragmatic considerations in conducting a randomized trial of PEP. Thus, the risks and benefits of PEP for sexual exposure remain uncertain. Efficacy of PEP is likely to be influenced by time to initiation of treatment, duration of treatment, size of inoculum, and drug characteristics.

Individual providers who are approached by anxious patients who have recently had a high risk sexual exposure must weigh the likelihood of HIV infection in the contact, antiretroviral treatment history if the contact is known to be HIV infected, specific nature and timing of the exposure (since initiation of PEP within 48 hours may be important) and possible risks of drug toxicity or side effects in choosing whether to use PEP and which drugs to prescribe. The CDC guidelines recommend two drugs (generally zidovudine or stavudine and lamivudine) for four weeks for most cases of occupational exposure, and this approach has been adopted by many providers when selecting a regimen for "sexual PEP." (CDC, 1998c).

The source partner's likelihood of resistant virus, based on treatment history, stage of disease, and viral load can be factored into the choice of a PEP regimen. Other considerations should include evaluation for other STDs, emergency contraception when appropriate, and possible indication for hepatitis B vaccination. Informed consent is recommended when administering PEP.

PEP should not be administered routinely, with exposures at low risk of transmission, or when care is sought after 72 hours from the time of exposure. Situations in which PEP should be considered include condom breakage with serodiscordant couples and sexual assault. PEP is not a substitute for risk reduction and should not be considered a form of primary HIV prevention. Individuals presenting for possible PEP should have reinforcement of the importance of initiating, resuming, or improving risk reduction activities. Providers are requested to report non-occupational PEP use to a national registry maintained by the CDC at (877) 488 1737 or **http://www.hivpepregistry.org**.

XII. CONCLUSIONS

Prevention of HIV remains a critical priority, particularly midst increasing complacency related to enthusiasm about more effective treatments for HIV. The most effective available strategies for prevention are HIV counseling and testing, behavioral interventions to reduce risk-taking, and condoms. Syndromic STD treatment has been shown to reduce HIV incidence in a large community-randomized trial, and ongoing studies are assessing other STD interventions. Topical microbicides may provide a prevention strategy directly under the control of women, although nonoxynol-9 has not been shown to have significant efficacy against HIV transmission in commercially available spermicidal concentrations. New microbicide products are early in pre-clinical and clinical trials testing. Several HIV vaccines are also currently in clinical trials, ranging from phase I safety and immunogenicity studies to phase III efficacy trials of a recombinant gp120 subunit HIV vaccine. Lastly, post-exposure prophylaxis is occasionally being prescribed for high-risk exposures, although there is very limited data on safety and efficacy. While these new strategies are being tested for their efficacy to prevent HIV infection, providers must continue to conduct risk assessments to identify women at risk for HIV and assist women in reducing their risk through setting achievable risk reduction plans.

REFERENCES

Ades AE, Gupta R, Gibb DM, et al. Selective versus universal antenatal HIV testing: epidemiological and implementational factors in policy choice. *AIDS* 13(2):271–8, 1999.

Anderson DJ, Politch JA, Martinex A, Van Voorhis BJ, Padian NS, O'Brien TR. White blood cells and HIV-1 in semen from vasectomised seropositive men. *Lancet* 338:573–4, 1991.

Bandura A. *Social Foundations of Thought and Action: A Social Cognitive Theory.* Englewood Cliffs, NJ: Prentice-Hall, 1996.

Bounds W. Female condoms. *European Journal of Contraception and Reproductive Health* 2(2):113–6, 1997.

Boyer CB, Barrett DC, Peterman TA, Bolan G. Sexually transmitted disease (STD) and HIV risk in heterosexual adults attending a public STD clinic: evaluation of a randomized controlled behavioral risk-reduction intervention trial. *AIDS* 11(3):359–67, 1997.

Branson BM, Peterman TA, Cannon RO, Ransom R, Zaidi AA. Group counseling to prevent sexually transmitted disease and HIV: a randomized controlled trial. *Sexually Transmitted Diseases* 25(10):553–60, 1998.

Carlin EM, Boag FC. Women, contraception, and STDs including HIV. *International Journal of STD & AIDS* 6:373–386, 1995.

Catania JA, Kegeles SM, Coates TJ. Towards an understanding of risk behavior: an AIDS risk reduction model (ARRM). *Health Education Quarterly* 17(1):53–72, 1990.

Celum C, Buchbinder S. Counseling and testing for HIV infection. In: Holmes KK, Sparling PF, Mardh PA, et al., eds. *Sexually Transmitted Diseases.* New York: McGraw-Hill,1999.

Centers for Disease Control. 1998 Guidelines for Treatment of Sexually Transmitted Diseases. *Mortality and Morbidity Weekly Report* 47(RR-1):1–111, 1998a.

Centers for Disease Control. HIV prevention through early detection and treatment of other STDs-United States: Recommendations of the advisory committee for HIV and STD prevention. *Mortality and Morbidity Weekly Report* 47(RR-12):1–111, 1998b.

Centers for Disease Control. Public Health Service guidelines for the management of health-care worker exposures to HIV and recommendations for postexposure prophylaxis. *Mortality and Morbidity Weekly Report* 47(RR-7):1–34, 1998c.

Centers for Disease Control. Update: HIV counseling and testing using rapid tests — United States, 1995. *Mortality and Morbidity Weekly Report* 47:211–215, 1998d.

Courey-Doniger P, Levenkron JC, Knox KL, Cowell S, Urban MA. Use of Stage of Change (SOC) to develop an STD/HIV behavioral intervention: phase 1. A system to classify SOC for STD/HIV sexual risk behaviors — development and reliability in an STD clinic. *AIDS Patient Care* 13:493–502, 1999.

Curtis JR, Holmes KK. Individual-level risk assessment for STD/HIV infections. In: Holmes KK, Sparling PF, Mardh PA, et al., eds. *Sexually Transmitted Diseases.* New York: McGraw-Hill,1999.

Elias CJ, Coggins C. Female-controlled methods to prevent sexual transmission of HIV. *AIDS* 10 (suppl 3):S43–51, 1996.

Fishbein M, Wolitski RJ, Doll LS. Behavioral interventions for sexually transmitted disease prevention at the individual level. In: Holmes KK, Sparling PF, Mardh PA, et al., eds. *Sexually Transmitted Diseases.* New York: McGraw-Hill,1999.

Fisher JD, Fisher WA. Changing AIDS-Risk Behavior. *Psychological Bulletin* 111(3):455–474, 1992.

Fontanet AL, Saba J, Chandelying V, et al. Protection against sexually transmitted diseases by granting sex workers in Thailand the choice of using the male or female condom: results from a randomized controlled trial. *AIDS* 12(14):1851–9, 1998.

Grady WR, Klepinger DH, Nelaon-Wally A. Contraceptive characteristics: the perceptions and priorities of men and women. *Fam Plann Perspect* 31:168–75, 1999.

Hayes BF. HIV vaccines: where we are and where we are going. *Lancet* 348:933–7, 1996.

Hayes R, Mosha F, Nicoll A, et al. A community trial of the impact of improved sexually transmitted disease treatment on the HIV epidemic in rural Tanzania: 1. Design. *AIDS* 9(8):919–26, 1995.

Kamb ML, Fishbein M, Douglas JM, et al. Efficacy of risk-reduction counseling to prevent human immunodeficiency virus and sexually transmitted diseases: a randomized controlled trial. Project RESPECT Study Group. *Journal of the American Medical Association* 280(13):1161–7, 1998.

Kamenga M, Ryder RW, Jingu M, et al. Evidence of marked sexual behavior change associated with low HIV-1 seroconversion in 149 married couples with discordant HIV-1 serostatus: experience at an HIB counselling center in Zaire. *AIDS* 5(1):61–67, 1991.

Kapiga SH, Shao JF, Lwihula GK, Hunter DJ. Risk factors for HIV infection among women in Dar-es-Salaam, Tanzania. *Journal of the Acquired Immune Deficiency Syndromes* 7:301–9, 1994.

Kassler WJ. Advances in HIV testing technology and their potential impact on prevention. *AIDS Education and Prevention* 9(Suppl 3):27–40, 1997.

Katz MH, Gerberding JL. Postexposure treatment of people exposed to the Human Immunodeficiency virus through sexual contact or injection drug use. *New England Journal of Medicine* 336:1097–1100, 1997.

Katz MH, Gerberding JL. The care of persons with recent sexual exposure to HIV. *Annals of Internal Medicine* 128:306–12, 1998.

Laga M., Manoka A, Kivuvu M, et al. Non-ulcerative sexually transmitted diseases as risk factors for HIV-1 transmission in women: results from a cohort study. *AIDS* 7(1):95–102, 1993.

Letvin NH. Progress in the development of an HIV-1 vaccine. *Science* 280:1875–80, 1998.

Martin HL, Nyange PM, Richardson BA, et al. Hormonal contraception, sexually transmitted diseases, and risk of heterosexual transmission of human immunodeficiency virus type 1. *Journal of Infectious Diseases* 178(4):1053–9, 1998.

Mayaud P, Mosha F, Todd J, et al. Improved treatment services significantly reduce the prevalence of sexually transmitted diseases in rural Tanzania: results of a randomized controlled trial. *AIDS* 11(15):1873–80, 1997.

NIMH Multisite HIV Prevention Trial: reducing HIV sexual risk behavior. The National Institute of Mental Health (NIMH) Multisite HIV Prevention Trial Group. *Science* 280(5371):1889–94, 1998.

Otten MW, Zaidi AA, Wroten JE, Witte JJ, Peterman TA. Changes in sexually transmitted disease rates after HIV testing and posttest counseling, Miami, 1988 to 1989. *American Journal of Public Health* 83(4):529–533, 1993.

Roddy RE, Schulz KF, Cates W. Microbicides, meta-analysis, and the N-9 question. Where's the Research? *Sexually Transmitted Diseases* 25:151–3, 1998a.

Roddy RE, Zekeng L, Ryan KA, et al. A controlled trial of nonoxynol-9 film to reduce male-to-female transmission of STDs. *New England Journal of Medicine* 339:504–10, 1998b.

Shain RN, Piper JM, Newton ER, et al. A randomized, controlled trial of a behavioral intervention to prevent sexually transmitted disease among minority women. *New England Journal of Medicine* 340(2):93–100, 1999.

Spielberg F, Kassler WJ. Rapid testing for HIV antibody: a technology whose time has come. *Annals of Internal Medicine* 125:509–511, 1996.

Stratton P, Alexander NJ. Prevention of sexually transmitted infections; physical and chemical barrier methods. *Infectious Disease Clinics of North America* 7(4): 841–59, 1993.

Taha TE, Hoover DR, Dallabeta GA, et al. Bacterial vaginosis and disturbances of vaginal flora: association with increased acquisition of HIV. *AIDS* 12(13):1699–706, 1998.

Temmerman M., Ndinya-Achola J, Ambani J, Piot P. The right not to know HIV-test results. *Lancet* 345(8955):969–70, 1995.

UNAIDS. Facts and figures: 1999 world AIDS campaign. Geneva: Joint United Nations Programme on HIV/AIDS (UNAIDS), 1999.

USPHS. Management of possible sexual, injecting-drug-use, or other non-occupational exposure to HIV, including considerations related to antiretroviral therapy. *Mortality and Morbidity Weekly Report* 47(RR-17) September 25, 1998.

Wang, C.C., Kreiss JK, Reilly M. Risk of HIV infection in oral contraceptive pill users: a meta-analysis. *Journal Acquired Immune Deficiency Syndrome* 21(1):51–8, 1999.

Wawer MJ, Sewankambo NK, Serwadda D, et al. Control of sexually transmitted diseases for AIDS prevention in Uganda: a randomised community trial. Rakai Project Study Group. *Lancet* 353:525–35, 1999.

Zenilman JM, Erickson B, Fox R, Reichart CA, Hook EW 3d. *Journal of the American Medical Association* 267(6):843–5, 1992.

This *Guide* is a PRELIMINARY EDITION.

We need YOUR HELP to make the NEXT EDITION as useful as possible!

Please send your
comments
criticisms
corrections
suggested changes, and
other guidance
to one of the addresses below. Be sure to include in your letter/note an address (fax, e-mail, or postal) where you can be reached for follow-up.

Translation Partners Needed

Write to us if you can help us find partners to help us have this *Guide* translated into your native language. For instance, provide us with a contact who works with translation in your country's Ministry of Health, or tell us about a group at a medical school that translates medical texts.

Send Us Your Comments

E-mail: womencare@hrsa.gov

Fax to the attention of "Womencare": 301-443-0791 (USA)

Postal address: Womencare
Parklawn Building, Room 11A-33
5600 Fishers Lane
Rockville, Maryland 20857
USA

Note that this and subsequent editions of
A Guide to the Clinical Care of Women with HIV
will be available online.

Go to the HIV/AIDS Bureau Web site
and click on the publication *Women's Guide*:
http://www.hrsa.gov/hab

IV. PRIMARY MEDICAL CARE
Judith Feinberg, MD and Janine Maenza, MD

I. INTRODUCTION

No field in medicine today is moving as swiftly as that of HIV/AIDS. The speed at which new developments occur and the rapidity with which they are superseded by newer data is nothing short of breathtaking. As a consequence, most studies are typically out of date at the time of publication. Because of the rapid turnover of key information, this chapter will focus on the essential principles of care for the HIV-infected woman. 'Cutting-edge' treatment strategies that are currently being studied will be mentioned but will not be described in detail. To be truly useful, we will indicate the general directions in which this field is moving and how to access updated information.

Several studies have demonstrated that positive clinical outcomes are a function of the clinician's experience in caring for HIV-infected individuals. (Kitahata, 1996) Nonspecialists are urged to seek expert advice and consultation whenever there is any question about the best way to manage a specific patient. This is especially important in the setting of antiretroviral treatment failure and in advanced HIV disease when patients are vulnerable to multiple simultaneous opportunistic processes.

There is as yet no compelling evidence that the clinical course of HIV infection in women differs significantly from that of men, with the obvious exception of the associated gynecological conditions and obstetrical issues which are described elsewhere. (Chapters VI and VII) Although recent data have indicated that women may have lower HIV viral loads than men with an equivalent degree of immunosuppression, no differences in overall survival or complication-free survival have been demonstrated. At present, the approach to management of HIV-infected women and men is the same. With prolonged survival now possible, general preventive strategies and health maintenance, such as smoking cessation, control of hypertension, minimizing cardiovascular risk factors and routine screening for malignancy (cervical, breast, colon) are all part of routine care for HIV-seropositive adults.

II. INITIAL EVALUATION

A. HISTORY

A comprehensive database is valuable to the primary caregiver in assessing the patient's current status and in formulating a management plan. It is critical to remember that most patients are anxious and frightened at their initial encounter for HIV care; the ability to empathize, to share knowledge without being patronizing, to provide reassurance and to remain non-judgmental are essential to gaining the patient's trust and to obtaining accurate information (see Chapter II: Approach to the Patient.) In addition to all the usual aspects of history-taking, the following areas are of particular importance in HIV disease and deserve special attention.

■ **HIV diagnosis:** When did you first test positive for HIV? Why were you tested? This neutral, open-ended start permits the patient to raise issues around HIV risk behaviors and possible route(s) of transmission, including sexual partners and practices and alcohol/drug use behaviors. Was the patient ever tested for HIV before? If prior test(s) were negative, it is valuable to assess whether HIV has been relatively recently acquired by looking for evidence of the acute seroconversion syndrome within the past 6–9 months. These symptoms are classically those of seronegative mononucleosis — fever, aches, pharyngitis, lymphadenopathy and frequently rash, although the range of possible clinical manifestations of acute HIV infection is very broad.

■ **HIV treatment history:** If the patient has already been treated for HIV disease, then it is extremely valuable to know the patientt's pre-therapy CD4 cell count and HIV viral load and specific treatment history. What was her prior antiretroviral therapy, including duration, any difficulties with adherence, response to therapy, adverse effects experienced and history of treatment-limiting intolerance to any agent? It is important to determine what, if any, obstacles she has experienced in taking antiretroviral therapy as prescribed. (See Chapter V on Adherence) Has she had any HIV-associated diagnoses and was she treated for these conditions? Has she taken any OI prophylaxis? Has she ever been hospitalized? For an HIV-related problem?

■ **History of sexually transmitted diseases and other infectious diseases:** including syphilis, gonorrhea, herpes simplex, pelvic inflammatory disease, anogenital warts; tuberculosis (PPD status, exposure to active case, prior prophylaxis or treatment for active disease); hepatitis A, B or C; prior vaccinations, including those for childhood illnesses, hepatitis A and/or B, pneumococcal infection and influenza; history of chicken pox or shingles; complete gynecologic history (See Chapter VI on Gynecologic Problems), including most recent evaluation, Pap smear and results.

■ **History of other medical diagnoses:** with particular attention to hypertension, type II diabetes, cardiovascular disease, premalignant or malignant conditions.

■ **Sexual practices:** including use of condoms (male and/or female versions) and/or other forms of birth control, consistency of use; number of current partners and their HIV status (if known); history of trading sex (oral or intercourse) for drugs or money; history of anal sex.

■ **Presence of HIV-associated signs and symptoms:** fatigue, lymphadenopathy, weight loss, skin problems, bacterial pneumonia, thrush (oral, vaginal), as well as signs/symptoms more typical of advanced HIV disease, including: fevers, night sweats, persistent diarrhea, severe headache, respiratory symptoms (especially progressive dyspnea on exertion and cough, whether productive or non-productive), mental status changes, difficulty swallowing, midline substernal discomfort with swallowing, and visual changes, particularly the presence of floaters or visual field deficits.

■ **Mental health history:** past and current problems, evidence of depression (trouble sleeping, early awakening, change in appetite, loss of interest in usual activities, anhedonia).

■ **Family history:** age and health of children, including HIV test results if performed; HIV in other familyy members; other medical diagnoses, especially hypertension, type II diabetes, cardiovascular disease, malignancy in family members.

■ **Medications taken regularly:** including prescription and over-the-counter remedies; history of and attitude to regular medication use; use of alternative (non-traditional) medications for HIV or other conditions; drug allergies.

■ **Social history:** place of birth, where patient was raisedd, where and with whom patient lives and relationship to others in the household; childcare responsibilities; history of domestic violence; pets, especially reptiles (risk of salmonellosis) and kittens (risk of toxoplasmosis); extent of formal education; occupational history and potential toxic exposures; travel history; cigarette, alcohol and illicit drug use in the past or continuing; misuse of prescription medications.

■ **Sources of support:** To whom has the patient disclosed her diagnosis and what were their reactions? Are there friends or family to whom disclosure seems possible either now or perhaps in the future? Are other family members HIV-positive? Are family or friends able to care for the patientt's children in the event of illness? Does she have a job and, if so, does it provide health insurance?

Just as important as the information that the clinician obtains in the history-taking process is the information about HIV disease that is shared with the patient. Counseling and education are important elements of the therapeutic bond with the caregiver, but because this entails an enormous amount of information, it is best broached initially and then reintroduced and reinforced at appropriate intervals.

Many patients are in a state of shock following diagnosis, or may be suffering from situational depression or fear of their partner's response. Be kind. Be patient. Schedule enough time (1 hour) for the initial visit. Make sure the patient knows your purpose is to support her and care for her. Another key bond is the one between the patient and the office/clinic nurse, which should be encouraged. Ensure that she has a path to reach you or the nurse for any questions, complaints, or symptomatic therapy, especially when starting antiretroviral therapy.

It is important to convey information in lay language at a level of complexity appropriate to the patient's level of comprehension (remembering that formal educational levels may not necessarily correlate with the patient's ability to understand complicated medical concepts). These include the following areas:

- **HIV pathogenesis:** What are CD4 lymphocytes and why are they important? How does HIV infection affect CD4 cells??

- **Natural history of HIV disease:** How is "AIDS" different from "HIV infection" (or "HIV disease")? What is the typical time course between acquisition of HIV and the development of HIV-associated problems? AIDS?

- **Monitoring the activity of HIV disease:** What do CD4 cell counts and HIV viral load tests measure? How are they used, and how often will they be repeated?

- **Goals of HIV disease management:** to maintain or improve the patient's immune system, control HIV replication; avoiding or minimizing side effects of medications; preventive care (vaccinations, OI prophylaxis, periodic Pap smears, other appropriate screening tests).

- **Principles of HIV treatment:** describe the available viral targets and classes of drugs used, and the value of combination therapy in preserving health and prolonging life.

- **Preventing spread of HIV infection:** notifying sexual partners and drug use contacts, safer sexual practices, safer needle use including needle exchange programs, ready availability of bleach in the household for cleaning up blood, appropriate wound care for accidental injuries, reassurance about the difficulty of transmitting HIV to casual contacts and to family members even in the close context of everyday family life.

Last, because a diagnosis of HIV infection remains a chronic, life-threatening disease and still carries a social stigma, the clinician plays a key role in exploring mental health and psychosocial needs, helping the patient identify potential sources of support, and referring the patient for additional medical, psychiatric and/or social services.

B. PHYSICAL EXAMINATION

The examination may yield clues to specific HIV-associated conditions. Vital signs should be tracked carefully, particularly temperature and weight. The discovery of hypertension, largely ignored in the past, should trigger appropriate attempts at control, including weight loss, reduction of salt intake and medication if necessary. Special attention should be paid to the following areas.

■ **General:** evidence of wasting, often prominent at the temples; fat redistribution syndromes including the development of a buffalo hump, enlarged breasts and truncal obesity which may coexist with or be separate fromm marked subcutaneous fat loss in the extremities, face and buttocks.

■ **Eyes:** The conjunctival surfaces should be examined for the purplish spots of Kaposii's sarcoma (KS) and for petechiae. Fundoscopy may reveal "cotton wool"spots (microinfarcts of the retinal nerve fiber layer due to occlusion of retinal capillaries). These must be differentiated from the typical 'eggs and ketchup' appearance of the infiltrates and hemorrhages caused by cytomegalovirus (CMV) retinitis in patients with very advanced HIV disease; visual field deficits are common in CMV retinitis and may be uncovered with simple field testing by confrontation.

■ **Oropharynx:** Oral examination often yields the earliest physical evidence of HIV infection with thrush (white plaques on buccal mucosa or posterior pharynx that are readily scraped with a tongue blade) and oral hairy leukoplakia (furry white plaques most often found on the lateral margins of the tongue which cannot be scraped off); purplish spots or plaques on mucosal surfaces, including the area under the tongue, typically indicate Kaposii's sarcoma but may also be consistent with bacillary angiomatosis. No examination of an HIV-infected person, regardless of disease stage, should be considered complete without a careful assessment of the oropharynx.

■ **Lymph nodes:** Non-tender or minimally tender generalized adenopathy may wax and wane and most often is related to HIV infection itself, but may also indicate lymphoma. Regional adenopathy is more frequently associated with local pathology, such as intrathoracic adenopathy in tuberculosis or abdominal adenopathy in disseminated Mycobacterium avium complex (MAC) infection. Extremely tender lymph nodes should trigger an evaluation for the etiology.

■ **Lungs:** fine dry "cellophane" rales are classic for Pneumocystis carinii pneumonia (PCP), but are a late finding and may be absent.

■ **Hepatosplenomegaly:** Organomegaly typically reflects disseminated infection with MAC, TB or histoplasmosis, or may be a sign of lymphoma.

■ **Pelvic examination:**
   ● **External genitalia/perineum:** sores or ulcers are usually indicative of sexually transmitted diseases, especially herpes simplex virus (HSV) or syphilis. In very immunosuppressed patients, ulcers may be caused

by other opportunistic pathogens, such as CMV, or may represent aphthous ulcers. Condyloma acuminata may appear as small fleshy papules or may be exuberant, florid growths reaching several centimeters in diameter; other HPV-associated lesions may be recognized only with magnification and/or application of acetic acid. Raised and pigmented lesions may represent premalignant changes (vulvar intraepithelial neoplasia).

- **Speculum and bimanual pelvic examination:** abnormal vaginal discharge can be caused by various forms of vaginitis (yeast, bacterial vaginosis, or trichomoniasis) or cervicitis. Pap smears should be obtained to rule out cervical dysplasia. Cervical motion, uterine, and adnexal tenderness suggest possible pelvic inflammatory disease (PID). (Gynecologic exam is discussed in detail in Chapter VI.)

■ **Neurologic:** Motor deficits may reflect space-occupying lesions of the central nervous system such as toxoplasmosis, CNS lymphoma and progressive multifocal leukoencephalopathy (PML), or may be due to neurosyphilis. Symmetrical, distal sensory deficits (especially decrease or loss of vibratory or proprioceptive sensation), typically affecting the feet more than the hands, indicate peripheral neuropathy, which may be due to HIV itself or to drug toxicity from the dideoxy nucleoside analogues. Poor short-term memory, diminished concentration and sensorimotor retardation are the hallmarks of AIDS dementia complex (HIV encephalopathy). Dysphoric mood or flat affect may reveal depression.

■ **Skin:** Like the oropharynx, careful examination of the skin often yields early clues about HIV infection, and should be performed regularly. Early manifestations include pruritic papular eruptions that may be bacterial folliculitis, eosinophilic folliculitis or scabies. Pearly papules, often with central umbilication, are typical of molluscum contagiosum. A painful vesicular rash may be HSV but in a dermatomal distribution is usually shingles (Varicella zoster virus). Seborrheic dermatitis may be severe and appears as scaly, erythematous areas on the face, especially the nasolabial fold and eyebrows, or may be confined to the scalp and hairline. Psoriasis is another common scaling lesion. Purplish macules or plaques may be either KS or bacillary angiomatosis, similar to their appearance on mucosal surfaces; however, in dark-skinned individuals, KS may appear more brown than purple.

III. LABORATORY TESTING

A. INITIAL DIAGNOSIS

HIV infection is usually diagnosed by serologic tests which detect antibody to the virus. Infection may also be detected by nucleic acid based assays that either measure the number of copies of the virus in plasma (RNA PCR) or detect the virus in cells (DNA). Informed consent, with pre- and post-test counseling, is legally mandatory for performing HIV serologic tests in most locations, and should be performed at all times when the test is offered.

■ **Serology:** The most common method of HIV detection is with an ELISA test for screening, followed by confirmation with a Western blot. For a positive Western blot, the CDC and Association of State and Territorial Public Health Laboratory Directors (ASTPHLD) require a band pattern indicating antibodies to two of the following proteins: p24, gp41, and gp120/160. A serologic test may be reported as positive if the ELISA is positive and Western blot criteria are met. The test may also be reported as indeterminate if the ELISA is positive, but only a single band is detected by Western blot. Serologic tests generally become positive 3–12 weeks after infection occurs. The interpretation of an indeterminate test during this window period may be clarified by the use of a quantitative virology assay with a PCR-based technique. (see Below) An indeterminate test may reflect the process of seroconversion, but may also be a constant finding in an uninfected individual. Causes of indeterminate results include:

- seroconversion;
- advanced HIV infection with decreased titers of p24 antibodies;
- HIV-2 (more common in West Africa);
- HIV subtype O (distinct from the more common subtypes A-I, collectively known as M) or non-clade B strains;
- autoantibodies due to autoimmune or collagen-vascular diseases or malignancy;
- cross-reactive alloantibodies from pregnancy, blood transfusions, or organ transplantation; and
- previous receipt of an experimental HIV vaccine.

The window period prior to seroconversion, agammaglobulinemia, and HIV subtype O are possible causes of false negative results.

ELISA assays are now available which detect HIV-2 and some ELISAs are designed to detect both HIV-1 and HIV-2; Western blot detection of HIV-2 remains inconsistent on standard assays, but there are also specific HIV-2 Western blots to confirm reactive HIV-2 ELISAs.

Accuracy of HIV serologic testing is quite high (with > 99% sensitivity and specificity), but the predictive value of a positive or negative test depends on the seroprevalence of HIV in the patient population. In a low prevalence population, the rate of false positive results of combined ELISA and Western blot testing is < .001%. The frequency of indeterminate results in a low prevalence population is .02%.

■ **Viral detection:**
- **Nucleic acid amplification:** May be used to clarify the diagnosis of HIV infection in acute infection, during the window period (after

exposure, prior to seroconversion), when serologic tests are indeterminant, or with neonatal infection.

> **plasma HIV-RNA:** routinely used to monitor the course and treatment of HIV infection. (See below) The three most common techniques are RT-PCR, a branched DNA (bDNA) technique, and nucleic acid sequence-based amplification (NASBA). These tests report the number of copies of virus per mL of plasma. The assays are considered equally reliable, but vary somewhat in lower levels of detection and dynamic range. Lower limits of detection for standard tests are 400 copies/ml, but ultrasensitive assays are now available which can detect as few as 20–50 copies/ml. Sensitivity is 90–95% overall, but is increased to 98–100% with CD4 counts < 200/mm³. False positive rates are 2–3%, usually with low HIV RNA titers. (Rich, 1999)

> **DNA PCR:** a qualitative test used to detect intracellular virus, and primarily used for viral detection with neonatal infection and with indeterminant serology. Sensitivity is > 99% at all stages of infection and specificity is approximately 98%.

● **Viral isolation:** qualitative or quantitative cultures are used primarily for diagnosis in neonatal HIV infection, and for more in-depth viral analysis. The procedure is expensive and labor intensive. Sensitivity is 95–100%.

■ **Alternative tests:**

● **Home testing:** Home Access Express Test is the only available home test for HIV as of April, 2000. Filter paper with a blood sample obtained with a lancet is mailed in to a laboratory in a coded, anonymous process. Dried blood samples are tested by the same ELISA and Western blot tests used on venous blood. Sensitivity and specificity approach 100%. Results are provided by phone (a recorded message for those with negative results, counseling for those with positive results).

● **Rapid tests:** There are three available tests that provide results in about 10 minutes: SUDS, Recombigen, and Genie. Sensitivity approaches 100%; specificity is also > 99%, but positive results should be confirmed with standard serology. Rapid tests may prove useful in STD clinics or emergency rooms (where patients often do not return for tests results) or on labor and delivery wards for high-risk pregnant women who have not previously been tested.

● **Saliva test:** The OraSure test uses ELISA and Western blot testing to detect antibodies to HIV in saliva. Sensitivity and specificity are similar to that with standard serology. This test is useful for people with poor venous access or those who want HIV testing, but refuse blood tests.

● **Urine test:** The only currently available urine test (Calypte HIV-1 Urine EIA) is licensed for screening only and must be administered by a physician; a positive result requires confirmation by another method.

B. BASELINE LABORATORY EVALUATION

After the diagnosis of HIV has been confirmed, a baseline laboratory evaluation is needed to establish the stage of disease, as well as exposure to other infectious diseases. In addition, routine tests of hematology, chemistry, and lipid profiles are needed at baseline, as HIV and other concomitant illness may affect these values, and detected abnormalities may also have an impact on the choice of therapy for the individual patient.

■ **CD4 lymphocyte count:** The hallmark of HIV infection is the progressive decline in CD4+ (helper) T lymphocytes. Normal laboratory ranges for CD4 lymphocyte counts are usually 500 to 1400/mm^3. CD4 counts may drop precipitously at the time of primary HIV infection, and then usually rebound to near-baseline levels. The natural history of HIV then involves a progressive loss of CD4 cells, averaging 30–60 cells/year. (See Figure 4-1on the following page) The risk of opportunistic infections increases with declining counts. (See Chapter I, Epidemiology and Natural History)

Knowledge of the baseline CD4 count is of vital importance in assessing the patient: staging of HIV infection (See Table 1-3 in Chapter I) as well as recommendations for antiretroviral treatment (see section IV.C) and prophylaxis against specific opportunistic infections (see section V.A) are based on the degree of immunosuppression as quantified by the CD4 count.

Many factors may cause variability in the CD4 count. These include:

■ inter-laboratory variations;

■ seasonal and diurnal variation (lowest levels at noon, highest in the evening)

■ the use of corticosteroids (decreases values)

■ intercurrent illness (decreases values)

■ HTLV-1 co-infection (increases values).

In addition, since the CD4 count is a value derived by determining the percentage of white blood cells that are lymphocytes, and then the percentage of lymphocytes that are CD4 receptor-positive, there may be variation in other WBC compartments (as may occur in pregnancy) that leads to variations in the CD4 count. Because the CD4 percentage is the directly measured value and the absolute CD4 count is the calculated one, it is more useful and accurate to focus on the CD4 percentage to assess trends in this important parameter.

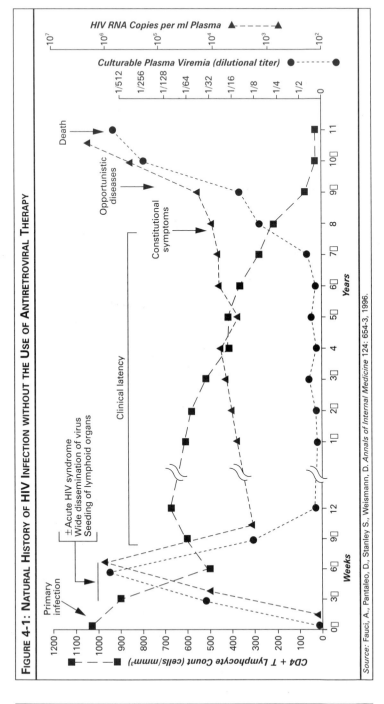

FIGURE 4-1: NATURAL HISTORY OF HIV INFECTION WITHOUT THE USE OF ANTIRETROVIRAL THERAPY

Source: Fauci, A., Pantaleo, D., Stanley S., Weismann, D. *Annals of Internal Medicine* 124: 654-3, 1996.

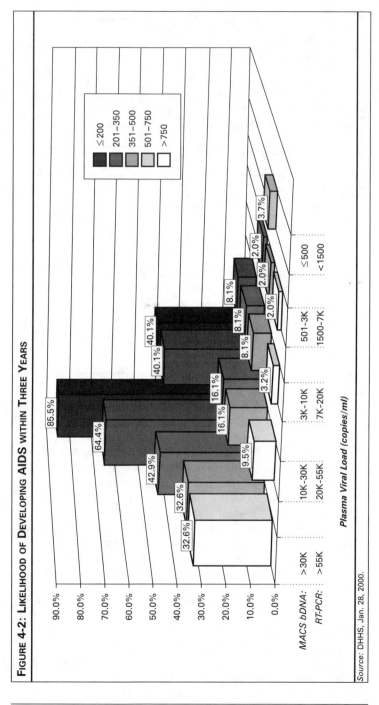

FIGURE 4-2: LIKELIHOOD OF DEVELOPING AIDS WITHIN THREE YEARS

Plasma Viral Load (copies/ml)

Source: DHHS, Jan. 28, 2000.

TABLE 4-1: INDICATIONS FOR PLASMA HIV RNA TESTING*

CLINICAL INDICATION	INFORMATION	USE
Syndrome consistent with acute HIV infection	Establishes diagnosis when HIV antibody test is negative or indeterminate	Diagnosis**
Initial evaluation of newly diagnosed HIV infection	Baseline viral load "set point"	Decision to start or defer therapy
Every 3-4 months in patients not on therapy	Changes in viral load	Decision to start therapy
2–8 weeks after initiation of antiretroviral therapy	Initial assessment of drug efficacy	Decision to continue or change therapy
3 – 4 months after start of therapy	Maximal effect of therapy	Decision to continue or change therapy
Every 3–4 months in patients on therapy	Durability of antiretroviral effect	Decision to continue or change therapy
Clinical event or significant decline in CD4+T cells	Association with changing or stable viral load	Decision to continue, initiate, or change therapy

* Acute illness (e.g., bacterial pneumonia, tuberculosis, HSV, PCP, etc.) and immunizations can cause increase in plasma HIV RNA for 2 – 4 weeks; viral load testing should not be performed during this time. Plasma HIV RNA results should usually be verified with a repeat determination before starting or making changes in therapy.

** Diagnosis of HIV infection made by HIV RNA testing should be confirmed by standard methods such as Western blot serology performed 2–4 months after the initial indeterminate or negative test.

Source: U.S. DHHS, Jan. 28, 2000.

■ **Quantitative virology/Viral load assays:** The HIV RNA level or "viral load" is also of pivotal importance in assessing the HIV-infected patient. Whereas the CD4 count indicates the current degree of immunosuppression, the viral load indicates the rapidity with which the disease is likely to progress: higher viral loads have repeatedly been shown to be associated with a more rapid rate of disease progression. (See Figure 4-2 on page 87.)

The most commonly used methods to quantify HIV RNA are RT-PCR, bDNA, and NASBA techniques (see Viral Detection section above). Standard tests have lower limits of detection of 400 copies/ml, but current ultrasensitive assays can detect as few as 20 copies/ml. Although results of different viral load assays correlate, absolute values differ and there is no standard multiplication factor to translate between results in the different assays. Therefore, the same assay should be used to follow an individual patient longitudinally. Intra-person variability on viral load assays is < 0.5 log, but this degree of variability is important to consider when determining clinical significance of a reported change in viral load values for an individual patient.

Indications for plasma HIV RNA testing are shown in Table 4-1. It is also critical to repeat any HIV RNA result that is being used as the basis for a change in patient management.

IV

■ **Hematology and Chemistry Panels:** The effects of HIV and related infections may involve hematologic, renal, or hepatic abnormalities. A complete blood count is necessary at baseline in order to evaluate for leukopenia, anemia, and thrombocytopenia. In addition, the total white count and lymphocyte count are needed in order to calculate an absolute CD4 count. A chemistry panel that includes an evaluation of renal and hepatic function is also necessary: HIV-associated nephropathy may be indicated by elevations in BUN/creatinine, and the effects of viral hepatitis, alcohol, or medications may cause abnormalities of liver function tests. Any of these findings provide important information in their own right, but will also have an impact on the patient's options for antiretroviral therapy.

■ **Other serologies:**

- **Syphilis:** High rates of co-infection with other STDs necessitate routine syphilis serology in all HIV-infected patients. A reactive non-treponemal assay (RPR or VDRL) must be confirmed with the treponemal-specific FTA or MTPA. CSF evaluation is indicated in HIV-infected persons with latent syphilis, treatment failure (when a non-treponemal test does not decline four-fold within 6–12 months after treatment), and those patients with neurologic signs or symptoms.

- **Toxoplasmosis:** Serologic evidence of latent toxoplasmosis infection, as detected by *Toxoplasma gondii* IgG, may be relevant for decisions on prophylaxis, evaluation of neurologic symptoms in patients with advanced immunosuppression, and avoidance of exposure in those who have not been previously infected. There is great worldwide variation in the prevalence of latent toxoplasma infection: in the U.S. the rate is approximately 30%.

- **Cytomegalovirus (CMV):** Latent CMV infection is present in the majority of HIV-infected adults. Knowledge of CMV antibody status is most useful in guiding the medical provider to the use of CMV-negative blood products if transfusions are required.

- **Varicella:** In patients who do not have a known history of chicken pox or of shingles, varicella serology should be obtained. The knowledge that a patient is varicella IgG-negative is important in the event of a subsequent exposure: post-exposure prophylaxis with varicella immune globulin could then be given.

- **Hepatitis:** Hepatitis A serology is not routinely performed, but given the newly available vaccine for those who are not immune, such testing may be appropriate to determine vaccine candidates. Hepatitis B serologies should be performed routinely: hepatitis B surface antigen (HBsag) and hepatitis B core and surface antibodies (anti-HBc and anti-HBs) allow determination of active hepatitis (HBsag-positive) and of those who are not immune to hepatitis B (anti-HBc-negative, anti-HBs-negative). Hepatitis B vaccination is then recommended in those who are not immune; and antiviral therapy, such as lamivudine (which

TABLE 4-2: LABORATORY TESTS FOR HEPATITIS VIRUSES

HEPATITIS VIRUS	LABORATORY TEST	INTERPRETATION
A	anti-HAV IgM	recent HAV infection
	anti-HAV IgG	immunity to HAV
B	Hbsag	current (acute or chronic) HBV infection
	Hbeag	current HBV infection with high risk of infectivity
	anti-HBc	past or present HBV infection
	anti-HBs	immunity to HBV (past infection or after vaccination)
C	anti-HCV IgG (ELISA)	past or present HCV infection
	anti-HCV IgG (RIBA)	confirms HCV ELISA
	HCV RNA	current HCV infection

has anti-hepatitis B activity), can be considered in those who are Hbsag-positive. Hepatitis C serology (anti-HCV IgG) is also routinely recommended. Recombinant immunoblot assays (RIBA) for HCV are also useful: both to confirm the diagnosis if a screening ELISA is positive and to clarify it if a first generation ELISA test is negative. HCV RNA, as detected by RT-PCR or bDNA assay, allows determination of active HCV infection. Knowledge of hepatitis C antibody status is needed to guide therapeutic decision for possible HCV treatment, and may also be relevant for decisions regarding antiretroviral therapy and other potentially hepatotoxic agents, as well as frequency of assessment of LFTs during such therapy. (See Table 4-2)

■ **Tuberculosis:** A baseline PPD should be obtained in all patients who do not have a history of a positive PPD in the past.

■ **G6PD:** A relative deficiency of glucose-6-phosphate dehydrogenase may be found in up to 2% of African-American women and an absolute deficiency is occasionally found in women of Mediterranean descent. Absolute G6PD deficiency predisposes to hemolytic anemia upon exposure to certain medications, including several that are commonly used in HIV treatment: dapsone, sulfonamides, primaquine. A relative deficiency is not usually clinically significant. Baseline testing in selected patients is helpful so that these agents may be safely administered at a later date without needing to determine G6PD levels at that point.

■ **Lipid Profile:** Many antiretroviral agents have been associated with the development of hypertriglyceridemia and hypercholesterolemia. A baseline fasting lipid profile should be performed to determine total cholesterol, triglycerides, HDL, and LDL levels prior to the initiation of any antiretroviral therapy.

TABLE 4-3: BASELINE LABORATORY EVALUATION

SUMMARY: BASELINE LABORATORY EVALUATION
❑ Confirm HIV diagnosis (usually with ELISA and Western blot)
❑ CD4 count
❑ Viral load
❑ Chemistry panel: including liver and renal function
❑ Hematology panel: including WBC differential
❑ Lipid profile: total cholesterol, HDL, LDL, triglycerides
❑ Serologies: Syphilis, Toxoplasmosis, CMV, VZV (if no history of chicken pox or shingles), Hepatitis A, Hepatitis B, Hepatitis C
❑ PPD
❑ G6PD (in selected patients)
❑ Pap Smear/STD screening

IV

■ **Pap smear/STD screening:** A Pap smear should be obtained, and testing done for gonorrhea and Chlamydia.

C. INTERVAL MONITORING

In an asymptomatic patient not on antiretroviral therapy with a high (> 500/mm³) CD4 count, follow-up every six months may be appropriate. For those patients who are symptomatic and/or receiving antiretroviral therapy, visits should occur at least every 3 months. For those who have just initiated or changed antiretroviral therapy, follow-up in 4–6 weeks may be appropriate. Laboratory evaluation at each of these visits should routinely include the following: complete blood count with differential, CD4 lymphocyte count, and viral load. Chemistry panels may be done less frequently (every six months) in a patient with prior normal values who remains clinically stable.

Hematology and chemistry values are needed to monitor possible medication toxicities, complications of HIV, and other possible illnesses. The CD4 count and viral load allow assessment of disease progression and effects of antiretroviral therapy. In following the CD4 count over time, it is important to recognize the causes of variability discussed above. Use of the CD4 percentage, rather than absolute CD4 count, may help eliminate some of this variability in order to clarify CD4 response to medications. In interpreting viral load changes over time, the variability of tests results must be noted: .3–.5 log. In a patient who has previously had a viral load below the limit of detection of the assay being used ("undetectable"), who now has quantifiable virus, a repeat test should be performed as soon as possible, rather than waiting until routinely scheduled follow-up.

The frequency with which lipid profiles are checked will vary by individual patient characteristics. In patients not taking antiretroviral therapy, a baseline lipid profile should be done with the initial evaluation or prior to the initiation of antiretroviral therapy. The profile should include total cholesterol, HDL, LDL, and triglycerides. If the baseline is normal, there is no need for interval

FIGURE 4-3: PATIENT INTAKE FLOW SHEET

Name			Provider/Attending			
History #			D.O.B.		Phone	
Dates	HIV+		AIDS		AIDS Reported	
	1st Visit		Psychosocial evaluation			
Immunizations	Pneumovax		dT (q 10yr)			
(dates)	Hep B vaccine #1		#2	#3	G6PD	
Serologies	HBsAg	HBsAb	HCV	Toxo	CMV	VZV
Year						
PPR						
PPD						
Pap smear						
Ophtho exam						
Flu vaccine						
Advance Directives			Family/Contacts			
Case Manager			Home Care			

Date	Wgt	CD4	RNA	Antiretrovirals	Other Meds	Diagnoses, S/Es, Comments

Source: Johns Hopkins Outpatient HIV Clinic. Reprinted with permission.

monitoring beyond that which would be done in an HIV uninfected adult. In patients taking combination antiretroviral therapy, general guidelines are:

1. get a baseline lipid profile (fasting) prior to initiation of therapy;

2. follow total cholesterol with routine chemistry panels;

3. obtain a complete fasting lipid profile annually or if the total cholesterol begins to increase on routine testing; and

4. follow complete lipid profiles every three–six months for patients in whom a lipid abnormality has been detected, both prior to initiation of any antihyperlipidemic therapy and once such therapy has been started.

Recommendations for management of hyperlipidemia may be found at **http://www.americanheart.org**.

Annual monitoring of syphilis serology for reactivation or new infection is generally recommended. PPDs should also be checked annually.

Baseline data and interval monitoring may be followed by the use of a flow sheet such as the one developed at the Johns Hopkins Outpatient HIV Clinic. (Figure 4-3)

IV. ANTIRETROVIRAL THERAPY

A. GENERAL PRINCIPLES

There are three characteristics of HIV infection that have significant implications for antiretroviral therapy:

1. between the time of initial infection and the development of clinical disease there is progressive immunosuppression as evidenced by a decline in CD4 lymphocyte counts;

2. viral replication is extremely rapid: the half-life of HIV in plasma is less than 48 hours and there is turnover of up to 1 billion virions per day (Ho, 1995); and

3. HIV has a high degree of inherent genetic mutability: mutations that may confer resistance to antiretroviral therapy arise rapidly.

Thus, there is a rationale for initiation of antiretroviral therapy prior to the onset of symptoms (i.e. to prevent immunosuppression), and therapy must be maintained to prevent viral replication. Strategies of antiretroviral therapy have therefore evolved to prevent the development of viral resistance. Although monotherapy with any of the antiretroviral agents will increase CD4 count, the clinical benefit of such therapy is very limited, largely due to the development of viral resistance. Combination antiretroviral therapy has been shown to have superior effectiveness in controlling viral replication and in limiting the emergence of resistant virus. These effects translate into greater clinical benefit: combination therapy reduces the risk of HIV progression and of death. In addition, patients with levels of circulating virus that are below 400–500 copies/mL (the limit of detection in the past few years), but greater than 20–50 copies/mL (the limit of detection in the newest generation of tests) will experience virologic failure sooner that those with viral loads that are below 20–50 copies/mL. (Raboud, 1998) Therefore, achievement of the lowest possible viral load should be a guiding principle in the selection of a treatment regimen.

The specific combination of antiretroviral therapy selected for an individual patient needs to take into account many factors. These include the specific side effects, dosing schedules, drug-drug interactions of different medications, as well as prior history of antiretroviral therapy. See Chapter XIV on Pharmacologic Considerations in HIV-infected Pregnant Patients for information on HAART in pregnancy and Chapter XV on Resources for sources of complete updated information on antiretroviral therapy.

B. ANTIRETROVIRAL AGENTS

NUCLEOSIDE ANALOGS

Nucleoside analog reverse transcriptase inhibitors (NRTIs) were the first class of agents shown to be effective in the treatment of HIV infection. The target enzyme for this group of drugs is HIV reverse transcriptase, an RNA-dependent DNA polymerase. (See Figure 4-4)

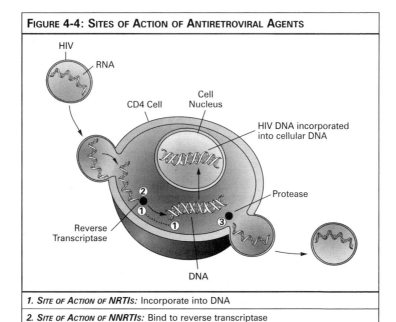

FIGURE 4-4: SITES OF ACTION OF ANTIRETROVIRAL AGENTS

1. SITE OF ACTION OF NRTIs: Incorporate into DNA
2. SITE OF ACTION OF NNRTIs: Bind to reverse transcriptase
3. SITE OF ACTION OF PIs: Bind to protease to inhibit viral protein cleavage and therefore release of virus from cell

TABLE 4-4: NUCLEOSIDE ANALOG REVERSE TRANSCRIPTASE INHIBITORS

GENERIC NAME	TRADE NAME	STANDARD DOSING	COMMON SIDE EFFECTS
zidovudine (AZT)	Retrovir	200 mg tid or 300 mg bid (2-6 pills/d)	anemia, nausea, headache
didanosine (ddI)	Videx	200 mg bid or 400 mg qd (125 mg bid if < 60kg) (4 pills/d)	GI symptoms (diarrhea), peripheral neuropathy, pancreatitis
zalcitibine (ddC)	Hivid	0.75 mg tid (3 pills/d)	peripheral neuropathy, pancreatitis
stavudine (d4T)	Zerit	40 mg bid (30 mg bid if < 60kg) (2 pills/d)	peripheral neuropathy, pancreatitis
lamivudine (3TC)	Epivir	150 mg bid (2 pills/d)	headache
lamivudine/ zidovudine	Combivir	1 pill bid	as for 3TC and ZDV
abacavir (ABC)	Ziagen	300 mg bid (2 pills/d)	hypersensitivity*, rash, GI symptoms

* 3-4% of patients will develop a hypersensitivity reaction to abacavir with symptoms that include fever, rash, myalgias. Re-challenge with abacavir after development of a hypersensitivity reaction may be life-threatening, and should never be done.

There are six NRTIs currently licensed in the U.S.: zidovudine (AZT), didanosine (ddI), zalcitibine (ddC), stavudine (d4T), lamivudine (3TC), and abacavir. (See Table 4-4)

In addition to the side effects listed for each medication, lactic acidosis with hepatic steatosis is a rare, but potentially life-threatening toxicity with the use of NRTIs.

NON-NUCLEOSIDE REVERSE TRANSCRIPTASE INHIBITORS

Non-nucleoside reverse transcriptase inhibitors (NNRTIs) noncompetitively inhibit HIV reverse transcriptase by binding to a site distant from the enzyme's active site. There are three NNRTIS currently available in the U.S.: nevirapine, delavirdine, and efavirenz. (See Table 4-5)

TABLE 4-5: NON-NUCLEOSIDE REVERSE TRANSCRIPTASE INHIBITORS

GENERIC NAME	TRADE NAME	STANDARD DOSING	COMMON SIDE EFFECTS
nevirapine	Virammune	200 mg qd x 14d, then 200 mg bid (2 pills/d)	Rash
delavirdine	Rescriptor	400 mg tid (12 pills/d)	Rash
efavirenz	Sustiva	600 mg qd (qhs administration may limit CNS side effects) (3 pills/d)	Headache, dizziness, cognitive effects, rash

TABLE 4-6: PROTEASE INHIBITORS

GENERIC NAME	TRADE NAME	STANDARD DOSING	COMMON SIDE EFFECTS
saquinavir (hard gel capsules)	Invirase	600 mg tid (9 pills/d)	diarrhea, nausea, abdominal discomfort
saquinavir (soft gel capsules)	Fortovase	1200 mg tid (18 pills/d)	diarrhea, nausea, abdominal discomfort
ritonavir	Norvir	600 mg bid (12 pills/d)	nausea, abdominal discomfort, circumoral paresthesias, hypertriglyceridemia
indinavir	Crixivan	800 mg q8h (6 pills/d)	nephrolithiasis, GI symptoms
nelfinavir	Viracept	750 mg tid (or 1250 mg bid) (9-10 pills/d)	diarrhea
amprenavir	Agenerase	1200 mg bid (16 pills/d)	GI symptoms, rash

PROTEASE INHIBITORS

Protease inhibitors (PIs) prevent maturation of virus protein by competitively inhibiting HIV protease, an enzyme essential for viral protein cleavage. When this enzyme is blocked, immature, non-infectious virus particles are produced. The other important properties which protease inhibitors share include their limited central nervous system penetration, and their metabolism by the cytochrome P450 enzyme system and resultant multiple drug-drug interactions. (See Table 4-6)

In addition to the medication-specific side effects listed here, there are a number of abnormalities associated with protease inhibitors as a class. Patients taking protease inhibitors may develop serum lipid abnormalities (hyperlipidemia, hypertriglyceridemia), redistribution of body fat (lipodystrophy), and/or glucose intolerance.

LIPODYSTROPHY (FAT REDISTRIBUTION SYNDROMES)

A dramatic increase in body shape changes has led some investigators to believe that some antiretroviral drugs may be associated with redistribution of body fat as well. Protease inhibitors, which may certainly produce hypertryglyceridemia, were the first agents associated with this syndrome, but other drug classes have recently been implicated as well, such as the nucleoside analog d4T (stavudine). However, the etiology of this syndrome (or syndromes) is unknown. Women seem particularly prone to developing truncal obesity (increased abdominal girth, increased breast size). Some patients may primarily lose subcutaneous fat in the face, buttocks and extremities, and a subset may have both fat loss and fat gain in different areas. Abnormal fatty deposits, which may be disfiguring, have been reported in the neck and the dorsocervical area ("buffalo hump"), although cortisol levels are normal. These body shape changes may or may not be accompanied by the development of hyperlipidemia and/or diabetes mellitus. Our current level of understanding of these syndromes and what causes them is fairly rudimentary.

It may be useful to obtain some standard measurements, such as minimum waist, maximum hips and neck circumference at an early visit, before antiretroviral therapy is started. It is important to question the patient at regular intervals about any perceived changes in body shape or changes in clothing and brassiere size, and anthropomorphic measurements may be repeated to document any changes. As yet there is no specific antidote to this poorly understood phenomenon.

Detailed descriptions of medications, drug-drug interactions, and medication use in pregnancy may be found in Chapter XIV on Pharmacologic Considerations in HIV-infected Pregnant Patients.

C. TREATMENT GUIDELINES

The Department of Health and Human Services (DHHS) Panel on Clinical Practices for Treatment of HIV Infection updates treatment guidelines on an ongoing basis. Updated recommendations are available at: **http://www. hivatis.org**. The guidelines detail indications for therapy in chronically infected patients, recommendations for initial therapy, considerations for changes in therapy, and possible regimens for such changes. (See Table 4-7)

TABLE 4-7: INDICATIONS FOR INITIATION OF ANTIRETROVIRAL THERAPY IN THE CHRONICALLY HIV-INFECTED PATIENT

CLINICAL CATEGORY	CD4 COUNT / HIV RNA	RECOMMENDATION
Symptomatic	Any Value	Treat
Asymptomatic	CD4 < 500/mm³, or HIV RNA > 10,000 (bDNA), or > 20,000 (RT-PCR)	offer treatment, with strength of recommendation based on prognosis for disease-free survival and willingness of patient to accept therapy
Asymptomatic	CD4 > 500/mm³, and HIV RNA < 10,000 (bDNA), or < 20,000 (RT- PCR)	many experts would delay therapy and observe, others would treat

Source: Adapted from DHHS Guidelines, Jan 28, 2000.

As indicated in this table, the strength of the recommendation for therapy in an asymptomatic patient must take into account prognosis for disease-free survival and the willingness of the patient to take, and adhere to therapy. (See Chapter V on Adherence) Prognosis for disease-free survival may be determined by utilizing the table in Table 4-8 (on the following page). In these considerations the potential benefits and risks of initiating therapy should be considered and reviewed with the patient.

TABLE 4-8: RISK OF PROGRESSION TO **AIDS** DEFINING ILLNESS IN A COHORT OF HOMOSEXUAL MEN PREDICTED BY BASELINE CD4 + T CELL COUNT AND VIRAL LOAD[1]

CD4 ≤350 PLASMA VIRAL LOAD (COPIES/ML)[2]		% AIDS (AIDS-DEFINING COMPLICATION)[3]			
bDNA	**RT-PCR**	*n*	*3 YEARS*	*6 YEARS*	*9 YEARS*
≤ 500	≤ 1,500	—[4]	—	—	—
501 — 3,000	1,500 — 7,000	30	0	18.8	30.6
3,001 — 10,000	7,001 — 20,000	51	8.0	42.2	65.6
10,001 — 30,000	20,001 — 55,000	73	40.1	72.9	86.2
> 30,000	> 55,000	174	72.9	92.7	95.6

CD4 351 — 500 PLASMA VIRAL LOAD (COPIES/ML)		% AIDS (AIDS-DEFINING COMPLICATION)			
bDNA	**RT-PCR**	*n*	*3 YEARS*	*6 YEARS*	*9 YEARS*
≤ 500	≤ 1,500	—	—	—	—
501 — 3,000	1,500 — 7,000	47	4.4	22.1	46.9
3,001 — 10,000	7,001 — 20,000	105	5.9	39.8	60.7
10,001 — 30,000	20,001 — 55,000	121	15.1	57.2	78.6
> 30,000	> 55,000	121	47.9	77.7	94.4

CD4 > 500 PLASMA VIRAL LOAD (COPIES/ML)		% AIDS (AIDS-DEFINING COMPLICATION)			
bDNA	**RT-PCR**	*n*	*3 YEARS*	*6 YEARS*	*9 YEARS*
≤ 500	≤ 1,500	110	1.0	5.0	10.7
501 — 3,000	1,500 — 7,000	180	2.3	14.9	33.2
3,001 — 10,000	7,001 — 20,000	237	7.2	25.9	50.3
10,001 — 30,000	20,001 — 55,000	202	14.6	47.7	70.6
> 30,000	> 55,000	141	32.6	66.8	76.3

[1] Data from the Multi-Center AIDS Cohort Study (MACS). (Mellors, 1996)

[2] MACS numbers reflect plasma HIV RNA values obtained by bDNA testing. RT-PCR values are consistently 2 – 2.5 fold higher than bDNA values, as indicated.

[3] In this study AIDS was defined according to the 1987 CDC definition and does not include asymptomatic individuals with CD4+ T cells < 200mm[3].

[4] Too few subjects were in the category to provide a reliable estimate of AIDS risk.

Source: U.S. DHHS, Jan. 28, 2000.

Among the benefits of therapy are:

- prevention of progressive immunosuppression by control of viral load;

- delayed progression of clinical disease/progression to AIDS;

- prolongation of life; and

- possible decreased risk of transmission. (Quinn, 2000)

The risks of initiation of therapy include:

- a decrease in quality of life associated with adverse drug effects and inconvenience of dosing;

- limitations of future options for therapy if resistance develops to current agents;
- unknown long-term toxicity of therapy;
- unknown duration of effectiveness of therapy; and
- possible transmission of drug-resistant virus.

RECOMMENDATIONS FOR INITIAL TREATMENT REGIMENS

Recommendations for antiretroviral treatment continue to evolve with the development of new medications and additional data from clinical trials. The most recent guidelines from the DHHS are shown in Table 4-9 on the following page.

Although these guidelines illustrate generally recommended regimens, nonspecialists should consider expert consultation regarding initiation of a specific regimen whenever there is any question about patient management.

The regimens listed in the preferred category are all considered highly active antiretroviral therapy or HAART. Although there are multiple possible HAART regimens, a comparison of several different example regimens will illustrate the principles used in selecting a regimen for a specific patient.

One possible HAART regimen is: AZT + 3TC + nelfinavir. This regimen could all be taken on a twice-daily basis, which may help with adherence, and the total pill burden is moderate: AZT and 3TC may be taken in combination as Combivir (1 pill bid) and nelfinavir requires 5 pills twice a day. In a patient with significant bone marrow suppression, the provider may wish to avoid AZT, and might instead select ddI + d4T + nelfinavir or d4T + 3TC+ nelfinavir. It is also possible to take a HAART regimen that does not utilize a protease inhibitor, such as: 2 NRTIs and efavirenz. In this example, the pill burden is lower than with PI-containing regimens (efavirenz is taken as 3 pills once a day), reductions in viral load are comparable to those with PI-containing regimens, and the potential class-specific side effects of protease inhibitors (e.g. lipid abnormalities) may be avoided, but the long-term effectiveness of an NNRTI-based regimen has been less well studied.

In addition to regimens designated as HAART, there may be instances in which alternative regimens are utilized. Such situations may occur, for example, when a patient states that she will only take a limited number of pills a day. Options for alternative regimens include AZT + 3TC + Abacavir. This regimen only requires 4 pills a day (Combivir bid, abacavir bid) and utilizes only NRTIs thus preserving both the NNRTIs and PIs for future regimens. Another possible alternative regimen containing only NRTIs is ddI + hydroxyurea, with or without a second NRTI. Hydroxyurea is not incorporated into most standardized guidelines, and has no antiretroviral activity on its own, but has been shown to increase the efficacy of ddI. It has most commonly been used in patients who have exhausted all standard regimens. There are recent

TABLE 4-9: RECOMMENDED ANTIRETROVIRAL AGENTS FOR INITIAL TREATMENT OF ESTABLISHED HIV INFECTION

This table provides a guide to the use of available treatment regimens for individuals with no prior or limited experience on HIV therapy. In accordance with the established goals of HIV therapy, priority is given to regimens in which clinical trials data suggest the following: sustained suppression of HIV plasma RNA (particularly in patients with high baseline viral load) and sustained increase in CD4+ T cell count (in most cases over 48 weeks), and favorable clinical outcome (i.e. delayed progression to AIDS and death). Particular emphasis is given to regimens that have been compared directly with other regimens that perform sufficiently well with regard to these parameters to be included in the "strongly recommended" category. Additional consideration is given to the regimen's pill burden, dosing frequency, food requirements, convenience, toxicity, and drug interaction profile compared with other regimens.

It is important to note that all antiretroviral agents, including those in the 'Strongly Recommended' category, have potentially serious toxic and adverse events associated with their use. The reader is strongly encouraged to consult Chapter XIV on Pharmacologic Considerations in HIV-infected Pregnant Patients while formulating an antiretroviral regimen.

Antiretroviral drug regimens are comprised of one choice each from columns A and B. Drugs are listed in alphabetical, not priority order.

	COLUMN A	COLUMN B
Strongly Recommended	Efavirenz	Stavudine + Lamivudine
	Indinavir	Stavudine + Didanosine
	Nelfinavir	Zidovudine + Lamivudine
	Ritonavir + Saquinavir (SGC* or HGC*)	Zidovudine + Didanosine

	COLUMN A	COLUMN B
Recommended as an Alternative	Abacavir	Didanosine + Lamivudine
	Amprenavir	Zidovudine + Zalcitabine
	Delavirdine	
	Nelfinavir + Saquinavir-SGC	
	Nevirapine	
	Ritonavir	
	Saquinavir-SGC	
No Recommendation; Insufficient Data**	Hydroxyurea in combination with other antiretroviral drugs	
	Ritonavir + Indinavir	
	Ritonavir + Nelfinavir	

	COLUMN A	COLUMN B
Not Recommended; Should Not Be Offered (All monotherapies, whether from column A or B***)	Saquinavir-HGC†	Stavudine + Zidovudine
		Zalcitabine + Lamivudine
		Zalcitabine + Stavudine
		Zalcitabine + Didanosine

* Saquinavir-SGC, soft-gel capsule (Fortovase): Saquinavir-HGC, hard-gel capsule (Invirase).

** This category includes drugs or combinations for which information is too limited to allow a recommendation for or against use.

*** Zidovudine monotherapy may be considered for prophylactic use in pregnant women with low viral load and high CD4 + T cell counts to prevent perinatal transmission, as discussed in Chapter VII on HIV and Reproduction.

† Use of Saquinavir-HGC (Invirase) is not recommended, except in combination with ritonavir.

Source: U.S. DHHS, Jan. 28, 2000.

concerns, however, about enhanced NRTI toxicity with hydroxyurea that may cause serious, and even life-threatening, pancreatitis. The role of hydroxyurea will likely be better defined after additional safety information is available.

RECOMMENDATIONS FOR ANTIRETROVIRAL THERAPY IN THE TREATMENT-EXPERIENCED PATIENT

The need for a change in antiretroviral therapy most commonly arises in two situations: medication toxicity and lack of therapeutic efficacy.

1. When the need to change therapy arises due to medication toxicity, it may be possible to simply change one component of a regimen. If the toxicity occurs in a regimen that has provided effective virologic control, the goal would be to continue effective therapy by changing the component that causes toxicity. For example, in a patient taking an effective regimen of AZT/3TC/PI, the development of anemia could be attributed to AZT. A different NRTI that does not commonly cause bone marrow suppression (e.g. d4T) could be substituted. The similar toxicities of certain agents must be remembered when making such changes: for example, in a patient taking ddI, the development of peripheral neuropathy, would not be expected to be alleviated by substituting d4T.

   There are other situations in which the toxicity is not as easily attributed to a single component of a regimen (e.g. rash, GI symptoms). In these instances, a "drug holiday" (temporary discontinuation) of the entire regimen may be necessary to allow symptoms to resolve, and a new regimen initiated with some change in components. With the exception of abacavir, which has caused hypersensitivity reactions (and should never be re-instituted after symptoms of such a reaction), re-initiation of antiretroviral therapy would not be expected to be associated with any increase in side effects.

2. Changes in regimen for lack of efficacy may be triggered by evidence of clinical progression, progressive decline in CD4 count, and, most commonly, for virologic "failure." Virologic failure is apparent when a regimen has failed to provide suppression to below the level of assay detection in 4–6 months after initiation, or when a patient with previously undetectable virus has a rebound to detectable levels. In these circumstances, (i.e. where viral load values will be used to determine a change in patient management), the test should always be repeated before a regimen change is made. Although some patients may derive continued clinical benefit and a sustained CD4 increase despite a detectable viral load, the possibility of development of viral resistance should lead the clinician to consider a change in regimen. The fact that continued exposure to an ineffective regimen will allow continued viral replication, and therefore the opportunity for development of additional resistance mutations, provides a rationale for changing therapy in this situation. Increased viral resistance may also lead to cross-resistance to other drugs in the same medication class, and therefore lower

chances of effectiveness of any future regimen. It is particularly important that the clinician use caution in this setting to avoid changing to an
even more complicated regimen in a patient who is demonstrating virologic failure due to difficulty with adherence. (See Chapter V on Adherence) In some circumstances, (e.g. prior exposure to multiple
medications) it may not be possible for the clinician to construct a new
regimen that is effective, and some experts choose to continue a viro-
logically failing, but well-tolerated, regimen under these circumstances

When a regimen is changed for lack of efficacy, the goal is to use
medications which are "new" to the patient to decrease the likelihood
of viral resistance. A general principle is that all medications should be
changed at the same time, and that a minimum of two new agents be
utilized. If there are two previously unused NRTIs that can be used
together, these should be part of a new regimen. There is significant
cross-resistance among NNRTIs, although efavirenz may sometimes
be used after delavirdine or nevirapine, depending on which mutations
have arisen; only resistance testing will enable the clinician to know
when this is possible. If an NNRTI was not used initially, it would be
beneficial to include one in a second regimen. For PIs, there are some
resistance mutations which are common to several agents in the class,
and others which may be distinct for an individual agent. In general, it
is has proven more effective to salvage a failing PI regimen, by using a
second regimen that contains a combination of two new PIs, rather
than just substituting one PI for another. (Hall, 1999; Tebas, 1999)
Recommendations for regimen changes may also be found at:
http://www.hivatis.org. Testing for resistance mutations may also
be a crucial factor when deciding on a regimen change. (See "Resistance Testing" below)

"Intensification" is a concept that some patients with a decrease in
viral load, but not complete viral suppression, from an initial regimen
may benefit from the early addition of just a single new agent. This
may also refer to the situation where a first rebound occurs after complete viral suppression. In these patients, low levels of detectable virus
(e.g. < 5000 c/mL) are present. This may be a unique situation where
it may be reasonable to add only a single medication, or to change only
a portion of the combination. However, it is important to realize that

TABLE 4-10: INDICATIONS FOR CONSIDERATION OF CHANGE IN THERAPY
■ Failure to suppress HIV RNA to undetectable levels within 4-6 months of initial therapy
■ Repeated detection of virus after initial suppression to undetectable levels
■ Increase (≥3X) from lowest HIV RNA (not due to other factors such as intercurrent illness, vaccination)
■ Medication side effects/toxicity
■ May also consider with: persistently declining CD4 counts and/or clinical deterioration

at the present time "intensification" represents an unproven hypothesis that is being evaluated in ongoing clinical trials.

A summary of situations in which a change of therapy should be considered is shown in Table 4-10.

RESISTANCE TESTING

There are two main techniques to assess the development of viral resistance to antiretroviral therapy. Phenotypic assays directly determine the amount of a medication required to inhibit HIV. These assays are not yet licensed for clinical use, and commercial availability is limited. Genotypic assays determine changes in the nucleotide sequences of the genes that code for the protease and reverse transcriptase enzymes. Interpretations of genotypic results require knowledge of which specific changes are associated with resistance. Results are reported as a string of three pieces of information or each mutation detected:

1. wild-type amino acid;

2. codon involved; and

3. amino acid coded for by mutated codon.

Figure 4-5 on the following page shows the mutations known to be associated with resistance to specific agents. (Hirsch, 1998) Updated listings of mutations and associated resistance can be found at: **http://hiv-web.lanl.gov** or **http://www.viral-resistance.com**.

Both phenotypic and genotypic assays are difficult to perform if the viral copy number is less than 1000 c/ml. Their utility is also limited by an inability to detect resistant virus that makes up less than 20% of the total viral burden in a sample. It is also critical to recognize that these assays will only reliably detect mutations conferring resistance to medications the patient is taking at the time the assay is performed: samples from patients who are off therapy at the time of resistance testing are likely to show reversion to wild-type (sensitive) virus as the predominant circulating viral strain. Thus, resistance testing is insensitive to mutations secondary to selective pressure that is no longer present after a change in regimen. Virions with these mutations likely still exist as a small percentage of circulating virus and may lead to clinical resistance if inactive drugs that test "sensitive" but are vulnerable to these resistance mutations are used; current assays will not detect their presence. A comparison of genotypic and phenotypic assays is shown in the Table 4-11 on page 105.

At least two studies have shown that patients for whom genotypic analysis is done prior to a change in antiretroviral therapy have a better virologic response to the new regimen than do patients in whom a change in therapy is based soley on antiretroviral history. (Durant, 1999; Baxter, 1999) Resistance testing may be useful in:

1. assessing NRTI resistance/cross-resistance in patients with virologic failure on a NRTI-containing regimen (e.g., to look for mutations associated with pan-NRTI-resistance)

FIGURE 4-5: MUTATIONS ASSOCIATED WITH RESISTANCE TO SPECIFIC AGENTS

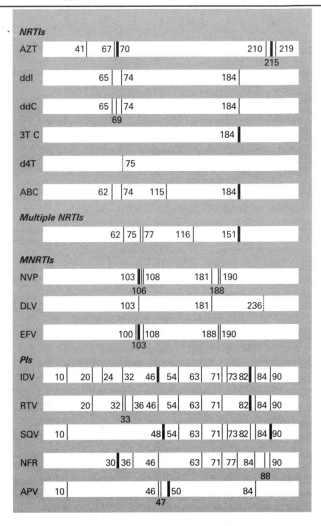

Mutations in the reverse transcriptase and protease genes that have been associated with drug resistance are depicted above. Bold lines represent major mutations, while thin lines indicate secondary mutations. Dotted lines represent mutations that have been identified in vitro though have not been associated with resistance in clinical isolates. Resistance mutations, along with more complete sequencing data, can be found at **http://www.viral-resistance.com** and at **http://hiv-web.lanl.gov.**

Source: Erbelding, 1999. (Adapted from *JAMA* 279(24) 1984–91, June 24,1998.)

TABLE 4-11: COMPARISON OF GENOTYPIC AND PHENOTYPIC ASSAYS

TYPE OF ASSAY	ADVANTAGES	DISADVANTAGES
Genotypic	■ easier to perform ■ more widely available ■ more rapid	■ only measures susceptibility indirectly ■ prior knowledge of mutations associated with resistance required ■ must have HIV RNA > 1000 c/ml ■ will not detect mutations if in less than 20% of total viral particles
Phenotypic	■ measures susceptibility directly ■ allows assessment of cross-resistance	■ complex assay: harder to perform, slower time to results, and less widely available ■ must have HIV RNA > 1000 c/ml ■ will not detect mutations if in less than 20% of total viral particles ■ clinically significant break-points for susceptibility/ resistance not yet defined

2. Assessing cross-resistance between NNRTIs

3. defining presence/extent of PI resistance in those with virologic failure on a PI-containing regimen

4. determining if there is drug-resistance in a patient with acute HIV who is considering antiretroviral therapy. (See "Treatment of Acutre HIV Infection" below.)

Patients with pan-sensitive virus in the face of virologic failure should be questioned carefully, but non-judgmentally, about their medication-taking behaviors.

D. TREATMENT OF ACUTE HIV INFECTION

In order to be able to consider treatment of acute HIV infection, the clinician must first recognize its presence. In more than half of all patients who acquire HIV infection, there are clinical symptoms two to six weeks after the exposure. The symptoms vary in severity, but commonly include fever, lymphadenopathy, fatigue, rash, myalgias, and pharyngitis – a symptom complex that mimics mononucleosis. HIV antibodies will not yet be present at this point, but techniques that detect viral nucleic acids (see "Initial Diagnosis" above) will confirm the diagnosis: a negative or indeterminate antibody test in conjunction with a positive HIV RNA or HIV DNA test is diagnostic of acute HIV infection. It is important to note, however, that a low level of HIV RNA (e.g. < 5000 c/ml) may be a false positive result, and should be repeated.

(Rich, 1999) In addition, an HIV DNA assay could be performed to clarify the diagnosis: this should almost always be positive in an infected person, regardless of RNA level. Relatively recent infection may also be diagnosed in a patient with negative HIV serologies in the previous 6–9 months and a first positive result, even in the absence of a seroconversion syndrome.

The benefits of treating acute HIV infection are not completely defined. The rationale for early treatment is that there will be early suppression of viremia, which may preserve CD4 cell number/function including HIV-specific CD4 cells. There are also risks associated with early treatment: these include the toxicities of the medications used and the possibility of the early development of resistance. These unanswered questions about risks and benefits of early therapy should be addressed with the patient; enrollment in clinical trials and observational studies of acute HIV should be considered. In treating acute HIV, it is always important to use a three- or four-drug regimen that would be expected to provide complete viral suppression. In addition, after considering the source of exposure and local epidemiologic information, genotypic resistance testing may prove useful in this setting. In acute HIV infection, the patient's predominant virus will be the strain that was transmitted, without reversion to the wild-type (pan-sensitive) virus seen in chronically infected patients who have stopped treatment. The potential risks and benefits of treating acute HIV are summarized in Table 4-12.

TABLE 4-12: RISKS AND BENEFITS OF EARLY INITIATION OF ANTIRETROVIRAL THERAPY IN THE ASYMPTOMATIC HIV-INFECTED PATIENT	
POTENTIAL BENEFITS	■ Control of viral replication and mutation; reduction of viral burden ■ Prevention of progressive immunodeficiency; potential maintenance or reconstruction of a normal immune system ■ Delayed progression to AIDS and prolongation of life ■ Decreased risk of selection of resistant virus ■ Decreased risk of drug toxicity ■ Possible decreased risk of viral transmission
POTENTIAL RISKS	■ Reduction in quality of life from adverse drug effects and inconvenience of current maximally suppressive regimens ■ Earlier development of drug resistance ■ Transmission of drug resistant virus ■ Limitation in future choices of antiretroviral agents due to development of resistance ■ Unknown long term toxicity of antiretroviral drugs ■ Unknown duration of effectiveness of current antiretroviral therapies
Source: U.S. DHHS, Jan. 28, 2000.	

POST-EXPOSURE PROPHYLAXIS

See Chapter XIII on Occupational Exposure.

TREATMENT IN PREGNANCY

Guidelines for optimal antiretroviral therapy in pregnancy are the same as those for non-pregnant adults. (See above) Particular concerns for fetal exposure to medications and for strategies to reduce the risk of viral transmission must also be considered. Please see Chapter VII on HIV and Reproduction. Information is also provided at: **http://www.hivatis.org**.

IMMUNE-BASED THERAPY

Therapy to augment the immune response to HIV may be possible through the use of HIV vaccines or cytokines, such as interleukin-2. Such strategies to enhance the control of HIV already provided by antiretroviral medications are being assessed in clinical trials, but are not part of current standard care.

ALTERNATIVE/COMPLEMENTARY THERAPY

Some patients may present with knowledge or questions about alternative or complementary therapy, or may indicate that they are already taking such therapy. Specific complementary therapies change rapidly, and their use varies widely with geography and patient demographics. For patients who do choose such therapies it is important to make sure that agents that have overlapping toxicities with a patient's prescribed therapy are avoided, and that discussions of alternative therapy are held in way that does not alienate the patient from her involvement in medical care.

V. COMPLICATIONS: OPPORTUNISTIC DISEASES

The risk for various opportunistic processes — so called because they take advantage of patients with a weakened immune system — is defined by the total CD4 lymphocyte count. They include opportunistic infections (OIs) and certain malignancies, and are similar to the diseases seen in other immuno-compromised hosts such as recipients of solid organ transplants. In fact, AIDS was first recognized as a new entity by the characteristic pattern of opportunistic diseasess — especially pneumocystis pneumonia and Kaposi's sarcoma — that were being diagnosed in young, previously healthy gay men. The pattern and sequence of OIs that are seen as the total CD4 cell count decreases is so reliable that in most cases the total CD4 cell count limits the differential diagnosis. (See Table 4-13)

At total CD4 cell counts above 500, illnesses are rarely specifically associated with the patient's HIV serostatus. Non-Hodgkin's lymphoma (NHL) and muco-cutaneous KS are occasional exceptions; they can occur at varying CD4 cell counts, but are more frequently diagnosed at lower values. Infections that are virulent among HIV-seronegative individuals, such as tuberculosis and bacterial pneumonia, may of course occur at any CD4 cell count but are increasingly more common and more severe as the CD4 count declines. Between 200-500

TABLE 4-13: CORRELATION OF COMPLICATIONS WITH CD4 CELL COUNTS

CD4 CELL COUNT*	INFECTIOUS COMPLICATIONS	NON-INFECTIOUS** COMPLICATIONS
> 500/mm³	■ Acute retroviral syndrome ■ Candidal vaginitis	■ Persistent generalized lymphadenopathy (PGL) ■ Guillain-Barré syndrome ■ Myopathy ■ Aseptic meningitis
200–500/mm³	■ Pneumococcal and other bacterial pneumonia ■ Pulmonary TB ■ Herpes zoster ■ Thrush ■ Candidal esophagitis ■ Cryptosporidiosis, self-limited ■ Kaposi's sarcoma ■ Oral hairy leukoplakia	■ Cervical intraepithelial neoplasia ■ Cervical cancer ■ B-cell lymphoma ■ Anemia ■ Mononeuronal multiplex ■ Idiopathic thrombocytopenic purpura ■ Hodgkin's lymphoma ■ Lymphocytic interstitial pneumonitis
< 200/mm³	■ P. carinii pneumonia ■ Disseminated/chronic Herpes simplex ■ Toxoplasmosis ■ Cryptococcosis ■ Disseminated histoplasmosis and coccidioidomycosis ■ Cryptosporidiosis, chronic ■ Microsporidiosis ■ Miliary/extrapulmonary TB ■ Progressive multifocal leukoencephalopathy (PML) ■ Candidal esophagitis	■ Wasting ■ Peripheral neuropathy ■ HIV-associated dementia ■ CNS lymphoma ■ Cardiomyopathy ■ Vacuolar myelopathy ■ Progressive polyradiculopathy ■ Immunoblastic lymphoma
< 50/mm³	■ Disseminated CMV ■ Disseminated M. avium complex	

* Most complications occur with increased frequency at lower CD4 counts.

** Some conditions listed as "Non-infectious" are probably associated with transmissible microbes: examples are lymphoma (EBV) and cervical canver (HPV).

Source: Bartlett, 1999. (Adapted from Arch Intern Med 1995;155:1537.)

cells, less serious HIV-associated problems begin to manifest themselves, such as oral hairy leukoplakia, various skin problems, shingles and oral or vaginal candidiasis (thrush). Candida vaginitis, which is also common among women who do not have HIV, may be the first indication of HIV infection. (Imam, 1990)

According to the 1993 version of the CDC case definition, AIDS may be defined by a number of serious opportunistic illnesses or by a decline in the total CD4 cell count below 200. (See Table 1-3 in Chapter I.) This CD4 cell count criterion acknowledges an important threshold for OI risk. *Pneumocystis*

carinii pneumonia (PCP), the most common AIDS-defining OI and leading
cause of death, is usually diagnosed as patients approach and drift below this
critical number of total CD4 cells. Other OIs, such as toxoplasmosis, cryptococcal meningitis and disseminated histoplasmosis, tend to occur as the CD4
cell count declines from less than 200 to below 100 cells. Typically, end-stage
illnesses such as CNS lymphoma, CMV end-organ disease and disseminated
MAC, tend to occur at very low CD4 cell counts, often less than 25 cells.

IV

Antimicrobial therapy works in concert with the individual's immune system to clear infection. Before the advent of potent combination antiretroviral
therapy, HIV-associated opportunistic diseases could not be controlled without
ongoing suppressive therapy, because the patients' immune function was too
weak to effect that control. Once an OI was diagnosed and treated acutely
("induction" therapy, borrowing from the language of oncology), treatment
would be continued at lower "maintenance" levels or the OI would inevitably
recur. "Cure" of OIs was not part of the vocabulary of HIV disease management. With potent combination antiretroviral therapy resulting in dramatic
improvement in CD4 cell counts and immune function, both prophylactic and
chronic suppressive therapies are being withdrawn successfully in responders.
This has opened an entirely new era in the care of people with advanced HIV
(vide infra).

A. OI PROPHYLAXIS

One of the early significant advances in the management of HIV/AIDS was
the demonstration that chemoprophylaxis could prevent PCP and thereby
improve survival. Prior to the development of potent combination antiretroviral therapy an important focus of the clinical research effort was to identify
effective prophylactic agents for the other common OIs. The success of this
research was in part responsible for the slowing of the death rate from AIDS
that was first apparent near the end of 1995, just before the era of potent
combination antiretroviral therapy began. Recommendations for prophylaxis
for specific OIs depend on a number of factors: the CD4 threshold that
defines the greatest risk, the overall effectiveness of a given approach, the risk
of resistance development, the presence of pregnancy, toxicity and cost. The
USPHS/IDSA guidelines for OI prophylaxis are updated periodically to
reflect the most current understanding of disease risk and prevention. (Current recommendations for initiating OI prophylaxis can be found at
http://www.hivatis.org, or in *1999 Medical Management of HIV Infection* by
John Bartlett, listed in the Resources Appendix.) (USPHS, 1999)

B. PRESENTATION AND MANAGEMENT OF THE MOST
   COMMON COMPLICATIONS OF ADVANCED HIV
   DISEASE (AIDS)

Summaries are presented below. However, specific agents and dosing regimens
for acute conditions and secondary opportunistic infection prophylaxis,

respectively, can be found at **http://www.hivatis.org**, or in the *1999 Medical Management of HIV Infection* by John Bartlett. See Table 4-14 for primary prophylaxis of the most common OIs.

TABLE 4-14: PROPHYLAXIS TO PREVENT FIRST EPISODE OF OPPORTUNISTIC DISEASE IN ADULTS AND ADOLESCENTS INFECTED WITH HUMAN IMMUNODEFICIENCY VIRUS

PATHOGEN	PREVENTIVE REGIMENS		
	INDICATION	*FIRST CHOICE*	*ALTERNATIVES*
I. STRONGLY RECOMMENDED AS STANDARD OF CARE			
Pneumocystis carinii[1]	CD4+ count <200/µL *or* oropharyngeal candidiasis	Trimethoprim-sulfamethoxazole (TMP-SMZ), 1 DS po q.d. (AI) TMP-SMZ, 1 SS po q.d. (AI)	Dapsone, 50 mg po b.i.d. *or* 100 mg po q.d. (BI); dapsone, 50 mg po q.d. **plus** pyrimethamine, 50 mg po q.w. **plus** leucovorin, 25 mg po q.w. (BI); dapsone, 200 mg po **plus** pyrimethamine, 75 mg po **plus** leucovorin, 25 mg po q.w. (BI); aerosolized pentamidine, 300 mg q.m. via Respirgard II™ nebulizer (BI); atovaquone, 1500 mg po q.d. (BI); TMP-SMZ, 1 DS po t.i.w. (BI)
Mycobacterium tuberculosis Isoniazid-sensitive[2]	TST reaction ≥5mm *or* prior positive TST result without treatment *or* contact with case of active tuberculosis	Isoniazid, 300 mg po *plus* pyridoxine, 50 mg po q.d. x 9 mo (AII) or isoniazid, 900 mg po *plus* pyridoxine, 100 mg po b.i.w. x 9 mo (BI); rifampin, 600 mg *plus* pyra-zinamide, 20 mg/kg po q.d. x 2 mo (AI)	Rifabutin 300 mg po q.d. *plus* pyrazinamide, 20 mg/kg po q.d. x 2 mo (BIII); rifampin 600 mg po q.d. x 4 mo (BIII)
Isoniazid-resistant	Same; high probability of exposure to isoniazid-resistant tuberculosis	Rifampin 600 mg *plus* pyrazinamide, 20 mg/kg po q.d. x 2 mo (AI)	Rifabutin, 300 mg *plus* pyrazinamide 20 mg/kg po q.d. x 2 mo (BIII); rifampin, 600 mg po q.d. x 4 mo (BIII); Rifabutin, 300 mg po q.d. x 4 mo (CIII)
Table continues . . .			

TABLE 4-14: PROPHYLAXIS TO PREVENT FIRST EPISODE OF OPPORTUNISTIC DISEASE IN ADULTS AND ADOLESCENTS INFECTED WITH HUMAN IMMUNODEFICIENCY VIRUS (continued)

| PATHOGEN | PREVENTIVE REGIMENS | | |
	INDICATION	FIRST CHOICE	ALTERNATIVES
Multidrug-(isoniazid and rifampin) resistant	Same; high probability of exposure to multidrug-resistant tuberculosis	Choice of drugs requires consultation with public health authorities	None
Toxoplasma gondii[3]	IgG antibody to Toxoplasma and CD4+ count <100/μL	TMP-SMZ, 1 DS po q.d. (AII)	TMP-SMZ, 1 SS po q.d. (BIII): dapsone, 50 mg po q.d. *plus* pyrimethamine, 50 mg po q.w. *plus* leukovorin, 25 mg po q.w. (BI); atovaquone, 1500 mg po q.d. with or without pyrimethamine, 25 mg po q.d. *plus* leukovorin, 10 mg po q.d. (CIII)
Mycobacterium avium complex[4]	CD4+ count <50/μL	Azithromycin, 1,200 mg po q.w., (AI) or clarithromycin, 500 mg po b.i.d. (AI)	Rifabutin, 300 mg po q.d. (BI); azithromycin, 1,200 mg po q.w. *plus* rifabutin, 300 mg po q.d. (CI)
Varicella zoster virus (VZV)	Significant exposure to chickenpox or shingles for patients who have no history of either condition or, if available, negative antibody to VZV	Varicella zoster immune globulin (VZIG), 5 vials (1.25 mL each) im, administered ≤96 h after exposure, ideally within 48 h (AIII)	
II. GENERALLY RECOMMENDED			
Streptococcus pneumoniae[5]	All patients	Pneumococcal vaccine, 0.5 mL im (CD4+ ≥200/μL [BII]; CD4+ <200/μL [CIII])– might reimmunize if initial immunization was given when CD4+ <200/μL and if CD4+ increases to >200/μL on HAART(CIII)	None
Hepatitis B virus[6]	All susceptible (anti-HBc–negative) patients	Hepatitis B vaccine: 3 doses (BII)	None
Table continues . . .			

TABLE 4-14 PROPHYLAXIS TO PREVENT FIRST EPISODE OF OPPORTUNISTIC DISEASE IN ADULTS AND ADOLESCENTS INFECTED WITH HUMAN IMMUNODEFICIENCY VIRUS *(continued)*

PATHOGEN	PREVENTIVE REGIMENS		
	INDICATION	*FIRST CHOICE*	*ALTERNATIVES*
Influenza virus[6]	All patients (annually, before influenza season)	Whole or split virus, 0.5 mL im/yr (BIII)	Rimantadine, 100 mg po b.i.d. (CIII), or amantadine, 100 mg po b.i.d. (CIII)
Hepatitis A virus[6]	All susceptible (anti-HAV–negative) patients with chronic hepatitis C	Hepatitis A vaccine: two doses (BIII)	None
III. NOT ROUTINELY INDICATED			
Bacteria	Neutropenia	Granulocyte-colony–stimulating factor (G-CSF), 5–10 μg/kg sc q.d. x 2–4 w or granulocyte-macrophage colony–stimulating factor (GM-CSF), 250 μg/m^2 iv over 2 h q.d. x 2–4 w (CII)	None
Cryptococcus neoformans[7]	CD4+ count <50/μL	Fluconazole, 100–200 mg po q.d. (CI)	Itraconazole, 200 mg po q.d. (CIII)
Histoplasma capsulatum[7]	CD4+ count <100/μL, endemic geographic area	Itraconazole capsule, 200 mg po q.d. (CI)	None
Cytomegalovirus (CMV)[8]	CD4+ count <50/μL and CMV antibody positivity	Oral ganciclovir, 1 g po t.i.d. (CI)	None

NOTES: Information included in these guidelines might not represent Food and Drug Administration (FDA) approval or approved labeling for the particular products or indications in question. Specifically, the terms "safe" and "effective" might not be synonymous with the FDA-defined legal standards for product approval. The Respirgard II™ nebulizer is manufactured by Marquest, Englewood, Colorado.

Letters and roman numerals in parentheses after regimens indicate the strength of the recommendation and the quality of evidence supporting it. Categories reflecting the quality of evidence forming the basis for recommendations regarding the use of a product or measure for the prevention of opportunistic infection in HIV-infected persons: I — Evidence from at least one properly randomized, controlled trial; II — Evidence from at least one well-designed clinical trial without randomization, from cohort or case-controlled analytic studies (preferably from more than one center), or from multiple time-series studies or dramatic results from uncontrolled experiments; III — Evidence from opinions of respected authorities based on clinical experience, descriptive studies, or reports of expert committees.

Categories reflecting the strength of each recommendation for or against the use of a product or measure for the prevention of opportunistic infection in HIV-infected persons: A — Both strong evidence and substantial clinical benefit support a recommendation for use; B — Moderate evidence—or strong evidence for only limited benefit—supports a recommendation for use; C — Poor evidence supports a recommendation for or against use; D — Moderate evidence supports a recommendation against use; E — Good evidence supports a recommendation against use.

ABBREVIATIONS: Anti-HBc = antibody to hepatitis B core antigen; b.i.w.= twice a week; DS = double-strength tablet; HAART = highly active antiretroviral therapy; HAV = hepatitis A virus; HIV = human immunodeficiency virus; im = intramuscular; iv = intravenous; po = by mouth; q.d. = daily; q.m. = monthly; q.w. = weekly; SS= single-strength tablet; t.i.w. = three times a week; TMP-SMZ = trimethoprim-sulfamethoxazole; sc = subcutaneous; and TST = tuberculin skin test.

Table continues . . .

TABLE 4-14: PROPHYLAXIS TO PREVENT FIRST EPISODE OF OPPORTUNISTIC DISEASE IN ADULTS AND ADOLESCENTS INFECTED WITH HUMAN IMMUNODEFICIENCY VIRUS (continued)

[1] Prophylaxis should also be considered for persons with a CD4+ percentage of <14%, for persons with a history of an AIDS-defining illness, and possibly for those with CD4+ counts >200 but <250 cells/μL. TMP-SMZ also reduces the frequency of toxoplasmosis and some bacterial infections. Patients receiving dapsone should be tested for glucose-6 phosphate dehydrogenase deficiency. A dosage of 50 mg q.d. is probably less effective than that of 100 mg q.d. The efficacy of parenteral pentamidine (e.g., 4 mg/kg/month) is uncertain. Fansidar (sulfadoxine-pyrimethamine) is rarely used because of severe hypersensitivity reactions. Patients who are being administered therapy for toxoplasmosis with sulfadiazine-pyrimethamine are protected against *Pneumocystis carinii* pneumonia and do not need additional prophylaxis against PCP

[2] Directly observed therapy is recommended for isoniazid, 900 mg b.i.w.; isoniazid regimens should include pyridoxine to prevent peripheral neuropathy. Rifampin should not be administered concurrently with protease inhibitors or nonnucleoside reverse transcriptase inhibitors. Rifabutin should not be given with hard-gel saquinavir or delavirdine; caution is also advised when the drug is coadministered with soft-gel saquinavir. Rifabutin may be administered at a reduced dose (150 mg q.d.) with indinavir, nelfinavir, or amprenavir; at a reduced dose of 150 mg q.o.d. (or 150 mg three times weekly) with ritonavir; or at an increased dose (450 mg q.d.) with efavirenz; information is lacking regarding coadministration of rifabutin with nevirapine. Exposure to multidrug-resistant tuberculosis might require prophylaxis with two drugs; consult public health authorities. Possible regimens include pyrazinamide plus either ethambutol or a fluoroquinolone.

[3] Protection against toxoplasmosis is provided by TMP-SMZ, dapsone plus pyrimethamine, and possibly by atovaquone. Atovaquone may be used with or without pyrimethamine. Pyrimethamine alone probably provides little, if any, protection.

[4] See footnote 2 regarding use of rifabutin with protease inhibitors or nonnucleoside reverse transcriptase inhibitors.

[5] Vaccination should be offered to persons who have a CD4+ T-lymphocyte count <200 cells/μL, although the efficacy might be diminished. Revaccination 5 years after the first dose or sooner if the initial immunization was given when the CD4+ count was <200 cells/μL and the CD4+ count has increased to >200 cells/μL on HAART is considered optional. Some authorities are concerned that immunizations might stimulate the replication of HIV. However, one study showed no adverse effect of pneumococcal vaccination on patient survival (McNaghten AD, Hanson DL, Jones JL, Dworkin MS, Ward JW, and the Adult/Adolescent Spectrum of Disease Group. Effects of antiretroviral therapy and opportunistic illness primary chemoprophylaxis on survival after AIDS diagnosis. *AIDS* 1999 [in press]).

[6] These immunizations or chemoprophylactic regimens do not target pathogens traditionally classified as opportunistic but should be considered for use in HIV-infected patients as indicated. Data are inadequate concerning clinical benefit of these vaccines in this population, although it is logical to assume that those patients who develop antibody responses will derive some protection. Some authorities are concerned that immunizations might stimulate HIV replication, although for influenza vaccination, a large observational study of HIV-infected persons in clinical care showed no adverse effect of this vaccine, including multiple doses, on patient survival (J. Ward, CDC, personal communication). Hepatitis B vaccine has been recommended for all children and adolescents and for all adults with risk factors for hepatitis B virus (HBV). Rimantadine and amantadine are appropriate during outbreaks of influenza A. Because of the theoretical concern that increases in HIV plasma RNA following vaccination during pregnancy might increase the risk of perinatal transmission of HIV, providers may wish to defer vaccination until after antiretroviral therapy is initiated. For additional information regarding vaccination against hepatitis A and B and vaccination and antiviral therapy against influenza see CDC. Prevention of hepatitis A through active or passive immunization: recommendations of the Advisory Committee on Immunization Practices (ACIP). *MMWR* 1996;45(No. RR-15); CDC. Hepatitis B virus: a comprehensive strategy for eliminating transmission in the United States through universal childhood vaccination: recommendations of the Advisory Committee on Immunization Practices (ACIP). *MMWR* 1991;40(No. RR-13); and CDC. Prevention and control of influenza: recommendations of the Advisory Committee on Immunization Practices (ACIP). *MMWR* 1999; 48(No. RR-4).

[7] In a few unusual occupational or other circumstances, prophylaxis should be considered; consult a specialist.

[8] Acyclovir is not protective against CMV. Valacyclovir is not recommended because of an unexplained trend toward increased mortality observed in persons with AIDS who were being administered this drug for prevention of CMV disease.

Source: Gross PA, Barrett TL, Dellinger P, et al. Purpose of quality standards for infectious diseases. *Clin Infect Dis* 1994;18:421. Also: CDC. USPHS/IDSA Guidelines for the Prevention of Opportunistic Infections in Persons Infected with Human Immunodeficiency Virus: A Summary. United States, July 1995. *MMWR* 44 (RR-8), 1995.

PNEUMOCYSTIS CARINII PNEUMONIA (PCP)

The diagnosis of PCP can be challenging and requires a heightened index of suspicion. Although there are "classic" symptoms, findings on exam and chest X-ray manifestations, the presentation of PCP can be subtle and nonspecific. The classic triad of fever, exertional dyspnea and nonproductive cough occurs in only half of cases, although almost all have at least two of the following: fever, cough, dyspnea, lactate dehydrogenase greater than 460 U/L or an arterial partial pressure of oxygen (PaO2) less than 75 mmHg. A careful history may reveal long-standing exertional dyspnea that has worsened incrementally over weeks to months. Physical exam findings are also nonspecific. Fine dry "cellophane" rales may be heard or auscultation may be entirely normal. In 2–6%, PCP may present as spontaneous pneumothorax. The classic X-ray findings are diffuse interstitial or perihilar infiltrates, but a wide range of X-ray abnormalities is possible and radiography is normal in over one-third of cases. Extrapulmonary pneumocystosis is uncommon. PCP is suggested by oxygen desaturation with exercise, easily measured in the office or clinic with a pulse oximeter. This is particularly useful when symptoms are minimal, the patient does not appear acutely ill, and the chest x-ray is unimpressive. Severity of illness is indicated by hypoxemia or a widened alveolar to arterial oxygen difference ([A-a]DO2) on blood gas analysis.

Many diseases may have a similar presentation, including mycobacterial, fungal, viral or bacterial pneumonias, heart failure, pulmonary KS and pulmonary emboli. The definitive diagnostic test requires bronchoalveolar lavage of affected lung segments that is then concentrated and stained for Pneumocystis carinii organisms. Experienced sites can make a histologic diagnosis from an induced sputum sample that is concentrated and stained, but this less-invasive, cheaper diagnostic test should not be attempted where expertise in both obtaining and interpreting the smear is lacking.

Trimethoprim-sulfamethoxazole (TMP-SMX) is the mainstay of treatment for PCP; intravenous or oral administration depends on the severity of the episode. There are a number of alternative regimens for patients who experience treatment-limiting toxicity or who fail to respond to TMP-SMX. PCP should be treated for 21 days. After completing acute therapy, the patient should begin routine daily PCP prophylaxis to prevent recurrence. Patients with PaO2 less than 70 mm Hg or with an (A-a)DO2 greater than 35 on room air should receive adjunctive steroids, which have been shown to decrease the incidence of ventilatory failure and death. A 21 day course of prednisone (40 mg twice daily for 5 days, then 20 mg twice daily for 5 days, followed by 20 mg once daily for 11 days) is the most popular and cost-effective approach.

CANDIDIASIS

The appearance of mucosal candidiasis is often the first clinical indication of impaired T cell immunity in HIV-infected individuals. While oral and vaginal thrush are almost ubiquitous and candida esophagitis is the second most common OI after PCP, candidemia and tissue-invasive disease are rare. Pharyngitis may be asymptomatic or may cause dysphagia. White plaques can be easily scraped from the pharynx or buccal mucosa; severe cases will involve the tongue, gums and lips. Vaginitis causes a thick white discharge, pruritus and sometimes dyspareunia, and has a similar appearance on speculum exam. Intense erythema may be the most prominent finding in some patients with either pharyngitis or vaginitis. Scrapings will be KOH positive by microscopic exam and will grow readily in culture. These forms of candidiasis may be treated with topical or oral antifungals; topical agents are more cost-effective, and avoid the risk of systemic side effects or drug interactions.

Candida esophagitis is a more serious infection that may result in significant weight loss because of odynophagia. Esophagitis should be considered when the patient describes midline substernal chest discomfort with swallowing instead of pain limited to the throat. It may occur in the absence of oropharyngeal thrush, and can be diagnosed by endoscopy or by barium swallow. Topical agents should not be used for esophagitis. Oral fluconazole, 200 mg once daily for 10 days, is the treatment of choice.

Prolonged usage of oral azoles such as fluconazole can result in resistant candidiasis, so it is important to avoid chronic usage. Most experts try to use topical antifungals or intermittent courses of azole drugs, whenever possible. Prophylaxis for vaginal candidiasis with topical antifungals should be considered when systemic antibiotics are given. Some patients with fluconazole-resistant esophagitis may respond to itraconazole, especially the cyclodextrin solution, or to oral amphotericin B solution. However, most patients with resistant infection will require IV amphotericin for relief.

CRYPTOCOCCAL MENINGITIS

Cryptococcal meningitis may present as nothing more than the worst headache of the patient's life. Fever is common but meningismus may be minimal or absent. Altered mental status and elevated intracranial pressure above 180 mm of water portend a poorer prognosis. Cranial nerve deficits and seizures are only seen in patients who present very late in the course of their infection and are often antemortem events. The diagnosis is made by detection of cryptococcal capsular antigen in the cerebrospinal fluid (CSF); relying upon a positive India ink stain that demonstrates the organism's thick capsule is too insensitive. Cryptococcus neoformans may also be cultured from blood and CSF. CT or MRI scans may reveal basilar inflammation, and in patients with intracranial hypertension, the ventricles may be enlarged. Very mild cases may be treated from the outset with oral fluconazole, 400 mg once daily for 10 weeks, followed by chronic suppressive therapy (200 mg once daily). Most experts prefer using intravenous amphotericin B at a dose of 0.7-1.0 mg/kg/d for the first two weeks, with or without flucytosine, and then switching to fluconazole as described above if the patient is responding. Intracranial hypertension can be managed with frequent lumbar punctures to remove large volumes of CSF (20-30 ml at a time). Serum cryptococcal antigen may occasionally be positive before the onset of headache. It may also be detectable when extra-meningeal infection occurs, and in the evaluation of a fever of unknown origin. In these situations, oral fluconazole is appropriate therapy.

TOXOPLASMOSIS

Toxoplasmosis manifests almost exclusively as an encephalitis in AIDS patients. The patient presents with a neurologic deficit and classically one or more ring-enhancing space-occupying lesions can be seen on CT or MRI scan. However, the radiographic appearance of the lesions is not pathognomonic and may mimic other processes such as primary CNS lymphoma. Because serology may be negative and because it is often difficult to obtain a brain biopsy for a definitive diagnosis, the standard approach is a diagnostic trial of anti-toxoplasma therapy with pyrimethamine and sulfadiazine for at least two weeks. Both clinical and radiographic improvement should be evident in response to therapy if the patient has toxoplasmic encephalitis (TE). Clindamycin may be substituted for sulfidiazine if it is poorly tolerated. Although TE in AIDS patients results from reactivation of latent infection, a baseline negative IgG test for T. gondii does not exclude the diagnosis, and seronegative patients will routinely receive a trial of therapy regardless of their serostatus. For this reason, and because PCP prophylaxis with TMP/SMX will also prevent TE, obtaining a toxo IgG may not be very cost-effective. A situation where knowledge of toxo serostatus is helpful is when a patient cannot tolerate TMP/SMX prophylaxis; in this case pyrimethamine should be added to second-line PCP prophylaxis with dapsone in order to provide protection from TE as well.

HERPES SIMPLEX VIRUS

HIV-infected individuals may have recurrent genital HSV that can be suppressed with oral antiviral drugs such as acyclovir, valaciclovir and famciclovir. Both treatment and prophylaxis of HSV may require higher doses and, in the case of treatment, longer administration than is required in the management of HIV-negative patients; this is particularly the case in women with more advanced immunosuppression. (see Chapter VI on Gynecologic Problems) Definitive diagnosis is usually made by culturing HSV from the base of the lesions, although experienced clinicians will often rely on typical appearance, distribution and symptoms. When patients develop severe mucocutaneous lesions or ulcers that persist for more than 4 weeks, this unusually persistent form of HSV is considered an AIDS-defining illness. Similar to fluconazole-resistant candidiasis, injudicious chronic use of antiherpes drugs may result in drug-resistant infection, which in this case requires treatment with intravenous foscarnet. Varicella zoster virus, a related member of the herpesvirus family, causes shingles which responds to higher doses of antiherpes drugs than those needed for HSV. Shingles can be exquisitely painful and patients may have prolonged post-herpetic neuralgia. Secondary bacterial infection may occur, so it is important to keep the lesions clean and to use topical or systemic antibiotics as needed. Control of pruritus and pain is essential for patient comfort. Drug-resistant VZV has also been reported and is also treated with IV foscarnet.

Cytomegalovirus

Cytomegalovirus (CMV) causes retinitis in 80-85% of AIDS patients with end-organ CMV disease. Gastrointestinal disease anywhere from the mouth to the anus is diagnosed in another 12-15%. Other diagnoses, such as encephalitis and pneumonitis, are uncommon (~1%). CMV retinitis can cause visual loss, and untreated, progresses inexorably to blindness. Because retinitis is a necrotizing process, with effective antiviral treatment the lesions become quiescent and atrophic, but the affected areas do not regain function. Retinitis near critical structures such as the macula or optic nerve may cause catastrophic visual loss even when the total infected area is small. Patients may be completely asymptomatic, or may complain of floaters (due to inflammatory debris), diminished acuity or visual field defects when the lesion(s) is (are) in the periphery. Diagnosis is made by visual inspection of the entire retina using dilated indirect ophthalmoscopy by an experienced ophthalmologist. Extensive disease may lead to retinal detachment which may require surgical repair. Treatment is usually begun with intravenous ganciclovir, foscarnet or cidofovir for 2-3 weeks, followed by chronic suppression with either less frequent IV doses or oral ganciclovir. Chronic use of these agents requires the placement of an indwelling catheter for ease of administration, or IV therapy can be used briefly until an intraocular device can be inserted surgically that slowly releases small amounts of ganciclovir directly into the vitreous. Because CMV is a systemic infection with viremia, patients who receive the ganciclovir implant also need chronic suppressive therapy with oral ganciclovir to prevent the development of extraocular CMV disease. CMV can become resistant to antivirals. Refractory disease is often treated with intraocular injections, which, like the ganciclovir implant, deliver high concentrations of drug to the site of active viral replication. End-organ disease at nonocular sites is treated with 2-3 weeks of intravenous induction therapy. There is no clear agreement that CMV disease at sites outside the eye requires chronic maintenance therapy, but with the availability of oral ganciclovir it seems reasonable to provide continued anti-CMV treatment.

Disseminated Mycobacterium Avium Complex (MAC)

Like CMV, disseminated MAC is one of the OIs that appears at end-stage disease, when the total CD4 cell count is extremely low. It presents non-specifically with fever, weight loss, diarrhea, anemia and sometimes abdominal discomfort due to organomegaly and impressive intraabdominal lymphadenopathy. Mycobacterial blood culture provides a definitive diagnosis. Combination oral antimicrobial therapy is required and should include, at a minimum, an azalide (azithromycin or clarithromycin) and ethambutol, 15-25 mg/kg/day. Other drugs, such as ciprofloxacin and amikacin, have been used but do not routinely provide much additional benefit; clofazimine has been shown to have an adverse effect on survival and should not be used.

TUBERCULOSIS (TB)

There is a bi-directional interaction between Mycobacterium tuberculosis and HIV; each facilitates acquisition of the other, so it is critical to assess all HIV-infected patients for active TB and to test all patients with active TB for HIV. Because TB is virulent enough to cause disease in patients with intact immune systems, it may occur in HIV-infected individuals who still have high CD4 cell counts. TB is especially virulent in HIV seropositive individuals. Aspects of this virulence include the high frequency of positive blood cultures and of disseminated (miliary) infection. However, standard combination antimicrobial therapy is effective as long as the patient is adherent and the acquired strain is not multidrug resistant. It is essential to provide directly observed therapy (DOT) to ensure an adequate course of treatment and conversion of positive sputum cultures to negative. Until susceptibilities are known, all HIV-infected patients should be treated initially with at least 3 drugs expected to be active according to local susceptibility patterns. Subsequently, when the results of susceptibility testing are available, therapy for drug-sensitive infection can usually be narrowed to 2 agents (isoniazid and rifampin). Clinicians should work closely with their local health department to ensure that patients receive DOT, and to track and limit the spread of TB, especially resistant strains. All close contacts — especially young children — must be evaluated for TB so they may be treated promptly for active disease or given prophylaxis as indicated.

CRYPTOSPORIDIOSIS AND MICROSPORIDIOSIS

These enteric protozoa can cause debilitating diarrhea and weight loss in patients with advanced HIV disease. Diagnosis is made by special stool stains. Unfortunately there is no effective therapy (except for Septatis intestinalis, which may respond to albendazole), so care is supportive. Every effort should be made to optimize the patient's antiretroviral therapy, as there are reported cases of clinical resolution (and even clearing of the organism from stool) with potent combinatiuon antiretroviral therapy. Patients may develop severe dehydration due to voluminous watery diarrhea. In addition to volume reple-tion, attempts at slowing the diarrhea should be made as follows by adding (not substituting) each additional agent in a stepwise manner: 1) diphenoxylate or loperamide, increased to their maximum dose, plus 2) tincture of opium or paregoric, with the dose titrated gradually until the desired effect is achieved, and, if additional control is needed, 3) parenteral somatostatin.

PERIPHERAL NEUROPATHY

Distal, symmetrical polyneuropathy, typically affecting the feet more than the hands, may result from use of the neurotoxic dideoxy nucleoside analogues (didanosine, stavudine, zalcitabine) and much less commonly from dapsone, or may be a consequence of advanced HIV disease itself. Most patients present with paresthesias and/or numbness, but some experience pain that can be disabling. Examination reveals slow or absent ankle jerks, diminished vibratory and proprioceptive responses in both feet, and in patients whose primary complaint is pain, discomfort sometimes even with light touch. If drug toxicity is suspected, the offending agent(s) should be discontinued immediately and replaced. If this is accomplished quickly enough, symptoms may resolve entirely. When the nerve damage is not attributable to anti-HIV therapy or does not resolve after drug discontinuation, supportive care may be offered. Non-steroidal antiinflammatory drugs; agents useful in chronic pain syndromes such as amitryptiline, phenytoin, or carbamazepine; the neurotransmitter inhibitor gabapentin; mexilitene; and in refractory cases, long-acting narcotics, all have a role in the management of dysesthesias and pain due to peripheral neuropathy.

AIDS DEMENTIA COMPLEX (ADC)/HIV ENCEPHALOPATHY

In the pre-HAART era, frank dementia was the AIDS-defining illness in up to 10% of patients. The initial manifestations may be subtle, and can be uncovered by questioning the patient carefully about short-term memory loss and difficulty concentrating. Useful questions about the latter include the ability to balance a checkbook or to make change. In some patients, a depressed affect may be a prominent finding, and in others, unexplained seizures may bring the patient to medical attention. Psychomotor retardation — slowing of the impulses that match actions to thoughts and intentions — is another hallmark of ADC. CT and MRI scans show diffuse cortical loss with prominent sulci ("walnut sign"). A good sense of the patientnt's level of intellectual functioning can often be obtained at the bedside. In subtle or difficult cases, especially when there is a prior history of depression or subnormal IQ, the patient can be referred for a battery of neuropsychological tests that may clearly demonstrate the losses characteristic of ADC. There is no specific treatment for ADC other than effective antiretroviral therapy. Patients may demonstrate a remarkable degree of recovery with antiretroviral therapy even when they present with advanced dementia, so it is valuable to attempt treatment of all patients, even those initially referred for nursing home care. It may be particularly useful to include agents that achieve good CSF levels.

WASTING SYNDROME ("SLIM DISEASE")

Weight loss is common in HIV disease, especially in its advanced stages, but the Centers for Disease Control surveillance definition of wasting syndrome specifically refers to involuntary weight loss that exceeds 10% of the patient's baseline weight in the presence of diarrhea (≥2 loose stools per day) or chronic weakness and documented fever (intermittent or constant) for at least 30 days that is not attributable to a condition other than HIV itself. Typically wasting syndrome is accompanied by loss of muscle mass, for example in the temporal areas, and complaints of generalized fatigue and modest weakness. In severe cases the serum albumin level will be very low. Wasting can accompany any of the typical end-stage illnesses, such as disseminated MAC, or may occur by itself in the absence of any evident concomitant illness. Loss of weight, and especially, of lean body mass, portends poorer survival. Appetite stimulants, such as the progestin megestrol acetate or the marijuana derivative dronabinol, may be used although weight gain with these agents typically consists of fat and water, rather than an increase in lean body mass. However, the psychological benefit of an improved appetite and some weight gain cannot be underestimated, even if the gain is primarily fat. Recombinant human growth hormone has been used with some short-term success for improvement in lean body mass, but it is very expensive and must be given parenterally. Other approaches include enteral and parenteral feedings, anabolic steroids such as nandrolone or oxandrolone, and thalidomide or pentoxifyline for cytokine suppression. Men with symptoms of hypogonadism often respond to testosterone replacement, but this approach has not been evaluated in women.

KAPOSI'S SARCOMA (KS)

Kaposi's sarcoma is an endothelial cell tumor that, along with PCP, was the harbinger of the AIDS epidemic. It primarily affects gay and bisexual men, and is fairly uncommon among injecting drug users and women. It is most likely caused by human herpesvirus-8 (HHV-8). KS can occur at a range of total CD4 cell counts, but prognosis is poorer at lower values. Most commonly it is limited to mucocutaneous surfaces, where it is a cosmetic problem but not a threat to health. KS of the GI mucosa is very vascular and may lead to slow, chronic blood loss. When it involves the lymphatic system, KS can cause massive edema and woody induration, especially of the lower extremities; such patients are prone to severe, recurrent episodes of cellulitus. KS may also invade the viscera, especially lung parenchyma. Experienced clinicians can generally diagnose mucocutaneous KS by inspection, but a punch biopsy showing typical spindle-shaped cells is easy to obtain and is definitive. GI and bronchial mucosal lesions are also diagnosed by inspection; bronchial lesions may bleed profusely and are generally not biopsied for that reason. Visceral KS, which may occur in the absence of mucocutaneous disease, requires a tissue diagnosis.

Mucocutaneous KS may be treated with a number of local modalities including intralesional vincristine or vinblastine, radiation and topical retinoids. Gastrointestinal lesions can be cauterized endoscopically. Visceral disease requires systemic chemotherapy, with single cytotoxic agents or combinations.

SYSTEMIC LYMPHOMA

Several different types of lymphoma occur at increased frequency among HIV-infected individuals. These too may occur at any CD4 cell count although once again prognosis is worse at lower absolute numbers of CD4 cells. HIV seropositive patients may develop Hodgkin's disease, immunoblastic lymphoma and Burkitt's lymphoma as well as less common forms, but the most common type is an aggressive non-Hodgkin B cell lymphoma. There is a marked tendency for extranodal presentations, and AIDS patients have been described with NHL at a range of unusual sites. AIDS-associated lymphoma is diagnosed and staged in the same manner as in seronegative patients, and the same types of combination chemotherapy are used. However, HIV-infected patients may require somewhat lower doses or aggressive support with GCSF because of their baseline bone marrow fragility.

Central Nervous System (CNS) Lymphoma

CNS lymphoma occurs at total CD4 cell counts well under 100 cells and is a typical end-stage complication. Definitive diagnosis is made by brain biopsy or CSF cytology in the presence of a space-occupying lesion(s) on CT or MRI scan. A presumptive diagnosis may sometimes be made by nuclear SPECT scan. Because brain biopsy may be difficult to obtain, patients who fail a trial of therapy for toxoplasmosis are often assumed to have CNS lymphoma. There is no effective cytotoxic chemotherapy for this disease, and irradiation is considered palliative. Survival after a diagnosis of CNS lymphoma is usually limited, on the order of a few months.

Progressive Multifocal Leukoencephalopathy (PML)

PML is another end-stage complication of HIV disease, usually presenting as a focal neurologic deficit(s). It is caused by the JC virus, which can be detected by PCR performed on CSF. MRI scan of the brain demonstrate involvement of the white matter that can be focal or fairly diffuse, but is not associated with either mass effect or surrounding edema. Most commonly it affects areas adjacent to the cortex, but lesions can located anywhere. Definitive diagnosis is made by brain biopsy or positive PCR, which is highly specific in the appropriate clinical context. Where these diagnostic modalities are unavailable, the typical MRI picture usually suffices. There is no specific proven therapy for this condition, although there are a number of case reports describing clinical remission in patients begun on potent combination antiretroviral therapy. In the pre-HAART era, survival was very limited, but now there are patients alive more than a year after diagnosis.

Chronic Hepatitis B and C

Many of the same behaviors that put women at risk of acquiring HIV also result in hepatitis B and/or C infection. Both hepatitis B and C may become chronic, resulting in hepatocyte destruction that is manifested as intermittent transaminase elevation (especially ALT), and ultimately to fibrosis, scarring and end-stage liver disease. ALT levels may wax and wane, and may only be modestly elevated. Coinfection with viral hepatitis and HIV results in higher hepatitis B and C viral loads. Conversely, hepatitis C has been associated with acceleration of HIV disease, although hepatitis B has not. Branched-chain DNA (bDNA) tests for either form of hepatitis are more suitable for follow-up

FIGURE 4-6: GUIDELINES FOR USE OF ERYTHROPOIETIN IN THE ANEMIC HIV PATIENT

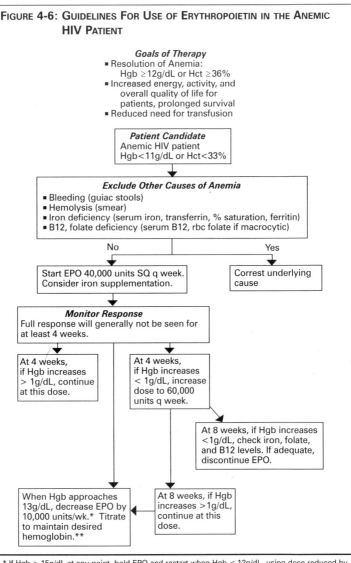

Goals of Therapy
- Resolution of Anemia:
  Hgb ≥12g/dL or Hct ≥36%
- Increased energy, activity, and overall quality of life for patients, prolonged survival
- Reduced need for transfusion

Patient Candidate
Anemic HIV patient
Hgb<11g/dL or Hct<33%

Exclude Other Causes of Anemia
- Bleeding (guiac stools)
- Hemolysis (smear)
- Iron deficiency (serum iron, transferrin, % saturation, ferritin)
- B12, folate deficiency (serum B12, rbc folate if macrocytic)

No → Start EPO 40,000 units SQ q week. Consider iron supplementation.

Yes → Correst underlying cause

Monitor Response
Full response will generally not be seen for at least 4 weeks.

At 4 weeks, if Hgb increases > 1g/dL, continue at this dose.

At 4 weeks, if Hgb increases < 1g/dL, increase dose to 60,000 units q week.

At 8 weeks, if Hgb increases <1g/dL, check iron, folate, and B12 levels. If adequate, discontinue EPO.

When Hgb approaches 13g/dL, decrease EPO by 10,000 units/wk.* Titrate to maintain desired hemoglobin.**

At 8 weeks, if Hgb increases >1g/dL, continue at this dose.

* If Hgb > 15g/dL at any point, hold EPO and restart when Hgb < 12g/dL, using dose reduced by 10,000/week.

** During dose adjustment phase, hemoglobin should be monitored every 2–4 weeks. Allow at lease 4 weeks to assess response to dose changes.

Source: Joel Gallant, MD.

of coinfected patients than PCR-based tests, which may be too sensitive. Both entities are treatable, and specific therapy should be considered to prevent or delay cirrhosis and liver failure. Hepatitis B responds to treatment with 3TC (lamivudine) and some investigational agents. Hepatitis C may respond to systemic alpha interferon, and better still, to a combination of interferon and ribavirin, although only a minority of patients achieve solid success rates.

ANEMIA

Modest anemia ($\geq$ 9–10 g/dL) is a hallmark of chronic HIV infection and may be complicated by menstrual losses in women of child-bearing age. Severe anemia ($\leq$ 9 g/dL) may occur as part of certain opportunistic diseases, especially MAC, disseminated histoplasmosis and lymphoma, and may also be the result of drug toxicity. Although severe anemia has been shown to be associated with a poorer prognosis for survival in a number of studies, diagnosis and treatment of the opportunistic process is often sufficient to improve anemia in these cases.

Patients who are symptomatic with exertional dyspnea and dizziness can be transfused acutely. Most HIV-infected patients become anemic gradually, and unconsciously limit their activities to control symptoms. These individuals can be managed with changes of antiretroviral or OI therapies known to be toxic to red blood cells, such as AZT (zidovudine) and trimethoprim-sulfamethoxazole. In patients refractory to conservative management, red blood cell production can be stimulated by using recombinant erythropoietin along with sufficient iron replacement to stimulate production of new red cells. (See Figure 4-6)

C. OPPORTUNISTIC DISEASE IN THE HAART ERA

The impact of highly active antiretroviral therapy on the natural history of opportunistic diseases has been profound, and the clinician must be familiar with at least the broad outline of these changes. There may be sufficient immune restoration that even patients with end-stage disease may become capable of mounting an inflammatory response to opportunistic pathogens. This can result in the atypical development of an acute OI in the first couple of months after initiating potent combination therapy, after CD4 cell counts have begun to improve. These cases may be marked by focal symptoms, such as the acute development of a tender, enlarged lymph node with negative blood cultures in the case of MAC lymphadenitis, where in the pre-HAART era the typical presentation would have been diffuse, with widespread nontender adenopathy and high-grade mycobacteremia. This seemingly paradoxical development of an OI with rising CD4 cell counts is likely due to an inflammatory response to an OI that was subclinical when HAART was begun.

Just as initial presentations may be altered as the result of HAART, continued disease activity may also be modified. Patients who recover pathogen-specific immunity in addition to the overall increase in CD4 cells may be able to discontinue chronic suppressive (maintenance) therapy, because the patient's immune system is now capable of containing the infection. Thus far this has been best demonstrated for discontinuing chronic suppression for CMV retinitis. However, there is no reason to think that other OIs will behave differently and multiple clinical trials are currently in progress. Last, patients with previously untreatable opportunistic processes, such as PML or cryptosporidiosis, have had clinical remissions after initiating HAART.

A number of studies have shown that patients receiving primary prophylaxis for PCP and MAC are at very low risk of developing these OIs if prophylaxis is withdrawn after total CD4 cell counts have improved above the threshold levels for risk of a specific OI for at least 3-6 months. Most of these studies have been performed among patients with reasonably well-controlled HIV viral loads, with the majority undetectable or at most, less than 10,000 copies. The 1999 revision of the USPHS guidelines on OI prophylaxis describe the data and rationale for discontinuing suppressive therapy and prophylaxis in the appropriate patient. These guidelines are likely to be revised in the near future, so it is wise to check the AIDS Treatment Information Service Web site listed in Chapter XV on Resources.

VI. ALGORITHMS FOR DIAGNOSIS AND MANAGEMENT OF SYMPTOMS

Figure 4-7: Fever of Unknown Origin in Patients with AIDS

Figure 4-8: Acute Diarrhea in Patients with AIDS

Figure 4-9: Chronic Diarrhea (CD4 Count $< 300/mm^3$)

Figure 4-10: Cough, Fever, Dyspnea

Figure 4-11: Headache in Patients with Aids

Figure 4-12: Advanced HIV Infection Plus Altered Status, New Seizures, Headache (Severe or Persistent), or Focal Neurologic Deficits

Figure 4-13: Lower Extremity Symptoms: Weakness and Numbness

Figure 4-14: Lower Extremity Symptoms: Pain

Figure 4-15: Lower Extremity Symptoms: Pain and Numbness

Figure 4-16: Odynophagia in Patients with AIDS

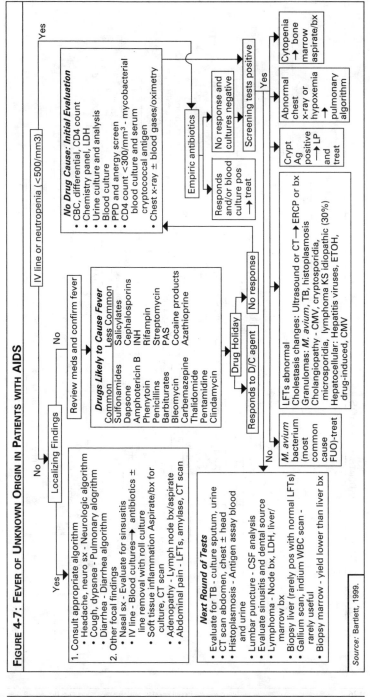

FIGURE 4-7: FEVER OF UNKNOWN ORIGIN IN PATIENTS WITH AIDS

Source: Bartlett, 1999.

IV

FIGURE 4-8: ACUTE DIARRHEA IN PATIENTS WITH AIDS

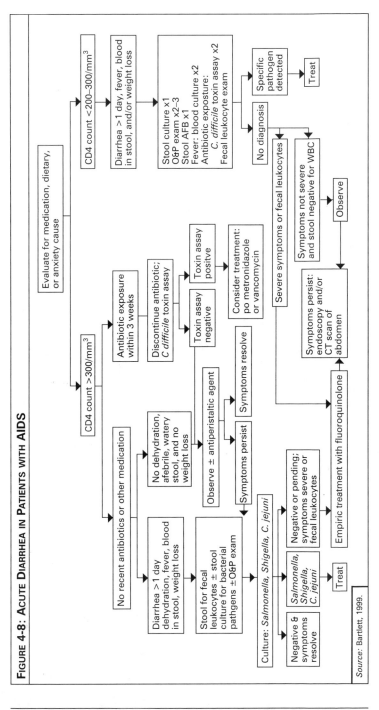

Source: Bartlett, 1999.

IV

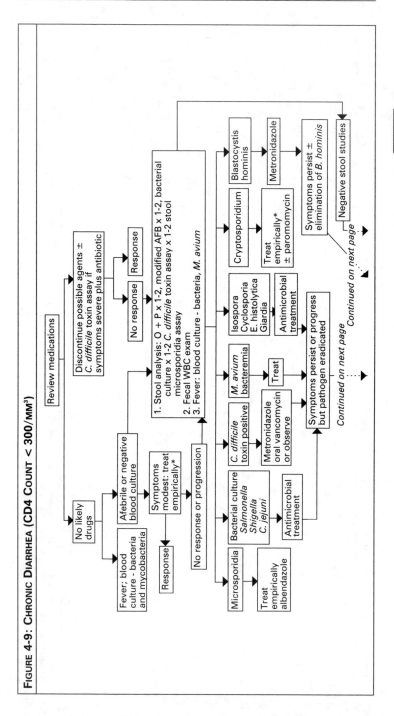

FIGURE 4-9: CHRONIC DIARRHEA (CD4 COUNT < 300/MM³)

Figure 4-9: Chronic Diarrhea (CD4 Count < 300/mm³) *(continued)*

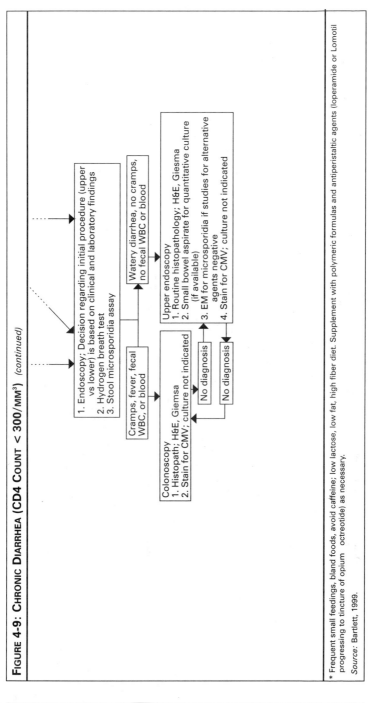

1. Endoscopy; Decision regarding initial procedure (upper vs lower) is based on clinical and laboratory findings
2. Hydrogen breath test
3. Stool microsporidia assay

Cramps, fever, fecal WBC, or blood

Watery diarrhea, no cramps, no fecal WBC or blood

Colonoscopy
1. Histopath; H&E, Giemsa
2. Stain for CMV; culture not indicated

No diagnosis

No diagnosis

Upper endoscopy
1. Routine histopathology; H&E, Giesma
2. Small bowel aspirate for quantitative culture (if available)
3. EM for microsporidia if studies for alternative agents negative
4. Stain for CMV; culture not indicated

* Frequent small feedings, bland foods, avoid caffeine; low lactose, low fat, high fiber diet. Supplement with polymeric formulas and antiperistaltic agents (Ioperamide or Lomotil progressing to tincture of opium octreotide) as necessary.

Source: Bartlett, 1999.

FIGURE 4-10: COUGH, FEVER, DYSPNEA

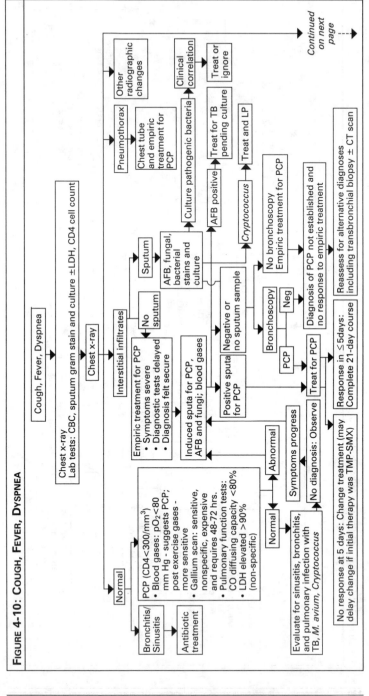

Continued on next page

FIGURE 4-10: COUGH, FEVER, DYSPNEA (continued)

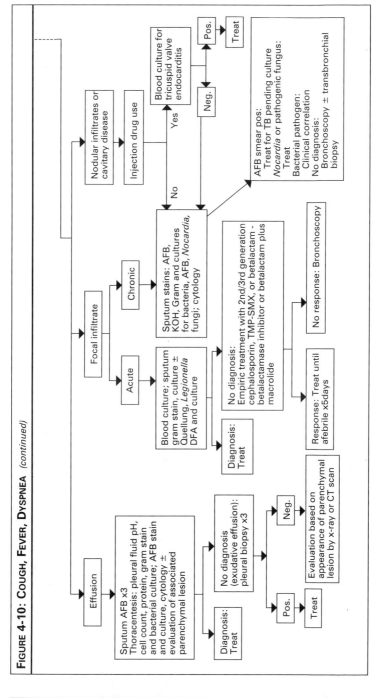

IV

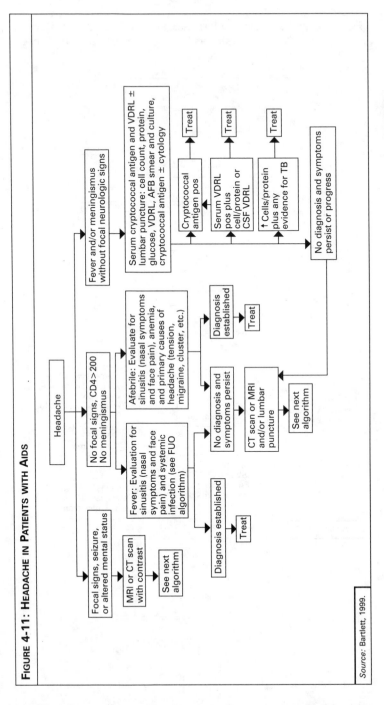

FIGURE 4-11: HEADACHE IN PATIENTS WITH AIDS

Source: Bartlett, 1999.

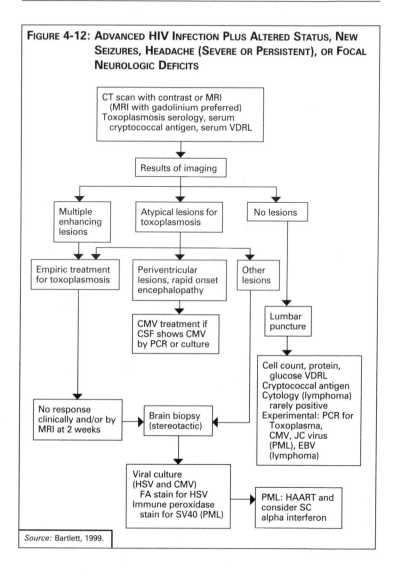

FIGURE 4-12: ADVANCED HIV INFECTION PLUS ALTERED STATUS, NEW SEIZURES, HEADACHE (SEVERE OR PERSISTENT), OR FOCAL NEUROLOGIC DEFICITS

Source: Bartlett, 1999.

IV

FIGURE 4-13: LOWER EXTREMITY SYMPTOMS: WEAKNESS AND NUMBNESS

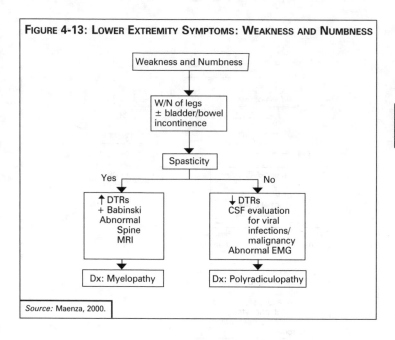

Source: Maenza, 2000.

FIGURE 4-14: LOWER EXTREMITY SYMPTOMS: PAIN

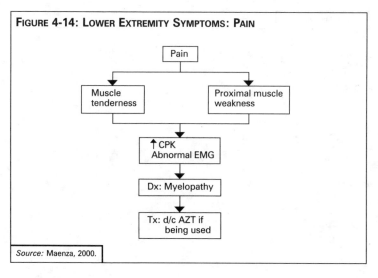

Source: Maenza, 2000.

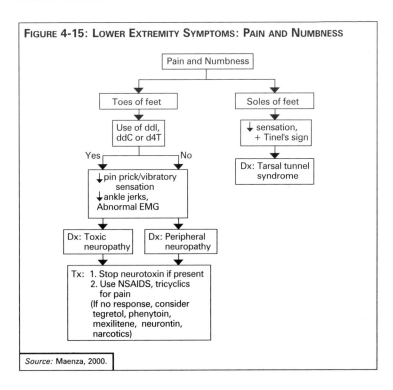

FIGURE 4-15: LOWER EXTREMITY SYMPTOMS: PAIN AND NUMBNESS

Source: Maenza, 2000.

Figure 4-16: Odynophagia in Patients with AIDS

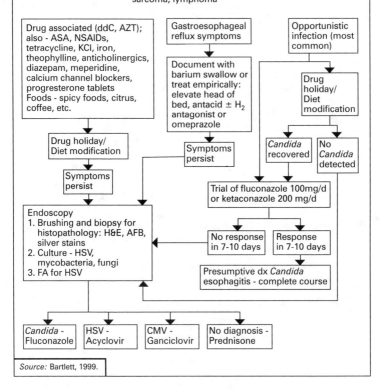

Evaluation

1. Medication or food related

2. Gastroesophageal reflux disease: (heartburn ± regurgitation and dysphagia)

3. Opportunistic infection or tumor

   Common: Candida sp.

   Less common: HSV, CMV, idiopathic (aphthous)

   Rare: TB, *M. avium,* histophasmosis, PCP, cryptosporidia, Kaposi's sarcoma, lymphoma

Drug associated (ddC, AZT); also - ASA, NSAIDs, tetracycline, KCl, iron, theophylline, anticholinergics, diazepam, meperidine, calcium channel blockers, progresterone tablets Foods - spicy foods, citrus, coffee, etc.

Gastroesophageal reflux symptoms

Document with barium swallow or treat empirically: elevate head of bed, antacid ± H$_2$ antagonist or omeprazole

Opportunistic infection (most common)

Drug holiday/ Diet modification

Drug holiday/ Diet modification

Symptoms persist

Candida recovered

No *Candida* detected

Symptoms persist

Endoscopy
1. Brushing and biopsy for histopathology: H&E, AFB, silver stains
2. Culture - HSV, mycobacteria, fungi
3. FA for HSV

Trial of fluconazole 100mg/d or ketaconazole 200 mg/d

No response in 7-10 days

Response in 7-10 days

Presumptive dx *Candida* esophagitis - complete course

Candida - Fluconazole

HSV - Acyclovir

CMV - Ganciclovir

No diagnosis - Prednisone

Source: Bartlett, 1999.

REFERENCES

Bartlett JG. *Medical Management of HIV Infection*. Baltimore, MD: Johns Hopkins University; 1999.

Baxter J, Mayers D, Wentworth D, et al. A pilot study of the short-term effects of antiretroviral management based on plasma genotypic antiretroviral resistance testing in patients failing antiretroviral treatment [LB8]. 6th Conference on Retroviruses and Opportunistic Infections, Chicago, IL, 1999.

Durant J, Clevenbergh P, Halfon P, et al. Drug-resistance genotyping in HIV-1 therapy: the VIRADAPT randomized controlled trial. *Lancet* 353: 2195-9, 1999.

Erbelding Emily J, Resistance Testing: A Primer for Clinicians. *The Hopkins HIV Report*. 11(3):1–12. May 1999.

Fauci A, Pantaleo D, Stanley S, Weismann D. Immunopathogenic mechanisms of HIV infection. *Annals of Internal Medicine* 124: 654-3, 1996.

Hall C, Raines C, Barnett S, Moore R, Gallant J. Efficacy of salvage regimens containing ritonavir and saquinavir after failure of single protease-inhibitor containing regimens. *AIDS* 13: 1207-12, 1999.

Hanson DL, Chusy, Farizo KM, Ward JW, and the Adult and Adolescent Spectrum of HIV Disease Project. Distribution of CD4+T Lymphocytes a+ diagnosis of Acquired Immunodeficiency Syndrome — defining and other Human Immunodeficiency-related Illnesses. *Arch Intern Med* 155:1537, July 24, 1995.

Hirsch MS, Conway B, D'Aquila RT, et al. Antiretroviral drug resistance testing in adults with HIV infection: implications for clinical management. International AIDS Society – USA Panel. *JAMA* 279 (24): 1984-91, 1998.

Ho D, Neumann A, Perelson A, et al. Rapid turnover of plasma virions and CD4 lymphocytes in HIV-1 infection. *Nature* 373:123-6, 1995.

Imam N, Carpenter CC, Mayer KH, Fisher A, Stein M, Danforth SB. Hierarchical pattern of mucosal candida infections in HIV-seropositive women. *Am J Med* 89(2): 142-6, 1990.

Kitahata MM, Koepsell TD, Deyo RA, Maxwell CL, Dodge WT, Wagner EH. Physicians' experience with the acquired immunodeficiency syndrome as a factor in patients' survival. *N Engl J Med* 334: 701-6,1996.

Mellors JW, Rinaldo CR, Gupta P, White RM, Todd JA, Kingsley LA. Prognosis in HIV-1 infection predicted by the quantity of virus in plasma. *Science* 272:1167–1170, 1996.

Quinn TC, Mawer MJ, Sewankambo N, et al. Viral load and heterosexual transmission of human immunodeficiency virus type 1. *N Engl J Med* 342: 921-9, 2000.

Rich JD, Merriman NA, Mylonakis SE, Greenough T, Flanigan T, Mady B, Carpenter CCJ. Misdiagnosis of HIV infection by HIV-1 plasma viral load testing: A case series. Ann *Int Med* 130 (1): 37-9, 1999.

Raboud J, Montaner J, Conway B, et al. Suppression of plasma viral load below 20 copies/ml is required to achieve a long term response to therapy. *AIDS* 12:1619-24, 1998.

Tebas P, Patrick A, Kane E, et al. Virologic responses to a ritonavir-saquinavir containing regimen in patients who have previously failed nelfinavir. *AIDS* 13: F23-8, 1999.

U.S. Department of Health and Human Services, *Guidelines for the Use of Antiretroviral Agents in HIV-Infected Adults and Adolescents,* January, 2000.

USPHS/ISDA Guidelines for the prevention of opportunistic infections in persons infected with human immunodeficiency virus. *MMWR* 1999; 48:1–67.

V. ADHERENCE TO HIV THERAPIES
Laura W. Cheever, M.D.

I. INTRODUCTION

Adherence to HIV therapies is critical if patients are to achieve and maintain undetectable viral loads and avoid preventable opportunistic infections. Initial clinical trials of highly active antiretroviral therapy demonstrated that 80–90% of patients receiving protease inhibitor therapy could achieve viral loads < 400 copies/ml. (Gulick, 1997) However, currently in real world clinical practice only 50% of patients achieve this goal. (Deeks, 1997; Lucas, 1999) The primary reason is nonadherence with therapy. Adherence with medications in any chronic disease is a challenge for most patients. As a general rule, only 50% of patients with chronic illnesses maintain "good adherence" (taking > 80% of medication doses) over time. Patients with HIV infection have similar rates of adherence. Unfortunately in this infection, "good adherence" is not good enough, and the consequences of nonadherence are severe.

This chapter addresses the important issues regarding adherence with HIV medications. Beyond this specific issue, there are other aspects of adherence with medical care, including adherence with recommendations for laboratory monitoring for toxicity and clinical response and adherence with appointment keeping, that are also critical factors in successful HIV treatment.

II. THE UNFORGIVING NATURE OF HIV AND THE MEDICATIONS TO TREAT IT

Adherence with medications is critical in HIV infections for several reasons involving both the nature of the virus and the drugs to combat it. First, the virus has a very high replication and mutation rate. If drug doses are intermittently missed, the virus quickly begins to replicate. In the presence of low levels of drug, viral mutations that confer drug resistance will thrive. Second, the most potent drugs, both protease inhibitors and nonnucleoside reverse transcriptase inhibitors, have broad class resistance. That is, when resistance to one drug in the class occurs, often resistance has developed to all the drugs in that class. Thus, nonadherence to one regimen can result in virus resistant to many antiretrovirals.

Finally, a patient needs to have near perfect adherence, as shown in Figure 5-1, to achieve an undetectable viral load necessary to prevent the develop-

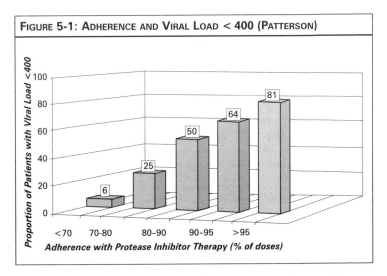

FIGURE 5-1: ADHERENCE AND VIRAL LOAD < 400 (PATTERSON)

ment of resistant virus. (Patterson, 1999) For most chronic diseases, 80% adherence is considered "good adherence." However, only 50% of patients achieved undetectable viral load with this level of adherence.

Thus, in HIV infection, patients must have exceptionally high levels of adherence to therapy to prevent the emergence of resistant virus. Additionally, unlike other chronic diseases, such as hypertension, if HIV-infected patients are nonadherent, even for a few weeks, they may severely limit their future treatment options due to broad class resistance.

III. PREDICTORS OF ADHERENCE

Adherence is a complex behavior. In analyzing predictors of adherence, it is important to consider factors related to the patient, the treatment regimen, the doctor-patient relationship, and the system of medical care. There are several patient related factors that are consistently predictive of adherence or nonadherence among HIV infected individuals. Depression and active substance abuse (including alcohol, cocaine, or heroin) correlate with nonadherence, whereas the patient's belief that they can both make HIV medication regimens fit into their life and be adherent with the regimen is predictive of adherence. (Table 5-1, Cheever, 1999) In addition, one of the best predictors of adherence is adherence with previous therapy.

In most chronic diseases, demographic characteristics, such as sex, race, income, education, and age are not predictive of adherence. (Haynes, 1979) However, in the initial studies of these factors of HIV-infected patients, the data are inconclusive. In the HIV Cost and Services Utilization Study (HCSUS), a national probability sample survey, the investigators found that

TABLE 5-1: PATIENT FACTORS ASSOCIATED WITH NON-ADHERENCE

STRONGLY ASSOCIATED

- Depression
- Alcohol/substance abuse
- Self Efficacy (Belief in one's ability to take medication as instructed)
- Belief medications can be fit into their day
- Understanding the relationship of viral resistance and adherence
- Previous adherence

INCONSISTENTLY ASSOCIATED

- Sex (F < M)*
- Race (AA < W)
- Age (younger < older)
- Stage of disease (Patients with higher CD4 < Patients with lower CD4)

NOT GENERALLY ASSOCIATED

- Education, Income, Employment
- HIV Risk Factor
- Belief that medications will improve health or cause symptoms

* In studies where an association is found, females are less adherent than males.

women, African Americans, Hispanics, younger adults, and patients with higher CD4 counts reported lower rates of adherence. (Wegner, 1999) Other studies report conflicting results, and the relationship between these demographic variables and adherence needs further exploration.

In terms of the treatment regimen, adherence decreases as the number of doses per day, pills, or medications increase. Likewise, medications with food restrictions are harder to take as directed. Length of time on therapy also impacts medication adherence. Adherence tends to wane over time, which is a compelling reason to delay therapy until the risk of progression to AIDS is significant. Pharmacy and social work counseling of patients whenever HAART is initiated or the regimen is changed can be helpful in ensuring that patients understand dosing and side effects and can assist in developing strategies to avoid missing doses.

The doctor-patient relationship is also an important variable in adherence and should not be overlooked. Several studies have shown that patients who trust their doctor are more likely to adhere to therapy, including one new study among HIV-infected patients. (Kaplan, 1999) Most medical providers believe that they can predict which patient will be able to adhere to a medical regimen. However, studies have repeatedly shown that physicians, nurse practitioners, and nurses *cannot predict* with reliability which patients will adhere to therapy.(Patterson, 1999) Table 5-2 lists the most common reason patients say they miss their medication.(Eldred, 1998; Chesney, 1997) These reasons vary significantly from the reasons that providers site as reasons their patients miss doses. (Gallant, 1998)

TABLE 5-2: Reasons Patients Cite for Missing Medication
■ Did not have medication at the time of the dose
■ Simply "forgot" to take it
■ Asleep at time of dose
■ Too busy at the time
■ Off usual daily schedule/routine
■ Ran out of medication
■ Using drugs/alcohol
■ Pills to difficult to take (too many, too big, schedule to complicated)
■ Didn't want to be reminded of HIV/AIDS
■ Didn't want to take pills in front of others

The system of care can impact adherence to a medication regimen. Situations that facilitate patients' access to medication, in terms of refill requests, reminders to refill medication, and mechanisms to obtain medications when gaps in medication insurance occur, can significantly impact a patient's ability to adhere. Similarly, systems that help patients overcome barriers to seeking medical care, including problems with transportation, childcare, and paying for services, also assist in the patient's adhere efforts. Finally, patient education is a critical part of improving adherence. Within the system of care, personnel and resources need to be dedicated to this important endeavor.

IV. ADHERENCE IN SPECIAL POPULATIONS

A. INCARCERATED PATIENTS

Incarcerated patients have unique challenges to medication adherence. Medical regulations vary significantly among correctional systems, and these regulations influence patients' medication adherence. Correctional institutions may provide directly observed therapy of each dose of medication which may result in excellent medication adherence. On the other hand, lockdowns and other security concerns supercede medical concerns and may result in missed doses. In correctional systems where HIV-infected inmates are identified and called by name to receive medications, many patients forego treatment rather than risk disclosure of their HIV infection. Additionally, the incarceration process itself provides many opportunities for potential disruption in access to medications. Most patients do not immediately access their antiretroviral medication on entry to the system or at times of transfer within the system. When patients are discharged from the penal system, they are provided with a limited supply of medication; often patients run out of medication prior to establishing medical care in their communities, resulting in nonadherence with their regimen.

B. HOMELESS PATIENTS

It is often assumed that homeless patients face insurmountable barriers to adherence with medications. Certainly, homelessness itself creates many challenges to adherence. Additionally, many homeless patients have mental illness or substance abuse that may further contribute to non-adherence. However, patients with homelessness can be successful in taking HAART. In a study of homeless and marginally housed patients from San Francisco, 38% of the 32 homeless patients taking protease inhibitors had high levels of adherence. (Bangsberg, 1999) However, the group appears to be highly selected since only 34 of 153 patients in this marginally housed cohort were prescribed HAART.

C. CHILDREN AND ADOLESCENTS

Young children are dependent on the adults around them for their medication adherence. As with many HIV-infected adults, HIV-infected children may be in tenuous social situations due to poverty and unstable housing, in addition to illness among their parents. In addition, many children are unable or unwilling to swallow unpalatable medication or pills, making dosing administration take hours each day. In one study, children with extreme problems around medication taking had gastric tubes placed with improvement in adherence, viral load, time necessary to administer doses, and interpersonal relationships with the persons administering the medication. (Shingadia, 1999) Adolescents who have not disclosed their HIV status may miss doses because of lack of a private place to take their medication. Furthermore, adolescence is a time of testing limits and feelings of invulnerability, both of which may contribute to the likelihood of nonadherence.

V. MEASURING ADHERENCE

There are many methods to measure adherence including electronic devises, pill counts, and drug assays. However, in clinical practice, the most efficient method to measure adherence is simply to ask the patient. (Icovicks, 1997) When asked in a nonjudgmental way, most patients (80% in several studies) are truthful about their medication taking. (Sackett, 1976) To get the most reliable information, patients should be given permission to have missed doses, asked in a nonjudgmental way, and given a specific time frame. For example, *"Everyone misses doses some of the time. In the last 2 weeks, how many doses have you missed?"*

Pharmacy records can also give important information regarding adherence when available to the clinical staff. Serum drug levels are now commercially available. These are most useful when patients professing adherence are not responding well to therapy; however, low drug levels may also be due to poor absorption or drug-drug interactions as well as to nonadherence.

VI. IMPROVING ADHERENCE

Given the importance of adherence in HIV infection and the relatively low rates of adherence in any chronic disease, it is of utmost importance to support efforts to increase patient adherence. Although there is little information specific to HIV infected individuals, many interventions have been shown to increase adherence with pill taking in chronic disease. Most interventions only have a modest effect on adherence. Those that work best are **multifaceted** (working on more than one aspect of the pill taking behavior) and **repetitive** (having the intervention reapplied over time). (Haynes, 1996; Roter, 1998) Also with antiretroviral medication, it is critical to start the intervention before non-adherence, and viral resistance, have occurred.

In initiating a successful regimen, the most important thing to consider is whether the patient is ready to start antiretroviral therapy. The patient is usually the best judge of when to start therapy as long as they are well informed regarding the rigors of antiretroviral therapy and the consequences of nonad-herence. Thus, a majority of patient education efforts should be made prior to initiation of therapy. Given that the patient's "first shot [of antiretrovirals] is the best shot," most patients benefit in the long run by delaying therapy if they are not ready to start. The urgency of therapy increases as the CD4 count falls and the viral load increases. Many physicians feel pressured by practice guide-lines for starting therapy. *The best time to start therapy is when the patient is ready.*

There are, however, a few "antiretroviral emergencies," pregnancy being one of them. Clearly, for the pregnant woman, the cost benefit considerations are different, as outlined in Chapter VII on HIV and Reproduction. In the case of pregnant women, the time permitted for the patient to prepare to start therapy is considerably compressed. Thus, even more intensive educational efforts are needed in this population.

Patient education is clearly important, with high returns on the investment made prior to starting therpy. Group education generally works better than one on one education, probably because of the support and practical peer advice that is shared. (Roter, 1998) Many patients resist groups, but many find them beneficial if they can be convinced to go. Specific interventions to improve adherence are outlined in Table 5-3.

Two controlled intervention trials to improve adherence in the HIV-infected population have been presented. In a pharmacy based trial from Spain, patients starting highly active therapy received education detailing the importance of treatment, adherence, and side effects management. (Knobel, 1998) They were engaged in tailoring the medication into their daily schedule and given a tele-phone number to call with problems. In follow up phone calls, the importance of adherence was stressed, and patients were engaged in problem solving around missed doses. At 48 weeks, in the intervention arm, 77% of patients were adherent with medication, compared with 52% in the control arm.

In a second controlled interventional trial, a nurse based intervention to improve adherence with PCP prophylaxis was also reported to be successful. (Cheever, 1998) Patients in the intervention group received a 10 minute nurse-

TABLE 5-3: INTERVENTIONS TO IMPROVE ADHERENCE

INTERVENTION	COMMENTS
THE PATIENT	
Start when the patient is ready	■ For pregnant women, the cost-benefit analysis of treatment is different.
Treat substance abuse and depression prior to initiating antiviral therapy	■ If there is no antiretroviral emergency, patients with active substance abuse and depression should have these comorbidities addressed prior to initiation of antiretrovirals.
Engage the patient in medication tailoring	■ Discuss with the patient in detail how the medications will fit into their daily routine- i.e. when (and if) meals are eaten, what the patient does on a daily basis that can be linked to dosing times.
Educate (group/individual) regarding: ■ The regimen ■ Side effects management ■ Consequences of nonadherence	■ Patient education is essential- both group and one-on-one education. ■ Involve caretakers and patient support network in educational efforts. ■ Patients need to know exactly how to take their medication. A daily calendar with pills on it will help a patient to visualize the regimen. ■ Prior to initiating therapy, patients should know which side effects to expect, what they can to do to manage them, and when to call the medical practice. ■ Patients need to understand the serious consequences of nonadherence and what to do in the event of a late or missed dose.
Increase support	■ Patients should enlist the aid of family and friends to promote their adherence. The HIV health care team staff can provide support through office visits, home visits, and telephone calls, especially in the first days and weeks of antiretroviral therapy.
Use skill building excercises	■ Have the patient use a trial of jellybeans in a pill box to accustom themselves to their pill taking schedule prior to initiating therapy.
Address barriers to adherence	■ Have the patient consider when medications are likely to be missed and make plans to decrease these events. ■ Some patients store a few doses in places where they spend a lot of time, such as at the houses of friends and relatives.
Use reminders	■ Alarm clocks, in the form of watch alarms or pill boxes, can decrease missed doses due to simply forgetting. ■ Patients can place medications in locations they will notice them at dosing times, such on the breakfast table.
THE REGIMEN	
Simplify as much as possible	■ Once or twice daily regimens are easiest for patients. ■ Use as few pills and medications as possible. ■ Try to use regimens than can be taken without regard to food intake.
Tailor the regimen to the patient's lifestyle (and not the patient's lifestyle to the regimen).	■ Ask the patient about her daily routine, comfort in taking medications in front of others and at work. ■ Construct a regimen that works for the patient.

Table continues . . .

TABLE 5-3: INTERVENTIONS TO IMPROVE ADHERENCE *(continued)*	
INTERVENTION	**COMMENTS**
THE REGIMEN *(continued)*	
Use pill boxes	■ Use of pill boxes allows the patient a mechanism to carry her daily medication. ■ Pill boxes allow for patients to easily recognize when they have missed a dose.
Make refills accessible	■ Develop policies to allow patients ready access to refills.
THE DOCTOR-PATIENT RELATIONSHIP	
Develop a trusting relationship	■ Rarely is initiation of antiretrovirals required at the first visit. Invest in the doctor-patient relationship prior to initiating therapy.
Ask about adherence	■ Medical providers cannot predict adherence- you must ask the patient. ■ Ask in a nonjudgmental way, with a specific time frame, to get good information. ■ Give permission for missed doses prior to asking. ■ Ask repetitively over time.
Use positive reinforcement	■ Share viral load and CD4 results and reinforce the relationship to adherence.
Listen to the patient	■ Individualize therapy based on patient preferences regarding fear of specific side effects or specific medication. Negotiate the regimen with the patient.
THE SYSTEM OF CARE	
Maintain close follow up at initiation of regimen.	■ Have telephone, office, or home contact with patient within first few days of therapy to assess for side effects and accurate understanding of regimen.
Develop patient education program	■ Consider use of nurses, case managers, pharmacists, and peers in patient education. ■ Have written materials accessible.
Incorporate the adherence message throughout the medical practice	■ All staff members need to understand and promote the importance of adherence. ■ Have pill boxes, alarms and other adherence aids available to patients.
Source: Adapted from Cheever 1999.	

based exit interview at the end of each regular clinic visit. During the exit interview, the nurse discussed the importance of PCP prophylaxis, stressed the importance of adherence, and engaged the patient in medication tailoring. Median adherence in the intervention group was 78%, 16% better than among the control group. More randomized trials are needed to define which interventions work best to improve adherence, and many are underway.

VII. CONCLUSION

Adherence with medications is critical in HIV infection. Whenever medications are prescribed, special emphasis needs to be placed on patient readiness and adherence. Many types of interventions can improve adherence, and it is vital that these are employed to give patients the best chance at an optimal response to HIV therapies.

REFERENCES

Bangsberg DR, Hecht FM, Charlebois EC, et al. Spontaneous adherence (ADH) audits (SAA) predict viral suppression in the REACH cohort. Program and Abstracts of the 6th Conference on Retroviruses and Opportunistic Infections, Chicago. Abstract 93, 1999.

Cheever LW, Barnes GL, Chaisson RE. A randomized educational intervention to improve adherence with medication. Abstracts of the 38th Interscience Conference on Antimicrobial Agents and Chemotherapy, San Diego, Abstract I-178, 1998.

Cheever LW, Wu AW. Medication adherence among HIV infected patients: understanding the complex behavior of taking this complex therapy. Current Infectious Diseases Report 1: 401–407, 1999.

Chesney MA. New antiretroviral therapies: adherence challenges and strategies. Abstracts of the 37th Interscience Conference on Antimicrobial Agents and Chemotherapy, Toronto, Canada. Evolving HIV treatments: advances and the challenge of adherence symposium. 1997.

Deeks S, Loftus R, Cohen P, et al: Incidence and predictors of virologic failure to indinavir (IDV) and/or ritonavir (RTV) in an urban health clinic. Abstracts of the 37th Interscience Conference on Antimicrobial Agents and Chemotherapy, Toronto, Canada, Abstract LB-2, 1997.

Eldred LJ, Wu AW, Chaisson RE, et al. Adherence to antiretroviral and pneumocystis prophylaxis in HIV disease. J *Acquir Immune Defic Syndr Hum Retrovirol* 18:117–125, 1998.

Gallant JE, Block DS. Adherence to antiretroviral regimens in HIV-infected patients: results of a survey among physicians and patients. *Journal of the International Association of Physicians in AIDS Care,* 1998.

Gulick RM, Mellors JW, Havlir D, et al. Treatment with indinavir, zidovudine, and lamivudine in adults with human immunodeficiency virus infection and prior antiretroviral therapy. *N Engl J Med* 337: 734–739, 1997.

Haynes RB. Determinants of compliance: the disease and the mechanics of treatment. In *Compliance in Health Care.* Edited by Haynes RB, Sackett DL. Baltimore: Johns Hopkins University Press 49–62, 1979

Haynes RB, McKibbon KA, Kanani R. Systematic review of randomized trials of interventions to assist patients to follow prescriptions for medications. *Lancet* 348:383–86, 1996.

Icovicks J. Behavioral measures. Adherence to New HIV Therapies: a Research Conference. Washington, D.C. NIH Office of AIDS Research 15–18, 1997.

Kaplan A, Golin C, Beck K, et al. Adherence to protease inhibitor therapy and viral load. Program and Abstracts of the 6th Conference on Retroviruses and Opportunistic Infections, Chicago. Abstract 96, 1999.

Knobel H, Carmona A, Grau S, et al. Strategies to optimise adherence to highly active antiretroviral treatment. Program and abstracts of the 12th World AIDS Conference, Geneva, Switzerland. Abstract 338/32322, 1998.

Lucas GM, Chaisson RE, Moore RD. Highly active antiretroviral therapy in a large urban clinic: risk factors for virologic failure and adverse drug reactions *Ann Intern Med* 131:81– 87, 1999.

Patterson D, Swindells S, Mohr J, et al. How much adherence is enough: a prospective study of adherence to protease inhibitor therapy using MEMS Caps. Program and Abstracts of the 6th Conference on Retroviruses and Opportunistic Infections, Chicago. Abstract 092, 1999.

Roter DL, Hall JA, Merisca R, et al. Effectiveness of interventions to improve patient compliance a meta-analysis. *Medical Care* 36:1138–1161, 1998.

Sackett DL, Haynes RB, Gibson ES, et al. Randomized clinical trial of strategies for improving medication compliance in primary hypertension. *Lancet* 1:1265–68, 1976

Shingadia D, Viani R, Dankner W, et al. Gastrostomy tube for improvement of adherence with HAART in pediatric HIV patients. Program and Abstracts of the 6th Conference on Retroviruses and Opportunistic Infections, Chicago. Abstract 436, 1999.

Wenger N, Gifford A, Liu H, et al. Patient characteristics and attitudes associated with antiretroviral (AR) adherence. Program and Abstracts of the 6th Conference on Retroviruses and Opportunistic Infections, Chicago. Abstract 98, 1999.

VI. GYNECOLOGIC PROBLEMS

Silvia Abularach, MD, MPH and Jean Anderson, MD

I. INTRODUCTION

Gynecologic problems are common among HIV-positive women and are frequently present at the time of initial presentation for evaluation and care. Minkoff et al found that 46.9% of 262 HIV-infected women had a least one incident gynecologic condition with serial assessment.(Minkoff, 1999) In a study of women admitted to an inpatient AIDS service, although only 9% were admitted with a primary gynecologic (gyn) problem, 83% had coexisting gynecologic disease when evaluated. (Frankel, 1997) Some gynecologic issues are unrelated to the patients' serologic status, whereas others are directly related to HIV disease and associated immunosuppression. Still others are associated epidemiologically with HIV because of common risk factors, such as sexual behavior or substance abuse.

From July 1998 to June 1999, women accounted for 23% of the adult AIDS cases and 32% of the adult cases of HIV infection reported in the United States. (CDC, 1999) Moreover, women have had the greatest increase in AIDS incidence in recent years when compared with other U.S. population groups . With this background and the fact that HIV infection primarily affects women during their reproductive years, gynecologic and reproductive health care will play an increasingly important role in the overall care of the HIV-infected woman. With improved longevity and quality of life, gynecologic problems will be encountered more commonly or may be more prominent. With these issues in mind, the goal of this chapter is to use a problem-oriented approach in reviewing the most common gynecologic complaints together with their differential diagnosis, evaluation, management, and relationship to HIV.

II. ABNORMAL UTERINE BLEEDING/AMENORRHEA

A. WHAT IS CONSIDERED "ABNORMAL" BLEEDING?

A normal menstrual period should occur every 21 to 35 days and last between 2 and 6 days. The average blood loss during menses is 20 to 60 ml., but up to 14% of healthy women have blood loss greater than 80 ml and are more likely to be anemic because of this. (Mishell, 1997)

Amenorrhea represents a sort of abnormal bleeding in that it is the lack of menstruation. Primary amenorrhea is defined as the absence of menses by age 16. Secondary amenorrhea is the absence of menses for a variable period of time, for at least 3 months and usually six months or longer, in a woman who has previously menstruated.

B. RELATIONSHIP TO HIV DISEASE

Menstrual disorders are frequently reported by HIV-positive women. However, controlled studies have yielded conflicting evidence regarding whether HIV or HIV-related immunosuppression exerts a clinically significant direct effect on these reported disturbances (Shah, 1994; Ellerbrock, 1996; Chirgwin, 1996) and more definitive studies are needed.

In the setting of HIV infection menstrual disorders may be related to confounding variables, such as weight loss, chronic disease, substance abuse, and progestational agents used for appetite stimulation or contraception. The impact of antiretroviral therapy on menstruation has not been well studied but hypermenorrhea, or excessive menstrual blood loss, has been reported with ritonavir. (Nielsen, 1999) The effect of HIV-RNA levels on menstrual function is unknown.

C. HISTORY

■ **Characteristics of bleeding:** date of last menstrual period, duration and frequency of menses, amount of bleeding (number of pads/tampons used per day); presence of clots or associated pain/cramping; duration of menstrual irregularities or amenorrhea; presence of intermenstrual or postcoital bleeding

■ **Other bleeding sources:** gastrointestinal (GI) or bleeding from the urinary tract versus a gyn source); history of easy bruising, nose or gum bleeds

■ **History of gynecologic problems/other symptoms:** abnormal Pap smears; uterine fibroids or polyps; prior ectopic pregnancy; abnormal vaginal discharge

■ **Medical history:** timing of diagnosis of HIV disease/AIDS and existing comorbid conditions; clinical symptoms of HIV; CD4 count and viral load; history of platelet disorders (thrombocytopenia is frequently diagnosed in HIV infection, particularly in individuals with more advanced stages of disease (Sloand, 1992); medications; history of substance abuse

■ **Sexual history:** last sexual intercourse and use of contraception and condoms

D. PHYSICAL EXAM

A careful and comprehensive abdominal and pelvic examination should be performed. The presence of abdominal tenderness or mass should be noted.

The external genitalia, vagina, and cervix should be inspected for evidence of actively bleeding lesions (e.g., lacerations, condylomata, polyps) or inflammation. A bimanual and rectovaginal examination assess the presence of pelvic tenderness, enlarged uterus or other pelvic mass.

E. DIFFERENTIAL DIAGNOSIS

■ **Pregnancy.** Pregnancy must be considered in any woman of reproductive age with irregular bleeding or amenorrhea. Pregnancy may be either intrauterine or ectopic (usually tubal); bleeding with an intrauterine pregnancy may indicate threatened or incomplete abortion or miscarriage or a serious obstetrical complication in later pregnancy.

■ **Anovulation.** Anovulation is the most common cause of abnormal uterine bleeding among reproductive-aged women. Typically, the woman has a history of menstrual irregularity and may go several months with no bleeding, followed by the onset of prolonged and heavy bleeding. Anovulatory bleeding is a diagnosis of exclusion and organic, systemic, and iatrogenic causes of bleeding must be ruled out. Anovulation and oligoovulation are more common among perimenopausal women and adolescents soon after menarche.

■ **Perimenopause.** In addition to anovulation/oligoovulation, women in the perimenopause may have irregular bleeding because of declining estrogen levels.

■ **Uterine fibroids.** Fibroids are common benign uterine tumors that are most often asymptomatic, but may cause heavy and/or prolonged periods.

■ **Cancer.** Malignant processes in every part of the female genital tract (vulva, vagina, cervix, uterus, fallopian tubes, and ovaries) can potentially present with abnormal bleeding; most common in postmenopausal women.

■ **Genital Tract Infections.** Cervicitis, vaginitis, endometritis, vulvitis, and pelvic inflammatory disease may present with abnormal vaginal bleeding or spotting. Associated symptoms, including pain/tenderness, discharge, fever, and other signs and symptoms of infection, will aid in making the diagnosis. In very immunosuppressed patients, consider opportunistic processes, including tuberculous or CMV endometritis.

■ **Medical conditions.** Thyroid disorders (hypothyroidism or hyperthyroidism), coagulopathy (including platelet disorders), cirrhosis, chronic illness/wasting.

■ **Substance abuse.** Drug use (including methadone) can lead to disturbances of the hyptothalamic-pituitary axis, with resulting irregular bleeding or amenorrhea.

■ **Medications.** Progestational agents, such as those used for contraception (e.g., Depo Provera, Norplant) or for appetite stimulation (e.g., Megace) frequently cause irregular vaginal bleeding. Consider antiretroviral agents as a potential cause of abnormal bleeding. Medications which can affect pro-lactin concentrations and possibly result in amenorrhea include psy-chotropic drugs (tricyclic antidepressants, pheothiazines, opiates) and metoclopramide.

F. EVALUATION

The basic evaluation includes the following:

- **Pregnancy test** (urine or serum): perform on all women with abnormal bleeding/amenorrhea within reproductive age range
- **Laboratory tests**:
    1. **CBC, platelet count**
    2. **Thyroid stimulating hormone (TSH), prolactin levels** — consider with any irregular bleeding/amenorrhea without apparent cause
    3. **Follicle stimulating hormone (FSH), estradiol** — with oligomenorrhea/amenorrhea and/or signs/symptoms of decreased estrogen production (hot flashes, vaginal atrophic changes). These tests are particularly helpful in distinguishing ovarian failure (low estradiol, high FSH) and hypothalamic amen-orrhea (e.g., with wasting) (low estradiol, low/normal FSH)
    4. **Coagulation profile** — if evidence of systemic bleeding, to rule out coagulopathy
- **Cervical testing** for gonorrhea and chlamydia
- **Pelvic ultrasound:** with abnormal exam (uterine enlargement, adnexal mass, significant tenderness)or positive pregnancy test
- **Endometrial biopsy:** indicated with postmenopausal bleeding, pro-longed amenorrhea followed by onset of irregular or heavy bleeding, per-sistently irregular bleeding. It is helpful in diagnosing endometritis, endometrial hyperplasia, and uterine cancer; endometrial tissue necessary to diagnose CMV or TB endometritis-alert your pathologist if these are considerations
- **Pap smear:** do not perform with active bleeding; if cervical lesion seen, biopsy is required.

Further evaluation or referral is indicated based on results of these tests, severity of the problem, and response to basic management.

G. MANAGEMENT

Management depends on the diagnosis and results of testing. All women with a positive pregnancy test require referral to a specialist. If anovulatory bleed-ing is suspected, medical management may be attempted with oral contracep-tive pills (OCPs) or cyclic progestins (medroxyprogesterone acetate 10 mg po QD for 10–14 days each month); these therapies help restore regular menstruation; reduce possible anemia; and protect the endometrium from prolonged estrogenic stimulation, which can cause hyperplasia or neoplasia. OCPs will also provide effective contraception, but are contraindicated in heavy smokers over the age of 35, with hypertension or other cardiovascular disease, and in diabetics and women with markedly abnormal liver function.

With severe bleeding and anemia, pelvic mass, findings suspicious for malignancy, or bleeding that is not resolved with conservative measures, referral is indicated.

III. ABNORMAL PAP SMEAR

In the setting of HIV infection 30–60% of pap smears exhibit cytologic abnormalities and 15–40% have evidence of dysplasia; these rates are ten to eleven times greater than those observed among HIV-negative women. (Maiman, 1998)

A. INTERRELATIONSHIP OF HIV AND HUMAN PAPILLO-MAVIRUS (HPV)

■ Human Papillomavirus (HPV) infection plays a causative role in genital intraepithelial and invasive neoplasia. The spectrum of HPV disease includes subclinical disease, classic genital warts and other HPV-related skin lesions, lower genital tract intraepithelial neoplasia, and invasive cancers of the lower genital tract. There are over 70 HPV subtypes, which are divided into low, intermediate or high risk, based on oncogenic potential; nevertheless, numerous exceptions exist and "low-risk" HPV types have been described in cervical carcinomas.

■ HPV is an extremely common infection; current evidence suggests that over 50% of sexually active adults have been infected with one or more genital HPV types, but most HPV infections are transient. (Evander, 1995; Ho, 1998) Studies have shown that HIV-infected women have higher prevalence of HPV (Sun, 1997; Shah, 1996; Palefsky, 1999; Minkoff, 1998); longer persistence of HPV (Sun, 1997); higher likelihood of multiple HPV subtypes (Brown, 1994); and greater prevalence of oncogenic subtypes (Minkoff, 1998; Uberti-Foppa, 1998) than in HIV-uninfected women.

■ In HIV-positive women the prevalence and persistence of HPV infection increases with decreasing CD4 count and increasing HIV RNA levels (Palefsky, 1999) and some studies show that oncogenic HPV types may be more common with lower CD4 counts and/or higher viral loads. (Minkoff, 1998; Luque, 1999)

■ Sun et al (Sun, 1995) have suggested that the presence of immunosuppression shifts the ratio of latent:clinically expressed HPV infections from 8:1 in the general population to 3:1 in HIV-positive women with CD4 > 500/mm^3 to 1:1 in HIV-positive women with CD4 < 200/mm^3.

B. HIV AND CERVICAL DYSPLASIA

■ Abnormal cervical cytology is more common among HIV-infected women and is associated with the presence of HPV infection and the degree of immunesuppression . Both frequency and severity of abnormal pap smears and histologically documented dysplasia increase with declining CD4 counts and have also been associated with higher HIV-RNA levels. (Shah, 1996; Garzetti, 1995)

■ In HIV-positive women dyspasia is associated with more extensive cervical involvement, and is more likely to involve other sites in the lower genital tract, such as the vagina, vulva, and perianal region (Maiman, 1990; Petry, 1996; Korn, 1995; Williams, 1994; Hillemans, 1996) as compared to HIV-negative women.

■ Recent studies have shown increased incidence of oncogenic HPV types (Minkoff, 1998) and increased incidence of biopsy proven cervical dysplasia (Ellerbrock, 2000) in HIV-positive women compared to HIV-negative controls. A French study found an increased likelihood of progression of cervical abnormalities in HIV-positive women, although analysis was based on pap smear results only. (Six, 1998) At the current time there is little evidence for increased rates of progression to invasive cancer, particularly if adequate screening and treatment programs are in place.

C. INVASIVE CERVICAL CANCER IN HIV DISEASE

■ In 1993, the CDC expanded the case definition of AIDS to include invasive cervical cancer.

■ There is little evidence to date that HIV infection is having a significant impact on cervical cancer rates. However, a review of New York City AIDS surveillance data 1990–1995 found that the observed cervical cancer cases were 2–3x higher than the expected number of cases. (Chiasson, 1997) One study reported a higher prevalence of invasive cervical cancer in HIV-positive as compared to HIV-negative hospitalized patients, particularly among those aged 20 to 34 and among African-American and Hispanic women. (Weber, 1998) Women with HIV and cervical cancer tend to be younger and less immunosuppressed as compared to HIV-positive women with other AIDS-indicator conditions.

■ HIV-positive women with invasive cervical cancer appear to present at more advanced stages, may metastasize to unusual locations (e.g. psoas muscle, clitoris, meningeal involvement), have poorer responses to standard therapy, and have higher recurrences and death rates, as well as shorter intervals to recurrence or death, as compared to HIV-negative women of similar stage. (Maiman, 1990; Klevens, 1996)

D. SCREENING TESTS

■ A single pap smear is associated with false negative rates of 10–25%; accuracy is significantly improved with regular periodic screening. Controlled studies have not demonstrated a decrease in sensitivity or specificity with standard cervical cytology in HIV-positive women as compared with HIV-negative controls. (Adachi, 1993; Spinillo, 1998)

■ Newer pap smear screening techniques using liquid-based media appear to increase sensitivity, decrease inadequate smears, and reduce, but do not eliminate, false negative results; they also offer the possibility of direct HPV testing on collected specimens. They are more expensive than conventional pap tests; there are no current data examining the utility of these tests in HIV-positive women.

■ HPV testing can identify both oncogenic and non-oncogenic viral types; such testing may play an important role in the evaluation of women with equivocal Pap smear results. (Manos, 1999)

■ The role of HPV-DNA testing as an alternative or addition to the pap smear in HIV-positive women is unknown. One small study found that HIV-positive women with normal paps and CD4 counts < 200/mm^3 and presence of HPV-DNA were more likely to have biopsy-proven abnormalities as compared to HIV-negative women or HIV-positive women with higher CD4 counts. (Anderson, 1996) A recent German study examining HPV-DNA testing as a primary screening method for cervical dysplasia in

TABLE 6-1: PAP SMEAR REPORT FORMAT FOR BETHESDA SYSTEM	
Statement on specimen adequacy	■ Satisfactory for interpretation ■ Less than optimal ■ Unsatisfactory
General categorization	■ Within normal limits □ Other/descriptive diagnosis
Descriptive diagnoses	■ Benign cellular changes (including infections) ■ Reactive and reparative cellular changes (including inflammation)
Epithelial cell abnormalities	■ Atypical squamous cells of undetermined significance (ASCUS) ■ Low-grade squamous intraepithelial lesion (SIL), including HPV changes and mild dysplasia/CIN 1 ■ High-grade squamous intraepithelial lesion, including moderate and severe dysplasia, CIN 2, CIN 3, carcinoma in situ ■ Squamous cell carcinoma ■ Glandular cell abnormalities
Nonepithelial malignant neoplasm	■ Specify
Hormonal evaluation (vaginal smears only)	■ Specify

94 HIV-positive women found that HPV-DNA testing identified high-grade cervical dysplasia more accurately than pap smear. (Petry, 1999)

■ Pap smear results are reported according to the Bethesda System. (National Cancer Institute Workshop, 1989)

E. RECOMMENDATIONS FOR PAP SMEAR SCREENING AND COLPOSCOPY (CDC, 1998):

■ Both the CDC and the Agency for Health Care Policy and Research recommend that HIV-infected women have a complete gynecologic evaluation, including a Pap smear and pelvic exam, as part of their initial evaluation.

■ A Pap smear should be obtained twice in the first year after diagnosis of HIV infection. If these results are normal, annual examinations are then indicated.

■ More frequent Pap smears should be obtained:
  - with previous abnormal Pap smear
  - HPV infection
  - after treatment for cervical dysplasia
  - in women with symptomatic HIV infection (including CD4 counts < 200/mm³)

■ The American College of Obstetricians and Gynecologists recommends Pap smears every 3–4 months for the first year after treatment of preinvasive cervical lesions, followed by Pap smears every six months. (ACOG, 1993)

■ The role of anal cytology is currently under study.

■ Indications for colposcopy are outlined in Table 6-2.

TABLE 6-2: INDICATIONS FOR COLPOSCOPY
■ Cytologic abnormality (atypia or greater, including ASCUS, AGCUS)
■ History of untreated abnormal Pap smear
■ Consider periodic colposcopy after treatment of cervical dysplasia
■ Consider with evidence of HPV infection
■ Consider screening colposcopy with CD4 < 200/mm³

TABLE 6-3: SUGGESTED FREQUENCY OF PAP SMEARS	
CLINICAL SCENARIO	*SCREENING FREQUENCY*
Normal Pap	One year
Symptomatic infection / CD4 < 200	6 months
ASCUS/LGSIL (evaluated and followed without treatment)	4–6 months
Following treatment of preinvasive lesions	3–4 months for first year, then 6 months

- ASCUS (atypical squamous cells of undetermined significance) represents the mildest cytologic abnormality in the Bethesda system; its significance, however, varies tremendously among different cytopathologists and laboratories. Various studies have found underlying dysplasia in 10–60% of women with ASCUS on pap. In a study of women with ASCUS, Wright (Wright, 1996) found that HIV-positive women were approximately twice as likely to have underlying dysplasia as compared to HIV-negative women; a recent cross-sectional analysis of 761 pap smears form HIV-positive women found that 27% were diagnosed as ASCUS; 15% had underlying high-grade dysplasia. (Holcomb, 1999) Immunesuppression did not appear to increase the frequency of dysplasia associated with ASCUS on pap. In the general population it is recommended that an initial report of ASCUS prompt repeat pap smear and referral for colposcopy be made with a second ASCUS report. However, given the frequency of cervical abnormalities and the possible increased likelihood of underlying dysplasia with ASCUS in the setting of HIV infection, many experts prefer to proceed with colposcopic evaluation with the initial report of atypical cells. The ability to do this may be limited by availability of colposcopic equipment and trained colposcopists.

- The risk of underlying pathology with a diagnosis of ACGUS (atypical glandular cells of undetermined significance) is significant: 17–34% have associated significant intraepithelial or invasive lesions. (Kennedy, 1996; Duska, 1998; Korn, 1998) Colposcopy is indicated with any AGCUS on pap, as well as endocervical and endometrial sampling.

- Biopsies should be obtained at the time of colposcopy to confirm cytologic abnormalities and/or if abnormal areas are visualized.

- Because of the multicentric nature of lower genital tract intraepithelial neoplasia in the setting of immunesuppression, it is recommended that the entire lower genital tract (vagina, vulva, and perianal region) be examined at the time of colposcopy.

F. MANAGEMENT OF CERVICAL LESIONS

Management of abnormal pap smears is outlined in Table 6-4. Documentation of a high grade cervical lesion requires treatment. Standard excisional or ablative treatment is recommended, although HIV-positive women have an increased incidence of recurrence after treatment (over 50% recurrence rate), correlated with degree of immunesuppression. (Fruchter, 1996; Holcomb, 1999) Cryotherapy has had the highest rate of recurrences and should be avoided, if other treatment methods are available.

Topical vaginal 5-fluorouracil (5-FU) cream (2 gm biweekly for six months) was shown to reduce recurrence rates after standard treatment for high-grade cervical dysplasia in HIV-positive women in a recent clinical trial; over 18 months of follow-up, 31% of women with observation only developed a

TABLE 6-4: RECOMMENDED MANAGEMENT FOR ABNORMAL PAP SMEARS

PAP SMEAR RESULT	MANAGEMENT (BASED ON HISTOLOGIC FINDINGS)
Severe inflammation	Evaluate for infection; repeat Pap if inadequate
Atypia, ASCUS	Colposcopy, biopsy if indicated; follow with Pap Q6 months
Low grade squamous intraepithelial lesion (LGSIL, LSIL, CIN 1)	Colposcopy, biopsy if indicated; follow with Pap Q6 months; consider repeat colposcopy annually
High grade squamous intraepithelial lesion (HGSIL, HSIL, CIN 2 or 3, carcinoma in situ)	Colposcopy, biopsy; treat with loop excision or conization
Invasive carcinoma	Colposcopy with biopsy or conization; treat with surgery or radiation (referral to gynecologic oncologist needed)

recurrent high-grade lesion as compared to 8% of women receiving 5-FU. Disease recurred more slowly in women who had received antiretroviral therapy, as compared to those who were antiretroviral-naïve. (Maiman, 1999)

5-FU may play a role in secondary prophylaxis of preinvasive cervical lesions in some cases. However, clinical experience with this therapy is too limited to provide a recommendation for routine use. 5-FU may have significant mucosal toxicity and concerns have been raised about the potential for increased risk for transmission of HIV or other STDs with this therapy.

The role of highly active antiretroviral therapy (HAART) and immune reconstitution in the management of lower genital tract precancerous lesions remains unclear. In one study use of HAART was associated with regression of cervical lesions over a median follow-up of 5 months. (Heard, 1998) However, Duerr and colleagues found no differences in pap smear results, HPV acquisition or persistence, number of HPV types, or the amount of HPV present after 6–12 months on HAART. (Duerr, 1998)

At the current time, HIV-positive women should continue to be followed closely for evidence of lower genital tract neoplasia, regardless of antiretroviral therapy or viral load.

IV. GENITAL ULCERS

A. HISTORY

Duration and location of lesion(s); previous history of genital ulcers, syphilis, or genital herpes (HSV); associated symptoms (pain, pruritus, fever, etc.); medications and timing of ulcers relative to initiation of new medication; sexual history (including condom use); and CD4 counts and HIV RNA levels.

B. PHYSICAL EXAM

Dimensions and location of lesion(s); presence of pigmentation, edema, erythema, or induration; presence of associated exudate or tenderness; presence of oral lesions; associated lymphadenopathy or rash.

C. EVALUATION

1. **Syphilis serology or darkfield examination**

2. **Culture or antigen test for HSV**

3. **Biopsy** — with unclear diagnosis, lack of response to treatment; consider special stains, if indicated (CMV, AFB)

4. **Culture for Haemophilus ducreyi** — not widely available commercially; diagnosis of chancroid generally made with typical clinical presentation, after excluding syphilis and HSV

D. DIFFERENTIAL DIAGNOSIS AND MANAGEMENT

INFECTIOUS

Herpes Simplex Virus (HSV)
- most prevalent infectious cause of genital ulcers in the U.S.
- two distinct serotypes of HSV (HSV-1 and HSV-2), most cases of recurrent genital herpes (60–95%) are caused by HSV-2
- since the late 1970s, the seroprevalence of HSV-2 infection has increased by 30%; infection is now detectable in 21.9% of people aged 12 or older nationwide (Fleming, 1997)
- typically lesions present as painful vesicles that ulcerate and heal without scarring
- primary infection often associated with systemic symptoms (fever, photophobia, headache); duration of lesions and viral shedding more prolonged with primary infection; after primary episode latency established in sacral dorsal root ganglia
- nonprimary first episode herpes occurs in individuals with antibodies to HSV-1 or HSV-1 but no previous clinical symptoms of HSV; milder, shorter episode
- recurrent episodes occur at variable frequency; more localized lesions, shorter duration as compared to first episodes (primary or nonprimary)
- viral shedding and sexual transmission can occur during asymptomatic periods
- HIV-positive patients:
  - more frequent, prolonged, and/or severe episodes common with progressive immunesuppression; lesions may be atypical in appearance or location

- viral shedding increases with declining CD4 counts (Augenbraun, 1995); may be more common in oral contraceptive or Depo-Provera users and in women with severe vitamin A deficiency (Mostad, 2000); most viral shedding asymptomatic
- HSV is associated with increased risk for HIV transmission/acquisition (Heng, 1994)

■ **Treatment:** See Table 6-5.

TABLE 6-5: RECOMMENDED MANAGEMENT FOR HSV		
	DRUG	**DOSE**
First clinical episode	Acyclovir	400 mg po three times a day for 7–10 days
	Acyclovir	200 mg po five times a day for 7–10 days
	Famciclovir	250 mg po three times a day for 7–10 days
	Valacyclovir	1 gm po twice a day for 7–10 days
Recurrent episodes	Acyclovir	400 mg po three times a day for 5 days
	Acyclovir	200 mg po five times a day for 5 days
	Acyclovir	800 mg po twice a day for 5 days
	Famciclovir	125 mg po twice a day for 5 days
	Valacyclovir	500 mg po twice a day for 5 days
Daily suppressive therapy	Acyclovir Famciclovir Valacyclovir Valacyclovir	400 mg po twice a day 250 mg po twice a day 500 mg po once a day 1000 mg po once a day
Severe disease	Acyclovir	5–10 mg/kg body weight IV every 8 hours for 5–7 days or until clinical resolution is achieved
Acyclovir-resistant HSV	Foscarnet	40 mg/kg body weight IV every 8 hours or 60 mg/kg IV every 12 hours for 3 weeks
	topical Cidofovir gel 1%	applied to lesions once a day for 5 consecutive days
Source: CDC, 1998.		

Syphilis

- ■ systemic disease caused by *Treponema pallidum*
- ■ definitive methods for diagnosing early syphilis are darkfield examination and direct fluorescent antibody test of lesion exudate or tissue
- ■ presumptive diagnosis is possible using two types of serologic tests for syphilis: VDRL or RPR (nontreponemal) and a confirmatory FTA-ABS or MHA-TP (treponemal)
- ■ nontreponemal test antibody titers usually correlate with disease activity and are used to assess treatment response
- ■ HIV-infected patients may have abnormal serologic test results (e.g., unusually high titers, false negatives or delayed seroreactivity). However, generally serologic tests can be interpreted in the usual manner. If clinical

findings suggest syphilis but serology is nonreactive, biopsy, darkfield examination, or direct fluorescent antibody staining of lesion material should be considered. The clinical presentation of syphilis is very variable at all stages; atypical manifestations may be seen in the setting of HIV disease. Neurosyphilis should be considered in the differential diagnosis of neurologic signs or symptoms in HIV-infected individuals (CDC, 1998)

■ **Treatment:** See Table 6-6.

TABLE 6-6: RECOMMENDED MANAGEMENT FOR SYPHILIS

STAGE	TREATMENT
Primary and Secondary Syphilis and Early Latent Syphilis	Benzathine penicillin G 2.4 million units IM (single dose); additional treatment recommended by some (i.e., three weekly doses of penicillin)
If penicillin-allergic (non-pregnant patients only)	Doxycycline 100 mg po twice a day for 2 weeks, OR tetracycline 500 mg po four times a day for 2 weeks
Late Latent Syphilis or Syphilis of Unknown Duration (including tertiary syphilis)	Examination of the CSF must be performed prior to initiation of treatment. If the CSF examination is negative, patients should be treated with 7.2 million units of benzathine penicillin G (three weekly doses of 2.4 million units each) IM
Neurosyphilis	Aqueous crystalline penicillin G 18–24 million units a day (administered as 3–4 million units IV every 4 hours) for 10-14 days. Administration of benzathine penicillin 2.4 million units IM after completion of the IV regimen recommended by some.

RECOMMENDED FOLLOW-UP	
STAGE	FOLLOW-UP
Primary and secondary syphilis	HIV-infected patients require clinical and serologic evaluation for treatment failure at 3, 6, 9, 12, and 24 months after treatment. Treatment failures necessitate a CSF examination and re-treatment (three weekly doses of 2.4 million units of benzathine penicillin G if CSF examination is negative). The latter regimen should also be considered for patients whose titers do not decrease fourfold within 6 to 12 months.

Table continues . . .

TABLE 6-6: RECOMMENDED MANAGEMENT FOR SYPHILIS *(continued)*	
STAGE	TREATMENT
RECOMMENDED FOLLOW-UP *(continued)*	
Latent syphilis	HIV-infected patients require clinical and serologic evaluation at 6, 12, 18, and 24 months after treatment. The CSF examination should be repeated and appropriate treatment instituted if clinical symptoms develop, titers rise fourfold, or if titers fail to decline fourfold between the evaluations at 12 and 24 months.
Neurosyphilis	CSF examination should be repeated every six months until the cell count is normal. Retreatment should be considered if the cell count has not decreased after six months or if the CSF is not entirely normal after two years.
Source: CDC, 1998.	

Chancroid

- caused by Haemophilus ducreyi
- endemic in some areas of the United States; also occurs in discrete outbreaks
- 10% of patients with chancroid have coinfection with *T. pallidum* or HSV
- initial presentation typically consists of a tender papule that becomes pustular and then ulcerative; the ulcer is usually well demarcated, with ragged undermined edges
- probable diagnosis can be made if: the patient has one or more painful ulcers, there is no evidence of *T. pallidum* or HSV infection, and the clinical presentation appearance of ulcers and regional lymphadenopathy is typical for chancroid .
- Response to treatment may be diminished in the HIV-infected patient: may require longer courses of therapy, increased risk for treatment failure
- **Treatment:**
  - Azithromycin 1 gm po (single dose), OR
  - Ceftriaxone 250 mg IM (single dose), OR
  - Ciprofloxacin 500 mg po twice a day for 3 days, OR
  - Erythromycin base 500 mg po four times a day for 7 days.
  - *Note*
    - ▶ In HIV-positive patients use single dose therapies only if follow-up can be ensured;
    - ▶ Some experts recommend the 7-day erythromycin regimen in the setting of HIV infection.

Cytomegalovirus (CMV)

- should be suspected in severely immunocompromised patients
- diagnosis requires biopsy of lesion with immunohistochemical stains
- cervical shedding of CMV is associated with low CD4 counts (Clarke, 1996)
- **Treatment:**
  - Ganciclovir 5 mg/kg IV twice a day for 2–3 weeks, OR
  - Foscarnet 60 mg/kg IV q 8 hours or 90 mg/kg q 12 hours for 2–3 weeks.

Other Infectious Causes of Genital Ulcers

- **Lymphogranuloma Venereum (LGV)**: rare in U.S.; associated with tender, usually unilateral inguinal or femoral lymphadenopathy, proctocolitis, rectal fistulas/strictures; diagnosis with serology and exclusion of other causes; treatment doxycycline or erythromycin for 3 weeks; HIV-positive individuals may require more prolonged treatment

- **Granuloma Inguinale** (Donovanosis): rare in U.S.; painless, progressive ulcers which bleed easily on contact, without regional lymphadenopathy; diagnosis with biopsy or tissue crush preparation; treatment trimethoprim-sulfamethox-azole or doxycycline for 3 weeks or until all lesions healed; CDC recommends adding aminoglycoside to regimen in HIV-positive patients

- **Tuberculosis** (Giannacopoulos, 1998): genital TB is generally a secondary manifestation of primary (usually pulmonary) disease. In the United States, the incidence of genital disease is < 1%. Diagnosis is established by biopsy. Genital tuberculosis should be treated as is extrapulmonary disease; expert consultation is necessary.

INFLAMMATORY CONDITIONS

Crohn's Disease

- This disease may be easily misdiagnosed since its principal clinical features (i.e., fever, abdominal pain, diarrhea, fatigability, weight loss) are often found in patients with HIV disease. Crohn's Disease may also present with genital ulcers, rectal fissures, perirectal abscesses, or intestinal fistulas. Sigmoidoscopy or barium enema is essential in making this diagnosis. Manage with expert consultation.

Behcet's Syndrome

- This is a multisystem disorder that presents with recurrent oral and genital ulcerations as well as uveitis, arthritis, and vasculitis. Vaginal ulcers are usually painless, whereas lesions on the external genitalia are generally painful. Ulcers range between 2 and 10 mm in diameter, and they can be shallow or deep with a central yellowish necrotic base; either a single lesion or crops of lesions may be evident. The diagnosis is established based on the clinical presentation and biopsy. Treatment consists of topical or systemic corticosteroids.

Hidradenitis Suppurativa. (Droegemueller, 1997)

■ This condition is a chronic, refractory infection involving the skin, subcutaneous tissues, and apocrine glands. Lesions are painful and are associated with a foul-smelling discharge. Eventually, a deep-seated chronic infection of apocrine glands develops, with multiple draining abscesses and sinuses. A biopsy is necessary to establish the diagnosis. In the early stages of disease, treatment options include antibiotics, topical steroids, antiandrogens, and isotretinoin. Treatment of advanced disease requires surgical intervention.

NEOPLASTIC

■ any nonhealing genital ulcer must be biopsied to rule out a neoplastic process

■ squamous cell carcinoma, basal cell carcinoma, adenocarcinoma, melanoma, lymphoma, Kaposi's sarcoma

■ refer to oncologist

DRUG REACTION

■ Has been described as rare side effect of treatment with ddC and foscarnet

APHTHOUS GENITAL ULCERATIONS (Anderson, 1996)

■ no specific etiology (typical or opportunistic organism) is identifiable

■ similar to aphthous ulcers seen in the gastrointestinal tract

■ most patients are significantly immunosuppressed (median CD4 count 50/mm^3)

■ lesions can be painful, multiple, deep, and extensive (size 1 to 6 cm)

■ associated morbidity includes immobility, bleeding, and superinfection

■ most have been reported to be chronic and/or recurrent or relapsing

■ oroesophageal ulcers coexist in about one third of cases and one fifth were associated with fistula formation

■ **Treatment:**
  - Consider empiric therapy for HSV.
  - If empiric therapy fails, systemic steroids (prednisone 40–60 mg/day for 1–2 weeks, then taper) have been moderately successful.

- Thalidomide (200 mg/day for 2–4 weeks) has been used in similar ulcers in the oropharynx or esophagus with complete healing in 55–73% of these ulcers (Jacobson, 1999; Jacobson, 1997); there has been similar success anecdotally in genital apththous ulcers. (Warning: this drug is a powerful teratogen and should only be used in women of reproductive age after appropriate counseling and pregnancy testing and in the setting of reliable contraception or abstinence.)

TRAUMA

- history of traumatic injury

- consider possibility of sexual violence

V. VAGINAL DISCHARGE

A. HISTORY

Duration and characteristics of discharge, associated symptoms (e.g., pruritus, malodor, burning, pelvic pain), sexual history (including condom and other contraceptive use), history of sexually transmitted diseases, history of douching, recent antibiotic use, CD4 counts and HIV-RNA levels, medications.

B. PHYSICAL EXAM

Complete genital inspection and bimanual pelvic examination; document the characteristics and amount of discharge as well as the presence of erythema, edema, and tenderness.

C. EVALUATION

- saline wet mount

- 10% potassium hydroxide (KOH) prep

- vaginal pH determination

- testing for gonorrhea and chlamydia

- fungal culture, if indicated (signs/symptoms of yeast infection with negative findings on microscopy; chronic/recurrent yeast infections)

D. DIFFERENTIAL DIAGNOSIS AND MANAGEMENT

BACTERIAL VAGINOSIS (BV)

- most prevalent cause of vaginal discharge or malodor

■ results from replacement of normal *Lactobacillus* dominant vaginal flora with increase in prevalence and concentration of mixed flora, including anaerobic bacteria, *Gardnerella vaginalis*, and *Mycoplasma hominis*

■ 18–42% prevalence among HIV-infected women; no significant difference as compared to HIV-negative controls and no difference by CD4 count (Cu-Uvin, 1999; Greenblatt, 1999)

■ some studies suggest that BV or BV-associated organisms (or lack of vaginal lactobacilli) may enhance HIV transmission (Olinger, 1999; Martin, 1999)

■ associated with increase in several obstetrical and gynecologic complications, including pelvic inflammatory disease (PID), post-abortal and posthysterectomy infections, preterm labor

■ standard diagnosis by clinical criteria; requires three of the following: 1) a homogeneous grayish or yellowish discharge (may coat vaginal walls); (2) clue cells on microscopic examination; (3) vaginal pH > 4.5; (4) a positive whiff test (i.e., fishy odor of discharge before or after addition of 10% KOH)

■ **Treatment:** See Table 6-7.

TABLE 6-7: RECOMMENDED MANAGEMENT FOR BACTERIAL VAGINOSIS

■ Metronidazole 500 mg po twice a day for 7 days

■ Clindamycin cream 2%, 5 gm intravaginally at bedtime for 7 days

■ Metronidazole gel 0.75%, 5 gm intravaginally twice a day for 5 days

Note: Clindamycin cream is oil-based and may weaken latex condoms and diaphragms.
  Alternative regimens: Metronidazole 2 gm po
      Clindamycin 300 mg po twice a day for 7 days

Source: CDC, 1998.

VULVOVAGINAL CANDIDIASIS

■ Most commonly caused by *Candida albicans*; the prevalence of infections due to nonalbicans species is increasing

■ 75% of all women will have at least one episode of candidiasis, and 40–45% will have two or more episodes; less than 5% of women experience recurrent episodes of candidiasis

■ typical symptoms: thick, white discharge and pruritus; other symptoms include vulvar burning, vaginal soreness, dyspareunia, and external dysuria

■ Prevalence among HIV-infected women is 3–15%; most studies suggest no significant difference in prevalence of infection between relatively immunocompetent HIV-positive women and HIV-negative controls; several other studies have found increasing infection rates with declining CD4 counts. (Cu-Uvin, 1999; Duerr, 1997) HIV-positive women may have higher incidence of infection (El-Sadr, 1997)

■ Possible confounding factor for HIV-positive women is more frequent use of antibiotics

■ Most studies show increased rates of vaginal (also rectal, oral) colonization in HIV-positive women, particularly with declining immune function; no data on relationship between HIV-RNA levels and candidiasis or colonization

■ In HIV-positive women 26–27% of vaginal isolates are non-albicans strains (NAS) (Schuman, 1998); available studies are conflicting re: proportion of NAS in HIV-positive as compared to HIV-negative women; most common is Torulopsis glabrata. No association found to date between strain diversity and HIV progression

■ diagnosis is made by identifying budding yeast or pseudohyphae on a wet mount or KOH prep or Gram stain of vaginal discharge; positive identification can also be accomplished by means of culture

■ **Treatment regimens:** See Table 6-8.

TABLE 6-8: RECOMMENDED MANAGEMENT FOR VULVOVAGINAL CANDIDIASIS
TOPICAL AZOLES
■ Butoconazole 2% cream 5 gm PV for 3 days*
■ Clotrimazole 1% cream 5 gm PV for 7–14 days*
■ Clotrimazole 100 mg vaginal tablet for 7 days
■ Clotrimazole 100 mg vaginal tablet, 2 tablets for 3 days
■ Clotrimazole 500 mg vaginal tablet x 1
■ Miconazole 2% cream 5 gm PV for 7 days*
■ Miconazole 200 mg vaginal suppository for 3 days*
■ Miconazole 100 mg vaginal suppository for 7 days*
■ Miconazole 1200 mg vaginal suppository x 1
■ Tioconazole 6.5% ointment 5 gm PV x 1*
■ Tioconazole 2% cream 5 gm PV for 3 days
■ Terconazole 0.4% cream 5 gm PV for 7 days
■ Terconazole 0.8% cream PV for 3 days
■ Terconazole 80 mg vaginal suppository for 3 days
* OTC.   *Note:* These creams are oil-based and may weaken latex condoms and diaphragms.
*ORAL AGENT**
■ Fluconazole 150 mg po x 1
* avoid concomitant use with terfenadine, astemizole, cisapride secondary to cardiotoxicity
OTHERS
■ Nystatin 100,000 unit vaginal tablet, one tablet for 14 days (less effective)
■ 1% Gentian violet applied to vagina 4 times at intervals of approximately 7 days*
■ Boric acid 600 mg intravaginal capsules BID for 2 weeks*
* may be useful in chronic/recurrent cases; gentian violet messy, causes mucosal exfoliation; encourage abstinence during treatment; reinforce condom use.

VI

- **Special considerations in HIV-positive women:**
  - ▶ Topical therapies may be more effective when given for at least 7 days
  - ▶ Consider prophylactic use of topical antifungals when antibiotics are given
  - ▶ Randomized, placebo-controlled trial of fluconazole 200 mg po weekly for prophylaxis of candidiasis in women with CD4 < 300/mm³ (median CD4 15/mm³): effective in preventing oropharyngeal candidiasis (RR 0.50, p < 0.001) and vaginal candidiasis (RR 0.64, p=0.05), but not esophageal candidiasis.(Schuman, 1997) Consider in selected cases with recurrent vaginal candidiasis.
  - ▶ Recent study found that ritonavir and indinavir (and possibly other protease inhibitors) strongly inhibited secretory aspartyl proteinase (proteolytic enzyme produced by pathogenic Candida species, considered a virulence factor) activity and production in a dose-dependent fashion, and exerted a therapeutic effect in an experimental model of vaginal candidiasis, with efficacy similar to fluconazole. (Cassone, 1999)

- **Azole resistance:**
  Concerns have been raised about extensive use of oral azoles and promotion of azole resistance, possibly limiting use of these agents for other HIV-related indications. Current information about development of resistance is limited:
  - ▶ ACTG 816: annual incidence of clinical failure to fluconazole (persistence of oral candidiasis after 200 mg/da or higher dose for 14 days) 5.8% (median CD4 15/mm³); C. albicans primary etiology
  - ▶ CPCRA-randomized, placebo-controlled trial of fluconazole 200 mg weekly for prophylaxis of candidiasis (described above) (median CD4 15/mm³): after median 29 months follow-up, fluconazole resistance < 5% resistance in both fluconazole and placebo groups (Schuman, 1997)
  - ▶ HIV Epidemiology Research Study (HERS): overall fluconazole resistance rare among C. albicans isolates, but frequent in non-albicans isolates from vagina and oral cavity; fluconazole resistance with non-albicans species more likely in HIV-positive women; not significantly related to CD4 count. Resistance among non-albicans species stable after 1 year of follow-up (Schuman, 1997)
  - ▶ 139 isolates from vulvovaginal candidiasis in HIV-positive women: 95–98% susceptibility of C. albicans to fluconazole, itraconazole, clotrimazole; Torulopsis glabrata-44% resistance to fluconazole, 72% resistance to itraconazole and clotrimazole. Twenty percent

of 90 relapses/persistence were with same organism; emergence of drug resistance was not observed between sequential isolates. Twelve percent had recurrent infection with different strains or species. (Li, 1997)

There are no current data to suggest that intermittent therapy with a single dose of fluconazole increases development of azole resistance. Similarly, weekly prophylaxis with fluconazole was associated with infrequent development of resistance, which was not significantly different from placebo recipients. Nevertheless, long-term use of fluconazole may select for more resistant and difficult-to-treat non-albicans species and should be used with caution. Further study is needed.

- **Recurrent candidiasis** (4 or more symptomatic episodes per year):
  - ▶ Evaluation:
    1. establish diagnosis –fungal culture may be needed
    2. identify/eliminate predisposing factors, if possible: uncontrolled diabetes, corticosteroid use, topical or systemic antibiotics, spermicides (conflicting data), tight-fitting synthetic underwear, douching, pregnancy, immunesuppression
    3. speciation/susceptibility testing
  - ▶ Management Options:
    1. longer duration of standard treatment regimen
    2. chronic intermittent therapy (e.g., with perimenstrual episodes)
    3. restriction of orogenital/anogenital sexual contact (anecdotal evidence only); double-blind, placebo-controlled trials of topical therapy for male sexual partners showed no benefit (Sobel, 1999)
    4. possible role for boric acid vaginal capsules, gentian violet
    5. maintenance therapy: initial intensive regimen for 10–14 days followed by a maintenance regimen for at least 6 months:
       a. fluconazole* 100–200 mg po q week
       b. itraconazole *50–100 mg po q week
       c. clotrimazole 500 mg suppository per vagina q week
       d. ketoconazole *100 mg po q day (associated with rare but significant hepatotoxicity-monitor liver function; significant drug interactions with some antiretrovirals (see Chapter XIV on Pharmacologic Considerations in HIV-infected Pregnant Patients)
    6. immune reconstitution; potential benefit with protease inhibitors

---

* Note: avoid concomitant use with terfenadine, astemizole, cisapride secondary to cardiotoxicity.

TRICHOMONIASIS

■ Caused by *Trichomonas vaginalis*

■ HIV-positive women: 5–23% prevalence; studies have not shown increased prevalence as compared to HIV-negative women; incidence in HIV-positive women 10–17% (Minkoff, 1999; Sorvillo, 1998)

■ Clinical features: profuse, malodorous, often frothy, yellow-green discharge and vulvar irritation; may have urinary symptoms or dyspareunia; signs of inflammation-vaginal erythema, "strawberry" vagina, cervix with punctate hemorrhages; may be asymptomatic in chronic cases

■ Diagnosis: saline wet mount (motile trichomonads seen in 50–70% culture + cases); Pap smear (60–70% sensitivity, false positives not uncommon); culture (95% sensitivity); DNA probes; monoclonal antibodies

■ T. vaginalis cysteine proteases degrade and render nonfunctional secretory leukocyte protease inhibitor, a substance thought to protect mucosal surfaces from HIV transmission by inhibition of HIV protease activity necessary for infection of monocytes and macrophages (Draper D, 1998)

■ **Treatment** (CDC,1998):
  - Metronidazole 2 gm po (single dose), OR
  - Metronidazole 500 mg po twice a day for 7 days.
  - *Note:*
    ➤ No change in treatment based on HIV status
    ➤ Sex partners should be treated with the same regimen (> 90% cure rates can be expected if partner is treated simultaneously); intercourse should be avoided until therapy is complete and patient and partner are asymptomatic
    ➤ Topical metronidazole less effective
    ➤ Metronidazole resistance is rare; organisms with decreased susceptibility usually respond to higher doses of metronidazole. If treatment failure occurs with either regimen, re-treat with metronidazole 500 mg po twice a day for 7 days. If treatment failure occurs repeatedly, treat with metronidazole 2 gm po once a day for 3–5 days. Patients with documented infection (with reinfection excluded) who have not responded to these measures should be managed in consultation with an expert.

GONORRHEA (GC)

■ caused by *Neisseria gonorrhoeae*

■ clinical presentation: commonly asymptomatic; vaginal discharge may be present; if untreated, 10–20% develop pelvic inflammatory disease (PID); urethra is primary site of colonization after hysterectomy and should be sampled with culture or DNA probe for testing in these patients; GC may also cause rectal infection, pharyngitis, and (rarely) disseminated infection

■ diagnosis: culture, DNA probe, polymerase chain reaction (PCR) or ligase chain reaction (LCR). PCR/LCR can be used with cervical, urethral, or urine specimens; may detect gonorrhea and chlamydia simultaneously; sensitivity 93–98%, specificity > 99%; able to detect 15–40% more infections than culture (Hook, 1999)

■ prevalence/clinical presentation/diagnosis/treatment in HIV-positive patients: no difference when compared to HIV-negative patients

■ **Treatment** (CDC,1998):

- Cefixime 400 mg po (single dose), OR
- Ceftriaxone 125 mg IM (single dose), OR
- Ciprofloxacin 500 mg po (single dose), OR
- Ofloxacin 400 mg po (single dose).
- **Alternative regimen:**
  - ➤ Spectinomycin 2 gm IM (single dose)
- *Note:*
  - ➤ It is recommended that women be presumptively treated for chlamydia, particularly in areas with high rates of coinfection, absence of chlamydial testing, and/or when patient may not return for results
  - ➤ Sex partners should be treated for both gonorrhea and chlamydia if their last sexual contact was within 60 days prior to the diagnosis or onset of symptoms. If a patient's most recent sexual contact occurred more than 60 days prior to the onset of symptoms, her most recent partner should be treated. Intercourse should be avoided until treatment is completed and symptoms have resolved.
  - ➤ Culture and susceptibility testing recommended after apparent treatment failure with standard regimen
  - ➤ Avoid use of quinolones and tetracyclines in pregnancy

CHLAMYDIA

■ caused by *Chlamydia trachomatis*

■ clinical presentation: asymptomatic infection common; abnormal discharge; symptoms of urethritis; if untreated, 10–40% develop PID

■ diagnosis: culture (cell based), antigen detection, DNA probe, PCR/LCR (90–100% sensitivity-see above) (Stamm, 1999)

■ prevalence/clinical presentation/diagnosis/treatment in HIV-positive women: no differences as compared to HIV-negative women

■ **Treatment** (CDC,1998):
- Azithromycin 1 gm po (single dose), OR
- Doxycycline 100 mg po twice a day for 7 days
- Alternative regimens:
  - Erythromycin base 500 mg po four times a day for 7 days OR
  - Erythromycin ethylsuccinate 800 mg po four times a day for 7 days, OR
  - Ofloxacin 300 mg po twice a day for 7 days.
- *Note:*
  - Recommendations for the management of sex partners are the same as for gonorrhea (see above)
  - Avoid use of doxycycline or quinolones in pregnancy

OTHER

■ Atrophic vaginitis: related to estrogen deficiency; irritative symptoms, vaginal dryness, and dyspareunia; the vaginal epithelium appears thin and a watery discharge may be present; treat with either topical or oral estrogen.

■ Foreign body (retained tampon, toilet paper, etc.)

■ Local irritants (spermicides, vaginal medications, toilet paper dye, hygeine sprays, soap, detergent, douches, etc.)

VI. PELVIC/ABDOMINAL PAIN

Abdominopelvic pain can be classified as acute, chronic, or cyclic. **Acute pain** is typically sudden in onset and short in duration, whereas **chronic pain** is of at least six months' duration. **Cyclic pain** is associated with the menstrual cycle.

A. HISTORY

Characteristics of pain: onset (rapid or gradual), character (crampy, colicky, sharp or dull), location (generalized or localized pain) and duration; associated symptoms: abnormal vaginal bleeding or discharge, gastrointestinal symptoms (e.g., nausea/vomiting, anorexia, constipation, diarrhea), and urinary (e.g., dysuria, frequency, urgency, hematuria) symptoms, fever or chills; history of other medical conditions; surgical history; gynecologic history: date of last menstrual period, use of contraception and condoms, history of STDs; medications; CD4 counts and HIV-RNA levels.

B. PHYSICAL EXAM

A complete set of vital signs should be obtained. The physical exam should focus on abdominal and pelvic findings. A complete abdominal exam should evaluate the presence and character of bowel sounds, distension, suprapubic or costovertebral angle tenderness, other abdominal tenderness (including rebound and guarding) and presence of masses. The pelvic exam should determine the presence of abnormal bleeding or discharge; reproducibility and location of tenderness (e.g., uterine, adnexal, or cervical motion tenderness); presence of a palpable abdominal or pelvic mass should be ruled out.

C. EVALUATION

■ Pregnancy test

■ Laboratory tests: CBC with differential, sedimentation rate, chemistry panel, others as indicated

■ Wet mount/STD testing

■ Urinalysis and urine culture

■ Stool studies (cultures, evaluation for ova and parasites, C. difficile toxin assay) — if indicated by GI symptomatology

■ Pelvic ultrasound, CT scans — if indicated

■ Blood cultures — bacteria, *M. avium*, if indicated

D. DIFFERENTIAL DIAGNOSIS AND MANAGEMENT

Includes but not limited to:

■ **Pregnancy:** refer

■ **Pelvic Inflammatory Disease (PID):** PID is an upper genital tract infection, usually polymicrobial in nature. Sexually transmitted organisms, including *N. gonorrhea* and *C. trachomatis*, are implicated in most cases of PID; bacterial vaginosis-associated organisms are also commonly present. Symptoms may be virtually absent or mild and nonspecific (e.g., abnormal bleeding, dyspareunia, vaginal discharge; less commonly right upper quadrant pleuritic pain secondary to perihepatitis). Current CDC—recommended criteria for diagnosis of PID are (CDC,1998):

  ● **Minimum criteria:**

    ▶ lower abdominal tenderness

    ▶ adnexal tenderness

    ▶ cervical motion tenderness

  Because of difficulty in diagnosis and the potential for long-term complications, empiric therapy should be initiated if these criteria are present and no other cause for symptoms is identified.

  ● **Additional criteria:**

    ▶ oral temperature > 101 F (> 38.3 C)

    ▶ abnormal cervical or vaginal discharge

    ▶ elevated erythrocyte sedimentation rate

> ➤ elevated C-reactive protein

> ➤ documented cervical gonorrhea or chlamydia infection

These criteria enhance specificity.

- **Definitive criteria:**

  > ➤ endometritis on endometrial biopsy

  > ➤ tubo-ovarian complex or thickened fluid-filled tubes on transvaginal ultrasound

  > ➤ laparoscopic abnormalities consistent with PID

  Warranted in patients who are severely ill and when diagnosis is uncertain.

- **PID in the HIV-positive woman:** Several studies have found increased seroprevalence of HIV in hospitalized PID patients. (Hoegsberg, 1990; Sperling, 1991) A recent analysis of hysterctomy specimens from HIV-positive women and HIV-negative women, matched for surgical indication, found chronic endometritis twice as commonly in the HIV-positive specimens; some degree of abnormal uterine bleeding had occurred in all cases. (Kerr-Layton, 1998) Moreover, the clinical presentation among these women may be more severe or otherwise altered (e.g., lower WBC counts than HIV-negative women) (Barbosa, 1997; Kamenga, 1995; Cohen, 1998); in African studies, more severe illness, including tubo-ovarian abscess, and longer hospital stays were required with significant immunosuppression. The microbiology of infection and response to standard antibiotic regimens are similar to HIV-uninfected women; however, some studies have reported a greater need for surgical intervention. (Korn, 1993) CMV and tuberculosis may cause upper genital tract infection in rare cases and should be considered in appropriate clinical situations. Current CDC recommendations call for managing immunosuppressed HIV-infected women with PID aggressively with a parenteral regimen. A more recent study from Kenya found similar efficacy of oral ambulatory therapy in HIV-positive and HIV-negative women with PID. (Bukusi, 1999) Decisions about oral versus parenteral therapy should be individualized.

- **Treatment** (CDC,1998):

  > ➤ **Parenteral regimens:**

  > > ◆ A. Cefotetan 2 gm IV every 12 hours, PLUS Doxycycline 100 mg IV, OR

  > > ◆ B. Cefoxitin 2 gm IV every 6 hours, PLUS Doxycycline 100 mg IV, OR

  > > ◆ C. Clindamycin 900 mg IV every 8 hours, PLUS Gentamicin loading dose IV or IM (2 mg/kg of body weight), followed by a maintenance dose (1.5 mg/kg) every 8 hours

➤ **Oral regimens:**

♦ A. Ofloxacin 400 mg orally twice a day for 14 days, PLUS
Metronidazole 500 mg orally twice a day for 14 days, OR

♦ B. Ceftriaxone 250 mg IM once, OR

♦ C. Cefoxitin 2 gm IM plus Probenecid 1 gm orally in a
single dose concurrently once, PLUS
Doxycycline 100 mg orally twice a day for 14 days.

For alternative oral and parenteral regimens, please see the CDC 1998
Guidelines for Treatment of Sexually Transmitted Diseases.
(**http://www.hivatis.org**)

Parenteral therapy may be discontinued 24 hours after there is evidence
of clinical improvement. Oral therapy with Doxycycline 100 mg every 12
hours (consider the addition of Metronidazole 500 mg every 12 hours, particularly with presence of tubo-ovarian abscess) or Clindamycin 450 mg
four times a day should then be instituted to complete a 14-day treatment
course. Sexual partners of women diagnosed with PID should be evaluated
and treated if they have had sexual contact within the sixty days preceding
the onset of symptoms.

VI

TABLE 6-9: INDICATIONS FOR HOSPITALIZATION IN PATIENTS WITH PID
■ Inadequate response to outpatient therapy
■ Uncertain diagnosis; surgical emergency cannot be excluded
■ Pregnancy
■ Inability to tolerate or follow outpatient regimen
■ Immunosuppression (low CD4 counts, clinical AIDS,on immunosuppressive drugs, other significant co-morbidity
■ Tubo-ovarian abscess or other evidence of severe illness, nausea and vomiting, or high fever

■ **Ruptured/hemorrhagic ovarian cyst rupture**: can cause acute abdominal pain; bleeding associated with rupture is usually self-limited but may
require surgical intervention.

■ **Ovarian torsion**: acute, severe, unilateral lower abdominal/pelvic pain,
often with history of previous similar episodes; palpable adnexal mass
usually present. Surgical intervention required.

■ **Uterine leiomyomas (fibroids)**: may cause pain with rapid enlargement,
degeneration, or torsion; referral indicated

■ **Endometriosis**: cause of acute or chronic pain, usually includes secondary dysmenorrhea and/or dyspareunia; referral to gynecologic specialist
indicated if endometriosis suspected

■ **Dysmenorrhea**: affects about half of all menstruating women; cyclic
pain with menses. Primary dysmenorrhea is menstrual pain in the
absence of pelvic pathology; secondary dysmenorrhea is associated with
underlying pathology (such as endometriosis). Treatment of primary

dysmenorrhea consists of nonsteroidal antiinflammatory drugs (NSAIDs) (80% effective) or OCPs (90% effective). Treatment of secondary dysmenorrhea is directed at the specific underlying problem.

■ **Mittelschmerz**: pain with ovulation, generally self-limited; manage with NSAIDs

■ **Gastrointestinal pathology**: includes appendicitis; diverticulitis (pain generally localizes to the left lower quadrant; usually seen at older ages); irritable bowel syndrome (pain is usually intermittent, cramp-like, and more common in the left lower quadrant; exacerbated by certain foods); inflammatory bowel disease; infectious enterocolitis (pain cramping, diarrhea); obstruction (colicky pain, distension, vomiting, obstipation). Opportunistic infections, including cryptosporidia, CMV and *M. avium* may be causes of chronic diarrhea in patients with AIDS and clinical features usually include abdominal pain.

■ **Urinary tract pathology**: renal/ureteral stones, cystitis, and pyelonephritis

■ **Medication-related**: indinavir (renal stones); ddI (pancreatitis)

VII. PELVIC MASS

A. HISTORY

Presence and duration of associated symptoms: pain, abnormal vaginal bleeding or discharge, urinary symptoms (e.g., frequency, urinary retention), gastrointestinal symptoms (e.g., nausea, vomiting, constipation, diarrhea), or constitutional symptoms (e.g., fever, chills, weight loss or gain).

B. PHYSICAL EXAM

A complete abdominal and pelvic examination should be performed, with particular attention given to the size, location, mobility, and characteristics of the mass (if palpable) as well as to signs of ascites; lymph node survey. With functional ovarian cysts, a normal ovary may be up to 5–6 cm in size for a woman in the reproductive age range. A palpable ovary in a postmenopausal woman is abnormal and requires further evaluation.

C. EVALUATION

■ Pregnancy test: if premenopausal

■ Laboratory tests: CBC with differential; chemistry panel; tumor markers, if indicated (e.g., CEA, Ca-125; frequent false positives and false negatives, should only be used in conjunction with other diagnostic procedures)

■ Radiologic studies: pelvic ultrasound (transabdominal/transvaginal), CT, and MRI, as indicated. Ultrasound is generally the first diagnostic modality employed in evaluating pelvic anatomy; concerning characteristics include complex or solid mass, presence of ascites. CT/MRI are better at imaging GI tract, retroperitoneal lymphadenopathy, liver

Additional evaluation involving procedures such as laparoscopy, colonoscopy, etc. require referral to appropriate specialists.

D. DIFFERENTIAL DIAGNOSIS

■ **Ectopic pregnancy**: the primary consideration in the setting of an adnexal mass and a positive pregnancy test.

■ **Ovarian functional cyst**: Functional cysts are the most common ovarian masses found among women of reproductive age; resolution occurs spontaneously in one to three months.

■ **Uterine leiomyomas (fibroids)**: often asymptomatic, but may be associated with heavy and/or prolonged menses, urinary frequency.

■ **Endometrioma**: consider in women with a documented or suspected history of endometriosis.

■ **Hydrosalpinx/Pyosalpinx and tuboovarian abscess**: consider with history suggestive of PID; initial management with broad-spectrum antibiotics.

■ **Benign or malignant ovarian neoplasm**: Surgical intervention is required. No evidence of increased prevalence in HIV-positive women; anecdotal reports suggest ovarian cancer may present at more advanced stage, with poorer response to cytoreductive surgery and chemotherapy. (Rojansky, 1996) Non-Hodgkins lymphoma of ovary described in an HIV-positive woman. (Neary, 1996)

■ **Retroperitoneal lymphadenopathy**: may present as pelvic mass; possible cause include tuberculosis, lymphoma

■ **Gastrointestinal masses**: includes diverticular abscess, bowel malignancy

In general, the presence of a pelvic or abdominal mass requires expert consultation and referral to an appropriate specialist.

VIII. URINARY SYMPTOMS

A. HISTORY

Duration and severity of urinary symptoms; specific symptoms: dysuria, frequency, urgency, hematuria, nocturia, incontinence; associated symptoms, including pain (suprapubic or flank), fever, chills, and weight loss; other medical conditions (e.g., diabetes, sickle cell disease); surgical history; medications; CD4 count and HIV-RNA level

B. PHYSICAL EXAM

Vital signs;document presence of suprapubic tenderness or flank or costovertebral angle tenderness

C. EVALUATION

- Microscopic exam of urine

- Urine culture and sensitivity

- GC/chlamydia testing, if indicated

- Cytology: consider in woman over the age of fifty who presents with irritative symptoms or hematuria and negative culture

- Urine for AFB culture, PPD: if indicated, urinary TB suspected

- Intravenous Pyelogram (IVP): if indicated; consider if stones, urinary tract anomalies, or urinary TB suspected

- Other tests: cystoscopy, urodynamics-refer to appropriate specialist

D. DIFFERENTIAL DIAGNOSIS AND MANAGEMENT

- **Bacterial urinary tract infection:** lower tract (cystitis) or upper tract (pyelonephritis); may be asymptomatic and clinical signs and symptoms cannot reliable distinguish between upper and lower tract infection. Classically cystitis characterized by the presence of dull, suprapubic pain; typical associated symptoms include dysuria, and urinary frequency and urgency, and occasionally hematuria. Pyelonephritis associated with flank or costovertebral pain and tenderness to percussion, as well as systemic signs/symptoms, including fever, chills,nausea, vomiting, tachycardia. Treat with appropriate antibiotics; severe pyelonephritis requires hospitalization for IV antibiotics and hydration.

- **Urethral syndrome:** dysuria, frequency with negative urine culture; rule out urethritis due to gonorrheal or chlamydial infection

- **Renal/ureteral stones:** severe, colicky pain; usually associated with urinary stasis or chronic infection, although may be related to metabolic abnormalities, such as gout or problems with calcium homeostasis; a significant side effect associated with indinavir therapy.

- **Interstitial cystitis:** symptoms include severe urinary frequency and urgency, (urinating as often as every 15 minutes daytime and nighttime) as well as suprapubic or perineal discomfort before, during, and after urination; refer for definitive evaluation

- **Urinary tuberculosis:** one of the most common sites of extrapulmonary TB; gross or microscopic hematuria and pyuria with negative bacterial culture should lead to consideration; manage with expert consultation

- **Tumors**: most common presenting complaint is gross or microscopic hematuria; hematuria without identifiable etiology (e.g., infection) requires referral to urologist

- **Urinary incontinence:** can be caused by many factors, including anatomic displacements related to aging and childbearing; bladder muscle (detrusor) instability; neurologic disease; infection; fistulas secondary to surgical injury, radiation, or cancer; and some medications. Rule out infection with culture and "overflow" incontinence (secondary to overdistended bladder) with post-void catheterization for residual urine determination. Further evaluation requires referral to urogynecologist or urologist..

- **Urinary retention:** may be caused by obstruction, neurologic disorders, or certain medications (e.g., antihistamines, antidepressants, antipsychotics, opiates, antispasmodics, terbutaline, over-the-counter cold remedies).

VI

IX. GENITAL WARTS

Genital warts are a common manifestation of HPV infection . HPV types 6 and 11 are usually the cause of visible genital warts. Oncogenic types (i.e., 16, 18, 31, 33, and 35) are occasionally found in visible warts and have been associated with squamous intraepithelial neoplasia of the external genitalia (see section on Abnormal Pap smear above).

A. HISTORY

Location of warts, duration, and the presence of associated symptoms (itching, irritation, pain, bleeding); history of prior occurrences of similar lesions and their treatment; history of abnormal Pap smear results

B. PHYSICAL EXAM

Complete examination of the external genitalia as well as of the cervix, vagina, and perianal region should be performed; location and size of warts should be documented. Genital warts can present as cauliflower-shaped growths (condyloma acuminata), smooth, dome-shaped, skin-colored papules, keratotic warts with a thick horny layer, or flat or slightly raised flat-topped papules.

C. RELATION TO HIV

HIV-infected women are more likely to have HPV coinfection and both prevalence and incidence of genital warts are increased as compared to HIV-negative women. (Chirgwin, 1995) Both prevalence and clinical expression of HPV increases with progressive clinical disease and immunologic decline. Immunosuppressed women may not respond as well to treatment and have more frequent recurrences after therapy. Squamous cell carcinomas that arise in or resemble genital warts may occur more commonly in the setting of immunosuppression, making confirmation of diagnosis with biopsy more frequently necessary.

D. EVALUATION

■ **Biopsy:** Typical condyloma accuminata are diagnosed by inspection and do not require biopsy. A biopsy of the lesion and histopathologic confirmation of the diagnosis are indicated in the following situations:

- diagnosis is uncertain
- . warts do not respond to therapy
- lesions worsen during therapy
- warts are pigmented, indurated, fixed, or ulcerated

■ **Colposcopy:** Colposcopy and directed biopsies of the entire lower genital tract should be considered in HIV-positive women with evidence of HPV infection. Colposcopy should be performed to rule out the presence of high-grade squamous intraepithelial lesions prior to initiating treatment of cervical warts.

■ **Treatment:** The primary goal of treatment is the removal of symptomatic lesions. When left untreated, visible warts may resolve spontaneously, may remain unchanged, or may increase in number or size. There is no evidence that currently available therapies eradicate HPV, have an effect on the natural history of infection, or affect the subsequent development of cervical cancer. Infectivity may or may not be decreased by the removal of visible warts.

The treatment modality depends on the number, size, and location of the warts. When there are a small number of lesions and they are fairly small, a

TABLE 6-10: RECOMMENDED MANAGEMENT FOR GENITAL WARTS

PROVIDER-APPLIED	PATIENT-APPLIED
80%-90% trichloroacetic acid (weekly if necessary); cryotherapy with liquid nitrogen or cryoprobe-repeat every 1–2 weeks; surgical removal	Podofilox 0.5% solution or gel applied twice a day for 3 days followed by 4 days of no therapy; may repeat application for up to 4 cycles; application should be limited to 0.5 ml per day and < 10 cm² area of warts
10%-25% podophyllin resin weekly if necessary; application should be limited to < 0.5 ml of podophyllin or < 10 cm² of warts per session and preparation should be thoroughly washed off 1–4 hours after application to reduce local irritation; because of concern about potential systemic absorption and toxicity, avoid use on mucosal surfaces	Imiquimod 5% cream applied three times per week for as long as 16 weeks; the treated area should be washed with mild soap and water 6–10 hours after application

Note: Avoid use of podophyllin, podofilox, and imiquimod during pregnancy topical agent may be employed. Table 6-10 displays provider-applied and patient-administered regimens recommended by the CDC (CDC,1998):

Most treatment modalities are associated with mild to moderate discomfort and local irritation. Intralesional interferon is an additional alternative treatment but is expensive and associated with a high frequency of systemic side effects. Treatment method should be changed if there is not substantial improvement after three provider-administered treatments or if there is not complete clearance after 6 treatments. Combining modalities does not appear to increase efficacy but may increase complications. Recurrence rates are significant with all modalities; frequent follow-up will allow re-treatment when new warts are small and few in number. When the number of warts is large or the lesions are very extensive, referral for possible laser surgery should be considered. In one study relapse rates of treated genital warts in HIV-positive patients was lower in those on combination antiretroviral therapy and was correlated with HIV-RNA levels (Giovanna, 1998)

X. GENITAL MASSES/NODULES

A. HISTORY

Duration; changes in size or appearance; associated symptoms (e.g., pain/tenderness, itching, edema); prior history of similar nodules and their treatment; sexual history (including presence of similar lesions on genitals of partner); medications; CD4 count and HIV-RNA level

B. PHYSICAL EXAM

Document anatomic location, number, and size of the nodules; presence of associated edema, erythema, induration, fluctuance, tenderness, discharge, or bleeding

C. EVALUATION

Biopsy indicated if etiology is unclear; culture of abscess contents

D. DIFFERENTIAL DIAGNOSIS AND MANAGEMENT

■ **Bartholin's abscess:** Bartholin's glands are normally non-palpable and located deep in the perineum at the 5 and 7 o'clock positions of the entrance to the vagina. Obstruction of a Bartholin's duct by nonspecific inflammation, infection (e.g., GC or chlamydia) or trauma can lead to the formation of an abscess; exquisitely tender. Treatment consists of incision and drainage.

■ **Molluscum contagiosum:** an asymptomatic viral disease that primarily affects skin of the vulva, although it can present as a generalized skin disease in immunosuppressed individuals; spread by close contact, both sexual and nonsexual. Clinical features: small nodules or domed papules, usually

1–5 mm in diameter; the more mature nodules appear to have an umbili-
cated center. This disease tends to be self-limited; however, treatment may
be complicated by repeat infection and autoinoculation of the virus. Treatment consists of serial applications of liquid nitrogen or of removal of the
nodules with a dermal curet and chemical cauterization of base with 85%
TCA or ferric subsulfate. Molluscum contagiosum affects 5–10% of HIV-
positive patients; extensive, severe lesions that show poor response to therapy are common; such unresponsive lesions, however, have been found to
regress with HAART. (Calista, 1999)

■ **Tumors, other masses:** biopsy required; expert consultation indicated.

XI. GENITAL ITCHING/IRRITATION

A. HISTORY

Duration, location, and severity of pruritis/irritation; associated symptoms
(erythema, edema, vulvar burning, dysuria, dyspareunia); prior episodes of
similar symptoms and treatment; exposure to particular agents (e.g., soaps,
sprays, vaginal contraceptives, douches, colored toilet tissue, etc.) coincident
with the beginning of symptoms; presence of similar symptoms in close contacts; medications, including antibiotics; CD4 counts and HIV-RNA level

B. PHYSICAL EXAM

Physical appearance and distribution of the irritated area (e.g., diffuse rash,
papular or vesicular lesions, skin burrows, etc.); associated findings, including
erythema, edema, and tenderness, vaginal discharge; if a more generalized
process is suspected (e.g., allergic reaction to detergent, scabies, etc.) a more
thorough inspection of the skin throughout the body may be indicated.

C. EVALUATION

■ Fungal culture/KOH prep: indicated if a fungal infection is suspected.

■ HSV culture: herpes may appear atypically and should be ruled out in the
presence of vesicular lesions, unexplained abrasions or fissuring, or if warranted by history .

■ Skin scrapings: scraping of skin papule is with a needle, and the crust is
placed under a drop of mineral oil on a slide; eggs, parasites, or fecal pellets
microscopically visualized by this technique are diagnostic of scabies or
pubic lice.

D. DIFFERENTIAL DIAGNOSIS AND MANAGEMENT

■ **Fungal infection:** although the primary symptom associated with fungal
infections is itching, women also complain of vulvar burning, dysuria, and

dyspareunia, particularly with involvement of vulvar skin. Examination often reveals edema, erythema, and excoriation; pustular lesions may be found to extend beyond the line of erythema when extensive skin involvement is present. Diagnosis is established by means of a KOH prep or fungal culture. Treatment is topical application of an antifungal preparation. (See vulvovaginal candidiasis in the Vaginal Discharge section above.)

■ **Allergic/irritative reaction:** Contact dermatitis frequently affects the vulvar skin, particularly the intertriginous areas; etiologic agents include urine or feces, latex, semen, cosmetic or therapeutic agents(including vaginal contraceptives, lubricants, sprays, perfumes, douches, fabric dyes, fabric softeners, synthetic fibers, bleaches, soaps, chlorine, dyes in toilet tissues, and local anesthetic creams); severe cases of dermatitis may be due to poison ivy or poison oak. Typical symptoms are itching, vulvar burning, and tenderness. Examination of the skin reveals erythema, edema, and inflammation; the skin may be weeping and eczematoid. Secondary infection may occur.

Treatment involves removing the offending agent. Severe lesions may be treated with wet compresses of Burow's solution diluted 1:20 for 30 minutes several times a day. If possible, the vulva should be dried with cool air from a hair dryer following the compresses. Lubricating agents such as Eucerin cream or petroleum jelly can help reduce the itching. Nonmedicated baby powders can be used to facilitate vulvar dryness. Symptomatic relief can be achieved with hydrocortisone (0.5% to 1%) or fluorinated corticosteroid (Valisone 0.1% or Synalar 0.01%) lotions or creams into the skin 2 to 3 times a day for a few days. Dermatitis due to poison ivy or poison oak nay require treatment with systemic corticosteroids. The use of white cotton undergarments is advisable, and tight-fitting clothing should be avoided.

■ **Scabies/lice**

● Scabies is a parasitic infection produced by the itch mite, *Sarcoptes scabiei*. The main symptom reported is severe, intermittent itching that tends to be more intense at night. Lesions can present as vesicles, papules, or burrows; any area of skin may be affected: the hands, wrists, breasts, vulva, and buttocks are most often infected. HIV-infected and other immunosuppressed patients are at increased risk for Norwegian scabies, a disseminated dermatologic infection; this can appear classically as hyperkeratotic, nonpruritic lesions or as crusting with pruritis, a pruritic, papular dermatitis, or lesions resembling psoriasis. (Schlesinger, 1994)

▶ CDC-recommended treatment for scabies (CDC,1998):

♦ Permethrin cream (5%) applied to all areas of the body from the neck down and washed off after 8 to 14 hours.

▶ Alternative regimens:

♦ Lindane (1%) one ounce of lotion or 30 grams of cream applied to all areas of the body from the neck down and washed off thoroughly after 8 hours OR Sulfur (6%) precipitated in ointment applied thinly to all areas nightly for 3 nights; previous applications should be washed off before new applications are applied. Thoroughly wash off 24 hours after last application.

♦ Lindane should not be used by pregnant or lactating women; or after a bath.

Itching may persist for days following treatment; antihistamine therapy should be considered for symptomatic relief. Norwegian scabies should be managed in consultation with an expert.

● Pediculosis pubis is due to infestation by the crab louse, *Phthirus pubis* or pubic louse. Transmission is by close contact, but the louse can also be acquired from bedding or towels. This infection is usually confined to the hairy areas of the vulva (eyelids are occasionally infested). The presenting symptom is constant itching in the pubic area. Eggs, adult lice, and fecal material can be seen upon close examination (without magnification). The diagnosis can be definitively established by microscopic visualization, as described above.

▶ The CDC-recommended treatment (CDC,1998) is permethrin 1% cream rinse applied to affected areas and washed off after 10 minutes. Alternatively, lindane 1% shampoo (applied for 4 minutes and thoroughly washed off; lindane not recommended for pregnant or lactating women) OR pyrethrins with piperonyl butoxide (applied to the affected area and washed off after 10 minutes). If symptoms do not resolve, patients should be re-examined in one week; if lice or eggs are seen at the hair-skin junction, the patient should be retreated. All clothing and bedding need to be decontaminated. Close household contacts and sexual contacts (within the previous month) should be treated.

XII. BREAST LUMP

A. HISTORY

If palpable by the patient, duration of the lump; any associated symptoms (e.g., tenderness, nipple discharge, cyclic pain); changes in the characteristics of the lump (e.g., increase in size); history of previous breast lumps; family history of breast disease or cancer.

B. PHYSICAL EXAM

Symmetry, contour, and appearance of the skin; presence of edema, erythema, skin dimpling, or nipple retraction; presence and size of dominant masses, nodularity, tenderness; nipple discharge (including color); and lymphadenopathy (axillary and supraclavicular).

C. EVALUATION

■ Mammogram: should be performed with any persistent palpable mass or other suspicious changes in the breast (e.g., bloody nipple discharge, skin retraction). A negative mammogram alone is not sufficient to rule out malignant pathology in a patient with a palpable breast mass; further evaluation and possible biopsy are indicated.

■ Ultrasound: most helpful to distinguish cystic and solid masses; useful initial test in younger women when simple cyst suspected.

■ Needle aspiration: for cystic lesion; fluid can be discarded if clear and if mass disappears; otherwise biopsy may be needed.

■ Biopsy: biopsy is indicated in cases of dominant mass (even with normal mammographic findings) or suspicious nonpalpable mammographic findings.

D. DIFFERENTIAL DIAGNOSIS AND MANAGEMENT

■ **Fibrocystic change**: Typically found among women who are 30 to 50 years old. Fibrocystic changes usually present as breast nodularity associated with cyclic bilateral pain or tenderness, which is worse premenstrually. Breast engorgement, increased density, and cyst formation are common and vary with menstrual cycle phase. The pain/discomfort associated with this condition can be relieved wearing a brassiere that gives adequate support. Analgesics can aid in symptomatic relief; some women have reported improvement of symptoms with vitamin E (400 IU a day) and decrease in caffeine consumption. Oral contraceptives are known to decrease benign breast disease. The appearance of a persistent dominant mass requires biopsy.

■ **Benign breast tumor**: most frequently diagnosed benign tumors of the breast are fibroadenomas, usually found in women aged 20 to 35. Typically, most masses are about 2 to 3 cm in diameter, although they can become much larger. Examination reveals a firm, smooth, rubbery mass that is freely mobile. Inflammation, skin dimpling, and nipple retraction are absent. On mammographic examination, the mass appears smooth with well-defined margins. Definitive diagnosis is established by means of biopsy. A fibroadenoma may simply be observed; however, a large, growing, or otherwise suspicious mass should be surgically excised.

■ **Breast cancer**: incidence of breast cancer increases with age; risk factors include positive family history, early menarche, late menopause, and nulliparity or late child-bearing. If a palpable mass is present, it is usually firm and nontender with irregular margins; it may be fixed to skin or underlying tissue. Definitive diagnosis is established by means of biopsy and referral to a surgeon is indicated. Although only a few cases of breast cancer have been reported among HIV-positive women, the unusual clinical presentations that have been noted, together with the rapid progression of disease that has been observed, have been suggestive of a "more virulent" course in the setting of HIV infection. (Guth, 1999)

XIII. MENOPAUSE

As HIV-positive women live longer and more women nearing menopause or postmenopausal become infected, menopausal issues become more important to consider and address. At the current time, there has been no documented association between HIV disease and premature ovarian failure.

Menopause is defined as the permanent cessation of menstruation caused by the loss of ovarian function. The mean age at which women undergo menopause is genetically predetermined and in the United States averages between 51 and 52 years of age. Certain medical conditions, such as osteoporosis and cardiovascular disease, have been linked to estrogen deficiency; associations have also been proposed between menopause and Alzheimer's disease and colon cancer. (Hurd, 1996; Mishell, 1997)

A. HISTORY

Last menstrual period and recent menstrual pattern (cycle length, duration and amount of flow); any irregular or intermenstrual bleeding or spotting; hot flashes; genitourinary dryness/atrophy; decreased libido; anxiety, irritability, sleep disturbances, and depression; difficulty with memory; urinary symptoms

B. PHYSICAL EXAM

Vagina appears smoother in contour, "drier"; may be more easily traumatized and more vulnerable to infection.

C. EVALUATION

If indicated, confirmation of menopause can be provided by an elevated serum follicle-stimulating hormone (FSH) level and a low estradiol level.

D. MANAGEMENT

■ **Hormone Replacement Therapy (HRT)**

The benefits and risks associated with HRT have been extensively studied among women who are HIV-negative. HRT is known to ameliorate symptoms of vasomotor instability (e.g., hot flashes, sleep disturbances, irritability, etc.) and urogenital atrophy (e.g., vaginal dryness, dyspareunia, etc.). More importantly, HRT is protective against cardiovascular disease and osteoporosis. Additional beneficial effects have been suggested with regards to prevention of Alzheimer's disease and colon cancer. One recent report found a trend towards increased survival among HIV-positive women on HRT and recommended that "HRT should be considered in the management of post-menopausal HIV-infected women who do not have an established contraindication as part of standard of care because of the documented known benefits among non-HIV-infected women." (Clark, 1997)

In addition to HRT, adequate calcium intake (1200 mg/day for menopausal women taking HRT; 1500 mg/day for women not on HRT) and the regular performance of weight-bearing exercise are important for bone protection.

Oral HRT can be administered in a continuous or cyclic fashion. The most commonly prescribed regimens are:

- Continuous therapy: Conjugated estrogens 0.625 mg po and medroxyprogesterone 2.5 to 5 mg po once daily (available in combined formulations).

- Cyclic therapy: Conjugated estrogens 0.625 mg po once daily and medroxyprogesterone 5–10 mg po once daily for 12–14 days per month.

Commonly used estrogen and progestin preparations are shown in Table 6–11. (ACOG, 1998)

TABLE 6-11: COMMONLY USED ESTROGEN AND PROGESTIN PREPARATIONS

ESTROGEN PREPARATIONS*	PROGESTIN PREPARATIONS**
Oral conjugated estrogen 0.625 mg	Medroxyprogesterone acetate 10 mg
Oral micronized estradiol 1 mg	Norethindrone 0.35 mg
Transdermal estradiol 0.05 mg/day	Micronized progesterone 200 mg
Oral esterified estrogen 0.625 mg	Progesterone vaginal suspension 90 mg
Estradiol vaginal ring	

* doses listed (with exception of vaginal ring) are approximately equivalent in terms of relative potency

** doses listed are approximately equivalent in terms of relative potency, with exception of noethindrone (approximately 0.5 relative potency)

The most common side effects associated with hormone replacement regimens are irregular vaginal bleeding and breast tenderness. There is an increased risk of endometrial cancer in women treated with estrogen-only hormone replacement. The addition of progestin to the regimen either cyclically or continuously (in women with a uterus) protects the endometrium and prevents the development of hyperplasia and cancer. There is a small increase in the risk of venous thromboembolism in women on HRT. The issue of the effects that HRT may have on the development of breast cancer remains controversial; although some studies have demonstrated an increase in risk that may be related to the duration of hormone replacement, other studies have found no increase in risk. Contraindications to HRT include: undiagnosed genital bleeding, active liver disease, recent myocardial infarction, active or prior history of thromboembolic disease, and breast or endometrial cancer.

■ **Alternatives to HRT**

- Progestin-only regimens (medroxyprogesterone acetate 10-30 mg or norethindrone 1–5 mg daily) may help relieve hot flashes in women who cannot or do not want to take estrogen-containing regimens.

- Non-hormonal lubricants or and moisturizers or Estring (vaginal ring with estradiol reservoir that is changed every 90 days — minimal systemic absorption) for the management of urogenital atrophy.

- Bisphosphonates (e.g., fosamax) for the prevention or treatment of osteoporosis.

- Selective Estrogen Receptor Modulators (SERMs) (Evista 60 mg po a day) offer bone and cardiovascular benefit without evidence of breast or endometrial stimulation; no effect on hot flashes, small increase in risk of venous thromboembolism.

XIV. HEALTH MAINTENANCE ISSUES (Hilliard, 1996)

■ **Gynecologic evaluation**: annually and as indicated by presence of symptoms, follow-up of ongoing problems, exposure to STDs, development of abnormal pap smear, or other need for referral based on primary care evaluation

■ **Pap smears**: twice within the first year of diagnosis and then annually; more frequent screening indicated with history of abnormal pap, HPV infection, after treatment for cervical dysplasia, and with symptomatic HIV disease

■ **STD screening**:
- annual syphilis screening or with development of neurologic signs/symptoms
- GC/chlamydia screening:offer annually at time of routine gynecologic visit; perform as indicated by the presence of relevant symptoms or findings on exam, with recent change in sexual partners, history of STD in sexual partner, periodically as indicated by sexual practices (commercial sex workers, multiple partners, inconsistent use of condoms), or with patient request

■ **Mammography**: baseline at 35–40 years; then every 1–2 years until age 50, then annually; women at increased risk (first degree family member(s) with breast cancer) should have annual screening after 40. Mammograph should be performed with presence of persistent palpable mass or other suspicious findings on exam

- **Sigmoidoscopy/colonoscopy**: sigmoidoscopy every 3–5 years after age 50; colonoscopy in women at increased risk (first-degree family member with colorectal cancer) every 3–5 years after age 40 or earlier with certain conditions (ulcerative colitis, familial polyposis, personal history of colon cancer)

XV. GUIDELINES FOR GYNECOLOGIC REFERRAL

In general referral to a gynecologic specialist should be considered under the following circumstances:

- Uncertain diagnosis with gynecologic condition part of differential diagnosis

- Inadequate response to standard treatment regimens for gynecologic conditions

- Possible need for surgical intervention

- A premalignant or malignant condition is suspected

REFERENCES

Adachi A, Fleming I, Burk RD, Ho GY, Klein RS.Women with human immunodeficiency virus and abnormal papanicolaou smears: a prospective study of colposcopy and clinical outcome. *Obstet Gynecol* 81:372–327, 1993.

American College of Obstetricians and Gynecologists. *Cervical cytology: Evaluation and management of abnormalities.* Technical Bulletin Number 183, August 1993.

American College of Obstetricians and Gynecologists. *Hormone replacement therapy.* Educational Bulletin Number 247, May 1998.

Anderson J, Clark RA, Watts DH, Till M, Arrastia C, Schuman P, et al. Idiopathic genital ulcers in women infected with Human Immunodeficiency Virus. *JAIDS* 3:343–7, 1996.

Anderson J, Cohen S, Kelly W, Shah K, Christensen C, Schuman P. Results of routine colposcopic examinations in women enrolled in the HIV epidemiology research study (HERS). Int Conf AIDS 11:309 (abst Tu.B.2255), Jul 7–12, 1996.

Augenbraun M, Feldman J, Chirgwin K, et al. Increased genital shedding of herpes simplex virus type 2 in HIV-seropositive women. *Ann Intern Med* 123:845–847, 1995.

Barbosa C, Macasaet M, Brockmann S, Sierra MF, Xia Z, Duerr A. Pelvic inflammatory disease and human immunodeficiency virus infection. *Obstet Gynecol* 89:65–70, 1997.

Brown DR, Bryan JT, Cramer H, Katz BP, Handy V, Fife KH. Detection of multiple human papillomavirus types in condylomata acuminata from immunosuppressed patients *J Infect Dis* 170:759–765, 1994.

Bukusi EA, Cohen CR, Stevens CE, et al. Effects of human immunodeficiency virus 1 infection on microbial origins of pelvic inflammatory disease and on efficacy of ambulatory oral therapy. *Am J Obstet Gynecol* 181:1374–1381, 1999.

Calista D Boschini A, Landi G. Resolution of disseminated molluscum contagiosum with Highly Active Anti-Retroviral Therapy (HAART) in patients with AIDS. *Eur J Dermatol* 9:211–3, 1999.

Cassone A, DeBernardis F, Torosantucci A, Tacconelli E, Tumbarello M, Cauda R. In vitro and in vivo anticandidal activity of human immunodeficiency virus protease inhibitors. *J Infect Dis* 180:448–453, 1999.

Centers for Disease Control and Prevention. 1998 Guidelines for treatment of sexually transmitted diseases. *MMWR* 47:1–116, 1998.

Centers for Disease Control and Prevention. *HIV/AIDS Surveillance Report,* Vol.11, No.1, Mid-year edition, 1999.

Chiasson MA. Declining AIDS mortality in New York City. New York City Department of Health. *Bull N Y Acad Med* 74:151–152, 1997.

Chiasson M, Ellerbrock TV, Bush TJ, Sun XW, Wright TC. Increased prevalence of vulvovaginal condyloma and vulvar intraepithelia neoplasia in women infected with the human immunodeficiency virus. *Obstet Gynecol* 89:690-694, 1997.

Chirgwin K, Feldman J, Augenbraun M, Landesman S, Minkoff H.. Incidence of venereal warts in human immunodeficiency virus-infected and uninfected women. *J Infect Dis* 172:235–238, 1995.

Chirgwin KD, Feldman J, Muneyyirci-Delale O, et al. Menstrual function in Human Immunodeficiency Virus-infected women without Acquired Immunodeficiency Syndrome. *Journal of Acquired Immune Deficiency Syndromes and Human Retrovirology* 12:489–94, 1996.

Clark RA, Bessinger R. Clinical manifestations and predictors of survival in older women infected with HIV. *J Acquir Immune Defic Syndr Hum Retrovirol* 15:341–345, 1997.

Cohen CR, Sinei S, Reilly M, Bukusi E, et al. Effect of human immunodeficiency virus type 1 infection upon acute salpingitis: a laparoscopic study. *J Infect Dis* 178:1352–1358, 1998.

Cu-Uvin S, Hogan JW, Warren D, et al. Prevalence of lower genital tract infections among human immunodeficiency virus (HIV)-seropositive and high risk HIV-seronegative women. HIV Epidemiology Research Study Group. *Clin Infect Dis* 29:1145–1150, 1999.

Draper D, Donohoe W, Mortimer L, Heine RP. Cysteine proteases of Trichomonas vaginalis degrade secretory leukocyte protease inhibitor. *JID* 178:815–9, 1998.

Droegemueller W. Benign gynecologic lesions in: *Comprehensive Gynecology,* 3rd Edition (Mishell DR, Stenchever MA, Droegemueller W, Herbst AL, eds.) St. Louis: Mosby, 1997.

Duerr A, Sierra MF, Feldman J, Clarke LM, Ehrlich I, DeHovitz J. Immune compromise and prevalence of Candida vulvovaginitis in human immunodeficiency virus-infected women. *Obstet Gynecol* 90:252–256, 1997.

Duerr A, Shah K, Schuman P, Klein RS, Cu-Uvin S. The effect of highly active antiretroviral therapy (HAART) on cervcial dysplasia and HPV infection among HIV-infected women. Int Conf AIDS 12:1052 (abst 60289), 1998.

Duska LR, Flynn CF, Chen A, Whall-Strojwas D, Goodman A. Clinical evaluation of atypical glandular cells of undetermined significance on cervical cytology. *Obstet Gynecol* 91:278–282, 1998.

Ellerbrock TV, Chiasson MA, Bush TJ, et al. Incidence of cervical squamous intraepithelial lesions in HIV-infected women. *JAMA* 282:1031–1037, 2000.

Ellerbrock TV, Wright TC, Bush TJ, et al. Characteristics of menstruation in women infected with Human Immunodeficiency Virus. *Obstet Gynecol* 87:1030-4, 1996.

El-Sadr W, Schuman P, Peng G, Capps L, Neaton J. Predictors of mucosal candidiasis among HIV-infected women. Natl Conf Women HIV :107 (abst 103.3), May 4–7, 1997.

Evander M, Edlund K, Gustafsson A, et al. Human Papillomavirus infection is transient in young women: a population-based cohort study. *J Infect Dis* 171:1026–1030, 1995.

Fleming DT, McQuillan GM, Johnson RE, Nahmias AJ, Aral SO, Lee FK, St. Louis ME. Herpes simplex virus type 2 in the United States, 1976 to 1994. *N Engl J Med* 337:1105–11, 1997.

Fruchter R, Maiman M, Sedlis A, Bartley L, Camilien L, Arrastia CD. Multiple recurrences of cervical intraepithelial neoplasia in women with the human immunodeficiency virus. *Obstet Gynecol* 87:338–344, 1996.

Frankel RE, Selwyn PA, Mezger J, Andrews S. High prevalence of gynecologic disease among hospitalized women with Human Immunodeficiency Virus infection. *Clin Infect Dis* 25:706–12, 1997.

Garzetti GG, Ciavattini A, Butini L, Vecchi A, Montroni M. Cervical dysplasia in HIV-seropositive women: role of human papillomavirus infection and immune status. *Gynecol Obstet Invest* 40:52–6, 1995.

Giannacopoulos KC, Hatzidaki EG, Papanicolaou NC, Relakis KJ, Kokori HG, Giannacopoulos CC. Genital tuberculosis in a HIV-infected woman: A case report. *Eur J Obstet Gynecol* Reprod Biol 80:227–9, 1998.

Giovanna O, Signori R, Fasolo MM, Schiavini M, Casella A, Gargnel A. Impact of HAART on clinical evolution of genital warts in HIV-positive patients. Int Conf AIDS 12:301 (abst 22192), 1998.

Greenblatt RM, Bacchetti P, Barkan S, et al. Lower genital tract infections among HIV-infected and high-risk uninfected women: findings fof the Women's Interagency HIV Study (WIHS). *Sex Transm Dis* 26:143–151, 1999.

Guth AA, Breast cancer and HIV: what do we know? *Am Surg* 65:209–211, 1999.

Heard I, Schmitz V, Costagliola D, Orth G, Kazatchkine MD. Early regression of cervical lesions in HIV-seropositive women receiving highly active antiretroviral therapy. *AIDS* 12:1459–1464, 1998.

Heng M, Heng S, Allen S. Coinfection and synergy of human immunodeficiency virus-1 and herpes simplex virus. *Lancet* 343:255–8, 1994.

Hillemanns P, Ellerbrock TV, McPhillips S, et al. Prevalence of anal cytologic abnormalities and anal human papillomavirus infections in HIV-seropositive women. *AIDS* 10:1641–1647, 1996.

Hillard PA. Preventive Health Care and Screening in: *Novak's Gynecology,* 12th Edition (Berek JS, ed.). Baltimore: Williams & Wilkins, 1996.

Ho GH, Bierman R, Beardsley L, Chang CJ, Burk RD. Natural history of cervicovaginal papillomavirus infection in young women. *N Engl J Med* 338:423–428,1998.

Hoegsberg B, Abulafia O, Sedlis A, et al. Sexually transmitted diseases and human immunodeficiency virus infection among women with pelvic inflammatory disease. *Am J Obstet Gynecol* 163:1135–1139, 1990.

Holcomb K, Abulafia O, Matthews RP, et al. The significance of ASCUS cytology in HIV-positive women. *Gynecol Oncol* 75:118–121, 1999.

Holcomb K, Abulafia O, Matthews RP, Chapman JE, Borges A, Lee YC, Buhl A. The significance of ASCUS cytology in HIV-positive women. *Gynecol Oncol* 75:118–21, 1999.

Holcomb K, Matthews RP, Chapman JE, et al. The efficacy of cervical conization in the treatment of cervical intraepithelial neoplasia in HIV-positive women. *Gynecol Oncol* 74:428–431, 1999.

Hook EW and Hansfield HH. Gonococcal infections in the adult. In *Sexually Transmitted Diseases* 3rd Edition. (Holmes, Sparling, Mardh, et al. Eds) NY: McGrawHill, 1999.

Hurd WW. Menopause in: *Novak's Gynecology*, 12th Edition (Berek JS, ed.). Baltimore: Williams & Wilkins, 1996.

Jacobson JM, Greenspan JS, Spritzler J, et al. Thalidomide for the treatment of oral aphthous ulcers in patients with human immunodeficiency virus infection. National Institutes of Allergy and Infectious Diseases AIDS Clinical Trials Group. *N Engl J Med* 336:1487–1493, 1997.

Jacobson JM, Spritzler J, Fox L, et al. Thalidomide for the treatment of esophageal aphthous ulcers in patients with human immunodeficiency virus infection. National Institutes of Allergy and Infectious Disease AIDS Clinical Trials Group. *J Infect Dis* 180:61–67, 1999.

Kamenga MC, De Cock KM, St Louis ME, et al. The impact of human immunodeficiency virus infection on pelvic inflammatory disease: a case-control study in Abidjan, Ivory Coast. *Am J Obstet Gynecol* 172:919–925, 1995.

Kennedy AW, Salmieri SS, Wirth SL, Biscotti CV, Tuason LJ, Travarca MJ. Results of the clinical evaluation of atypical glandular cells of undetermined significance (ACGUS) detected on cervical cytology screening. *Gynecol Oncol* 63:14–8, 1996.

Kerr-Layton JA, Stamm CA, Peterson LS, McGregor JA. Chronic plasma cell endometritis in hysterectomy specimens of HIV-infected women: a retrospective analysis. *Infect Dis Obstet Gynecol* 6:186–190, 1998.

Klevens RM, Fleming PL, Mays MA, Frey R. Characteristics of women with AIDS and invasive cancer. *Obstet Gynecol* 88:269–273, 1996.

Korn AP, Abercrombie PD, Foster A. Vulvar intraepithelial neoplasia in women infected with human immunodeficiency virus-1. *Gynecol Oncol* 61:384–386, 1995.

Korn AP, Judson PL, Zaloudek CJ. Importance of atypical glandular cells of uncertain significance in cervical cytologic smears. *J Reprod Med* 43:774–778, 1998.

Korn A, Landers DV, Green JR, Sweet RL. Pelvic inflammatory disease in human immunodeficiency virus-infected women. *Obstet Gynecol* 82:765–768, 1993.

Li RK, Frankel R, Kirkpatrick WR,et al. Mycology, molecular epidemiology, and drug susceptibility of yeasts from vulvo-vaginal candidiasis in HIV-infected women. *Am Soc Microbiol* 97:270 (abst F63) May 4–8, 1997.

Luque AE, Demeter LM, Reichman RC. Association of human papilomavirus infection and disease with magnitude of human immunodeficiency virus type 1 (HIV-1) RNA plasma level among women with HIV-1 infection. *J Infect Dis* 179:1405–1409, 1999.

Maiman M. Management of cervical neoploasia in human immunodeficiency virus-infected women. *J Natl Cancer Inst Monogr* 23:43–49, 1998.

Maiman M, Fruchter RG, Guy L, Cuthill S, Levine P, Serur E. Human immunodeficiency virus infection and invasive cervical carcinoma. *Cancer* 71:402–406, 1993.

Maiman M, Fruchter RG, Serur E, Remy JC, Feuer G, Boyce J. Human immunodeficiency virus infection and cervical neoplasia. *Gynecol Oncol* 38:377–382, 1990.

Maiman M, Watts DH, Andersen J, Clax P, Merino M, Kendall MA. Vaginal 5-fluorouracil for high-grade dysplasia in human immunodeficiency virus infection: a randomized trial. *Obstet Gynecol* 94:P954–961, 1999.

Manos MM, Kinney WK, Hurley LB, Sherman ME, Shieh-Ngai J, Kurman RJ, et al. Identifying women with cervical neoplasia: Using human papillomavirus DNA testing for equivocal Papanicolaou results. *JAMA* 281:1605–10, 1999.

Martin HL, Richardson BA, Nyange PM et al. Vaginal lactobacilli, microbial flora, and risk of human immunodeficiency virus type 1 and sexually transmitted disease acquisition. *J Infect Dis* 180:1863–1868, 1999.

Minkoff HL, Eisenberger-Matityahu D, Feldman J, Burk R, Clarke L. Prevalence and incidence of gynecologic disorders among women infected with human immunodeficiency virus. *Am J Obstet Gynecol* 180:824–836, 1999.

Minkoff H, Feldman J, DeHovitz J, Landesman S, Burk R.. A longitudinal study of human papillomavirus carriage in human immunodeficiency virus-infected and human immunodeficiency virus-uninfected women. *Am J Obstet Gynecol* 178:982–986, 1998.

Mishell DR. Abnormal uterine bleeding in: *Comprehensive Gynecology,* 3rd Edition (Mishell DR, Stenchever MA, Droegemueller W, Herbst AL, eds.) St. Louis: Mosby, 1997.

Mishell DR. Menopause in: *Comprehensive Gynecology,* 3rd Edition (Mishell DR, Stenchever MA, Droegemueller W, Herbst AL, eds.) St. Louis: Mosby, 1997.

Mostad SB, Kreiss JK, Ryncarz AJ, et al. Cervical shedding of herpes simplex virus in human immunodeficiency virus-infected women: effects of hormonal contraception, pregnancy, and vitamin A deficiency. *J Infect Dis* 181:58–63, 2000.

National Cancer Institute Workshop. The 1988 Bethesda System for reporting cervical/vaginal cytological diagnoses. *JAMA* 262:931–4, 1989.

Neary B, Young SB, Reuter KL, Cheeseman S, Savarese D. Ovarian Burkitt lymphoma: pelvic pain in a woman with AIDS. *Obstet Gynecol* 88:706–708, 1996.

Neilsen H. Hypermenorrhea associated with ritonavir. *Lancet* 353:811–812, 1999.

Olinger GG, Hashemi FB, Sha BE, Spear GT. Association of indicators of bacterialvaginosis with a female genital tract factor that induces expression of HIV-1. *AIDS* 13:1905–1912, 1999.

Palefsky JM, Minkoff H, Kalish LA et al. Cervicovaginal human papillomavirus infection in human immunodeficiency virus-1 (HIV)-positive and high risk HIV-negative women. *J Natl Cancer Inst* 91:226–236, 1999.

Petry KU, Bohmer G, Iftner T, Femming P, Stoll M, Schmidt RE. Human papillomavirus testing in primary screening for cervical cancer of human immunodeficiency virus-infected women, 1990-1998. *Gynecol Oncol* 75:427–431, 1999.

Petry KU, Kochel H, Bode U et al. Human papillomavirus is associated with the frequent detection of warty and basaloid high-grade neoplasia of the vulva and cervical neoplasia among immunocompromised women. *Gynecol Oncol* 60:30-34, 1996.

Reyes M, Graber J, Reeves W. Acyclovir-resistant HSV: preliminary results from a national surveillance system. Abstract presented at International Conference on Emerging Infectious Diseases; March 10, 1998, Atlanta, Georgia.

Rojansky N, Anteby SO. Gynecological neoplasias in the patient with HIV infection. *Obstet Gynecol* Surv 51:679–683, 1996.

Schuman P, Capps L, Peng G, et al. Weekly fluconazole for the prevention of mucosal candidiasis in women with HIV infection. A randomized, double-blind, placebo-controlled trial. Terry Beirn Community Programs for Clinical Research on AIDS. *Ann Intern Med* 126:689–696, 1997.

Schuman P, Sobel J, Ohmit SE, et al. Mucosal candidal colonization and candidiasis in women with or at risk for human immunodeficiency virus infection. HIV Epidemiology Research Study (HERS). *Clin Infect Dis* 27:1161–1167, 1998.

Schuman P, Sobel J, Ohmit S, Mayer K, Klein R, Rompalo A, et al. Fluconazole resistance among oral and vaginal Candida isolates, the HER study. Natl Conf Women HIV, 1997;107 (abstract no. 103.2).

Schuman P, Sobel J, Ohmit S, et al. Fluconazole resistance among oral and vaginal Candida isolates. The HER study. Natl Conf Women HIV 107 (abst # 103.2), 1997.

Shah KV, Munoz A, Klein RS, et al. Prolonged persistence of genital human papillomavirus infections in HIV-infected women. Int Conf AIDS 11:345 (abst Tu.C.2466), July 7–12,1996.

Shah PN, Smith JR, Wells C, et al. Menstrual symptoms in women infected by the Human Immunodeficiency Virus. *Obstet Gynecol* 83:397–400, 1994.

Six C, Heard I, Bergeron C, et al. Comparative prevalence, incidence and short-term prognosis of cervical squamous intraepithelial lesions amongst HIV-positive and HIV-negative women. *AIDS* 12:1047–1056, 1998.

Sloand EM, Klein HG, Banks SM, Vareldzis B, Merritt S, Pierce P. Epidemiology of thrombocytopenia in HIV infection. *Eur J Haematol* 48:168–72, 1992.

Sobel, J. Chapter on treating candida. In *Sexually Transmitted Diseases* 3rd Edition. (Holmes, Sparling, Mardh, et al. Eds) NY: McGrawHill, 1999.

Sorvillo F, Kovacs A, Kerndt P, Stek A, Muderspach L, Sanchez-Keeland L. Risk factors for trichomoniasis among women with human immunodeficiency virus (HIV) infection at a public clinic in Los Angeles County, California: implications for HIV prevention. *Am J Trop Med Hyg* 58:495–5000, 1998.

Sperling RS, Friedman F, Joyner M, Brodman M, Dottino P. Seroprevalence of human immunodeficiency virus in women admitted to the hosptial with pelvic inflammatory disease. *J Reprod Med* 36:122–124, 1991.

Spinillo A, Capuzzo E, Tenti P, De Santolo A, Piazzi G, Iasci A. Adequacy of screening cervical cytology among human immunodeficiency virus seropositive women. *Gynecol Oncol* 69:109–113, 1998.

Stamm WE. Chlamydia trachomatis infections of the adult. In *Sexually Transmitted Diseases* 3rd Edition. (Holmes, Sparling, Mardh, et al. Eds) NY: McGrawHill, 1999.

Sun XW, Ellerbrock TV, Lungu O, Chiasson MA, Bush TJ, Wright TC. Human papillomavirus infection in HIV-seropositive women. *Obstet Gynecol* 85:680-686, 1995.

Sun XW, Kuhn L, Ellerbrock TV, Chiasson MA, Bush TJ, Wright TC. Human papillomavirus infection in women infected with the human immunodeficiency virus. *N Engl J Med* 337:1343–1349, 1997.

Uberti-Foppa C, Origoni M, Maillard M, et al. Evaluation of the detection of human papillomavirus genotypes in cervical specimens by hybrid capture as screening for precancerous lesions in HIV-positive women. *J Med Virol* 56:133–137, 1998.

Weber T, Chin K, Sidhu JS, Janssen RS. Prevalence of invasive cervical cancer among HIV-infected and uninfected hospital patients, 1994–1995. Conf Retroviruses Opportunistic Infect 1998, 5th:213 (abstract no. 717).

Williams A, Darragh TM, Vranizan K, Ochia C, Moss AR, Palefsky JM. Anal and cervical human papillomavirus infection and risk of anaol and cervical epithelial abnormalities in human immunodeficiency virus-infected women. *Obstet Gynecol* 83:205–211, 1994.

Wright T, Sun XW. Anogenital papillomavirus infection and neoplasia in immunodeficient women. *Obstet Gynecol* Clin N Am 23:861–893, 1996.

Wright TC, Moscarelli RD, Dole P, Ellerbrock TV, Chiasson MA, Vandevanter N. Significance of mild cytologic atypia in women infected with human immunodeficiency virus. *Obstet Gynecol* 87:515–519, 1996.

COLOR PLATES

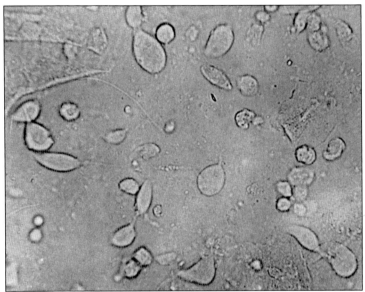

PLATE 1. Tricholmonads in a saline wet mount (high power). (Monif, 1982; Fig. 22-2)

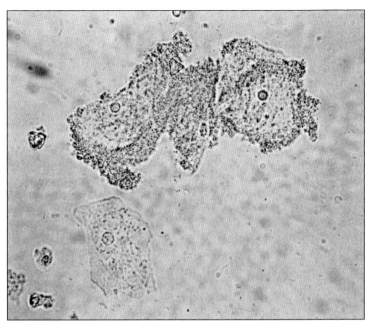

PLATE 2. Clue cells of *G vaginalis* vaginitis on a saline wet mount (high power). (Monif, 1982; Fig. 22-3)

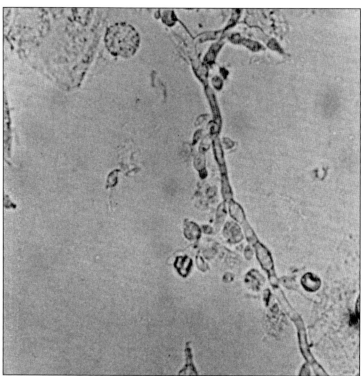

COLOR PLATE 3. *Candida* in a saline wet mount (high power). (Monif, 1982; Fig. 22-4B)

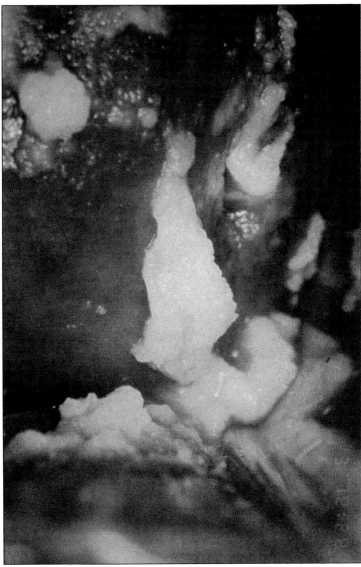

COLOR PLATE 4. Vaginal candidiasis: thrush patches on the vaginal wall of a patient with candidiasis. (J, Anderson, MD, ed.)

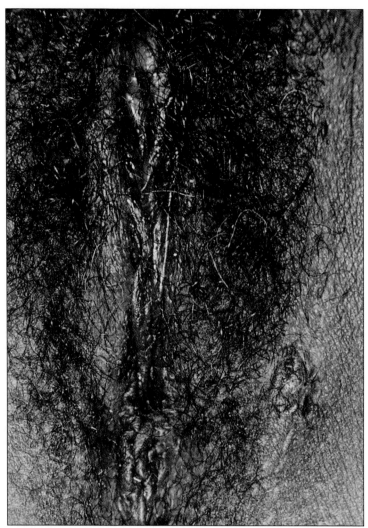

COLOR PLATE 5. Severe vulvar intraepithelial neoplasia (VIN3). (Wilkinson and Stone, 1995; Fig 6.27)

COLOR PLATES

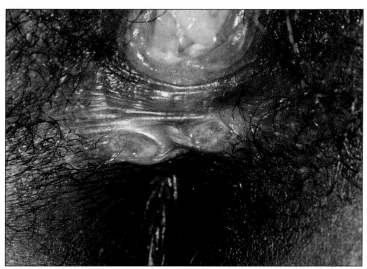

COLOR PLATE 6. Nontender chancres (Kissing lesions) in a woman with primary syphilis. (Wilkinson and Stone, 1995; Fig 8.46)

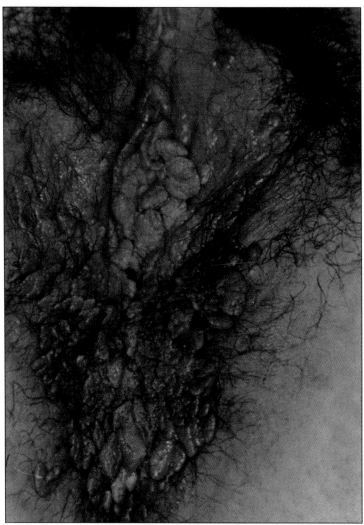

COLOR PLATE 7. Extensive vulvar condylomata accuminata (HPV). (Wilkinson and Stone, 1995; Fig 9.3)

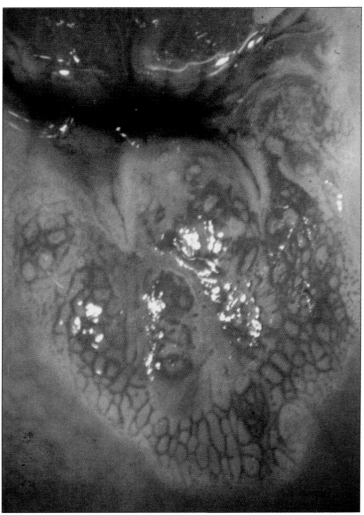

COLOR PLATE 8. Cervical intraepithelial neoplasia (CIN3) demonstrating coarse mosaicism and punctuation on posterior lip. (Burghardt, 1991; Fig. 11.37)

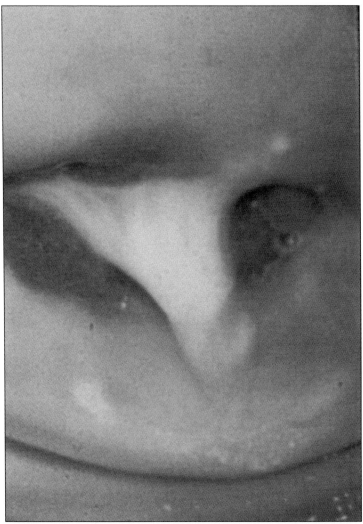

COLOR PLATES

COLOR PLATE 9. Mucopurulent cervicitis caused by *C. trachomatis*. (Holmes, 1999; Plate 16)

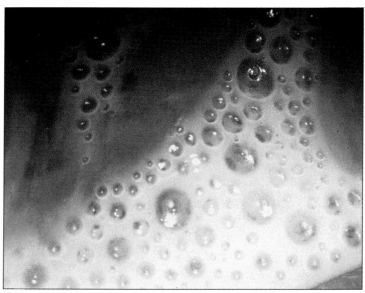

COLOR PLATE 10. Profuse purulent frothy vaginal discharge due to trichomonas. (Holmes, 1999; Plate 21)

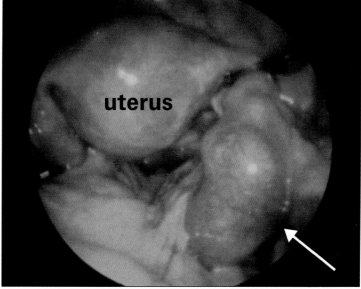

COLOR PLATE 11. PID, proven chlamydial pyosalpinx. Right tube is swollen and tortuous (arrow). (Holmes, 1999; Plate 17)

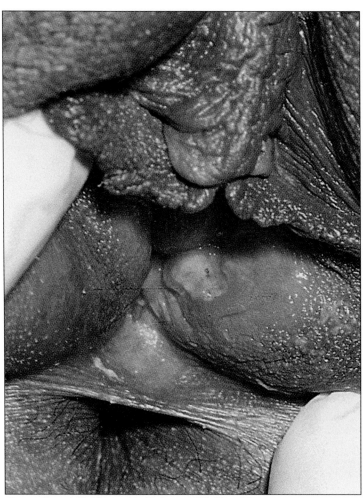

COLOR PLATE 12. Chancroid. (Holmes, 1999; Plate 32)

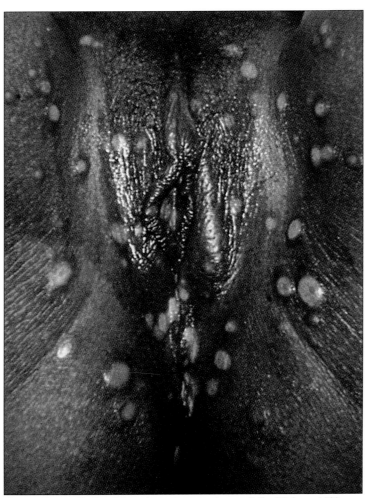

COLOR PLATE 13. Condyloma latum in secondary syphilis. (Holmes, 1999; Plate 47)

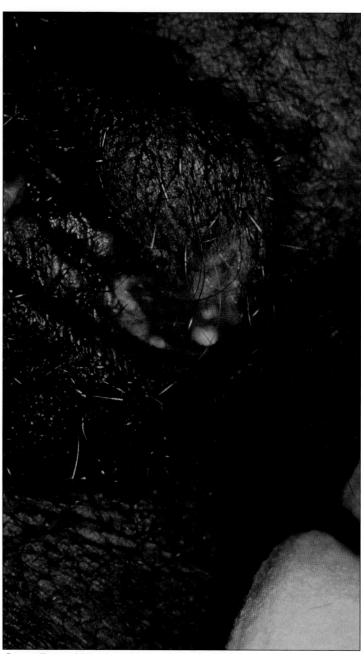

Color Plate 14. Lesion of herpes simplex. (J, Anderson, MD, ed.)

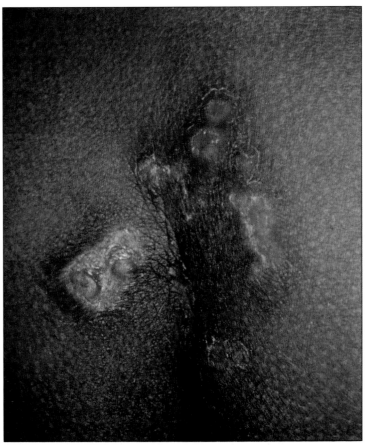

COLOR PLATE 15. Herpes simplex (HSV) in woman with AIDS, CD4<50.
(J, Anderson, MD, ed.)

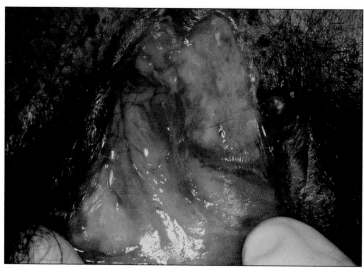

COLOR PLATE 16. Apthous genital ulceration. (J, Anderson, MD, ed.)

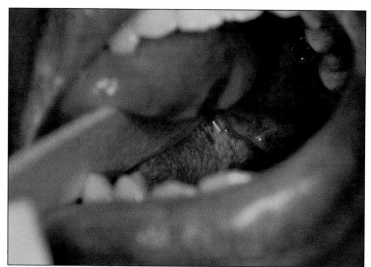

COLOR PLATE 17. Apthous oral ulceration. (J, Anderson, MD, ed.)

REFERENCES

Burghardt, Erich. *Colposcopy – Cervical Pathology – Textbook and Atlas,* 2nd Revised and Enlarged Edition. NY: Thieme Medical Publishers Inc, 1991.

Holmes, King K, Sparling, P Frederick, Mardh, per-Anders, et al. *Sexually Transmitted Diseases,* 3rd Edition. NY: McGraw Hill, 1999.

Monif, Gilles RG. *Infectious Diseases in Obstetrics and Gynecology.* Philadelphia: Harper and Row Publishers, 1982.

Wilkinson, Edward J and Stone, I Keith. *Atlas of Vulvar Disease.* Baltimore: Williams & Wilkins, 1995.

VII: HIV AND REPRODUCTION
Jean Anderson, MD

I. INTRODUCTION

The ability to become pregnant and to bear children is uniquely female. With increasing numbers of HIV-infected women, 80% of whom are of childbearing age, and concerns about perinatal transmission of HIV, pregnancy in the setting of HIV infection has been a focus of much interest, research, and often discrimination. From 1989–1994 it was estimated that 1.5 to 1.7/1000 U.S. childbearing women were HIV-positive (Davis, 1998); however, this number may grow as more women become infected through sexual exposure, often unaware of their risk, and as more women who know they are infected choose to become pregnant because of therapeutic advances in care and prevention of vertical transmission.

This chapter will review issues related to contraception and pregnancy and will discuss guidelines for care during pregnancy to optimize the health of both the mother and and the fetus and infant.

II. COUNSELING

For women known to be HIV-infected, education and counseling about pregnancy and HIV should be done early in the course of HIV care, not delayed until the woman is pregnant, so that decisions about contraception and if or when to get pregnant can be most informed and carefully considered. Over one-half of pregnancies in US women are unplanned and many of the risk factors for unintended pregnancy also place women at increased risk for HIV. These include:

- substance abuse (patient or partner)
- mental illness
- domestic violence

Women with advanced HIV disease and HIV dementia may be at increased risk for unintended pregnancy if they are dependent on a contraceptive method (such as condom use or oral contraceptives) which requires negotiation with a sexual partner or other ongoing patient action (i.e., remembering to take pills).

Issues to discuss when counseling about reproductive issues are listed in Table 7-1.

TABLE 7-1: HIV AND PREGNANCY COUNSELING ISSUES
■ Impact of HIV on pregnancy course/outcome
■ Impact of pregnancy on HIV progression
■ Other reproductive issues based on maternal factors
• coexisting drug/alcohol
• advanced maternal age
• hypertension, diabetes, etc.
■ Long term health of mother and care for children (guardianship issues)
■ Perinatal transmission
■ Use of antiretrovirals and other medications in pregnancy
■ Safe conception if partner HIV negative

III. CONTRACEPTION

The majority of HIV-infected US women use some form of contraception, most commonly condoms. (Wilson, 1996; Watts, 1999) Women using no form of contraception do not necessarily intend to become pregnant but may lack significant power in their sexual relationship, be under pressure from partner or family to have children, be unaware of their options concerning contraception or believe they cannot become pregnant, have a disorganized lifestyle that precludes consistent use of contraception, or simply have decided to take their chances. Unplanned also does not necessarily mean unwanted; several studies show low rates of elective pregnancy termination in HIV-positive women (Smits, 1999; Greco, 1999) and no significant difference in repeat pregnancy rates in HIV-positive compared to HIV-negative women from an inner-city population. (Lindsay, 1995) Table 7-2 outlines currently available methods of contraception, their effectiveness, side effects and contraindications, and non-contraceptive benefits.

Hormonal methods of contraception, particularly oral contraceptives, can have significant drug interactions, resulting in either decreased contraceptive effectiveness or increased or decreased concentrations of the co-administered drug. Use of nelfinavir, ritonavir, amprenavir, and efavirenz may be associated with decrease in effectiveness of oral contraceptives (and possible increase in break-through bleeding); an alternative or additional method should be used. (CDC, 1998) Other medications which are known to interact with oral contraceptives (and in some cases with progestin-only contraceptives) include tetracyclines, penicillin, oral hypoglycemic agents, rifampin, tricyclic antidepressants, oral anticoagulants, beta-blockers, methyldopa, vitamin C, benzodiazepines, and seizure medications. Clinicians treating women who are at risk for drug interactions should review the need for possible use of alternative methods of contraception or dose adjustment for the interacting agent.

Concerns have been raised about possible increased risk of HIV transmission or acquisition in hormonal contraceptive users. There is evidence that both combined oral contraceptives and progestin-only contraceptives may increase genital tract HIV shedding; furthermore, oral contraceptives have

TABLE 7-2: CONTRACEPTIVE METHODS

METHOD	FAILURE RATES % PREGNANCIES IN FIRST YEAR OF TYPICAL AND PERFECT USE		CONTRAINDICATIONS	BENEFITS	POTENTIAL SIDE EFFECTS	CONVENIENCE	DISADVANTAGES	COST (PUBLIC PROVIDER-MANAGED CARE SETTING)
	TYPICAL	PERFECT						
HORMONAL								
Oral Contraceptive Pill	3	.1	hx/o of CVD, DVT, stroke hypertension high LDL/HDL ratio > 35 and heavy smoker markedly impaired liver function hepatocellular adenoma headache with focal neurologic symptoms diabetes with nephro--pathy, retinopathy, neuropathy, or vascular disease breast cancer major surgery with immobilization	decreased menstrual pain, PMS and blood loss may reduce acne decreased benign breast disease decreased functional ovarian cysts decreased ovarian and endometrial cancers decreased pelvic inflammatory disease (PID)	nausea headache weight gain dizziness breast tenderness vaginal spotting chloasma depression	use independent from sexual intercourse	no STD protection may increase susceptibility to some STDs	$17.70–$21.00

Table continues . . .

Table 7-2: Contraceptive Methods *(continued)*

Method	Failure Rates % Pregnancies in First Year of Typical and Perfect Use		Contraindications	Benefits	Potential Side Effects	Convenience	Disadvantages	Cost (Public Provider-Managed Care Setting)
	Typical	Perfect						
Depo-medroxy-progestone acetate (DMPA)	.3	.3	unexplained vaginal bleeding breast cancer	decreased risk of seizures may have protective effects against PID and ovarian & endometrial cancer decreased blood loss, anemia amenorrhea	menstrual changes (spotting, irregular bleeding, amenorrhea) weight gain breast tenderness headache adverse effect on lipids depression	often causes amenorrhea requires only 4 injections a year requires no ongoing action by user use independent from sexual intercourse.	same as above	$30.00 q 3 months plus visit cost
Norplant	.09	.09	same as above	same as above	tenderness or infection at site menstrual changes hair loss weight gain breast tenderness depression	provides 5 years of contraception requires no ongoing action by user use independent from sexual intercourse	same as above	Implant — $365.00 Insertion — $62.00–$333.00 Removal — $79.64–$100.00

Table continues . . .

TABLE 7-2: CONTRACEPTIVE METHODS *(continued)*

METHOD	FAILURE RATES % PREGNANCIES IN FIRST YEAR OF TYPICAL AND PERFECT USE		CONTRAINDICATIONS	BENEFITS	POTENTIAL SIDE EFFECTS	CONVENIENCE	DISADVANTAGES	COST (PUBLIC PROVIDER-MANAGED CARE SETTING)
	TYPICAL	PERFECT						
Progestin only pill	1.1–13.8	.5	same as above	same as above	menstrual changes (spotting, irregular bleeding, amenorrhea) breast tenderness depression weight gain	use independent from sexual intercourse	no STD protection ectopic pregnancy more likely among progestin only pills than other forms of hormonal contraception	$100.00–$300.00 a year
BARRIER METHODS								
* Condom — male	12	3	latex allergy	protects against STDs, including HIV delays premature ejaculation	allergy or sensitivity to latex decreased sensitivity	inexpensive and readily available does not require a prescription	requires partner possible cooperation loss of spontaneity during sex	$.33–$1.00

Table continues . . .

VII

TABLE 7-2: CONTRACEPTIVE METHODS *(continued)*

| METHOD | FAILURE RATES % PREGNANCIES IN FIRST YEAR OF TYPICAL AND PERFECT USE | | CONTRAINDICATIONS | BENEFITS | POTENTIAL SIDE EFFECTS | CONVENIENCE | DISADVANTAGES | COST (PUBLIC PROVIDER-MANAGED CARE SETTING) |
	TYPICAL	PERFECT						
Condom — female	21 limited data	5	polyurethane allergy	protects against STDs, including HIV	allergy or sensitivity to polyurethane	woman controlled less likelihood of breakage can be inserted up to 8 hrs before intercourse does not require a prescription	may be awkward to use aesthetically unappealing to some	$1.25–$3.66

Table continues . . .

TABLE 7-2: CONTRACEPTIVE METHODS (continued)

METHOD	FAILURE RATES % PREGNANCIES IN FIRST YEAR OF TYPICAL AND PERFECT USE		CONTRAINDICATIONS	BENEFITS	POTENTIAL SIDE EFFECTS	CONVENIENCE	DISADVANTAGES	COST (PUBLIC PROVIDER-MANAGED CARE SETTING)
	TYPICAL	PERFECT						
Cervical cap — Parous	36	26	latex allergy	limited STD protection	pelvic pressure	woman controlled	efficacy based on high motivation	$19.00–$31.00 q 3 years + office visit & spermicide
			abnormal cervical/ vaginal anatomy		vaginal irritation	can be inserted ahead of time	spermicide re-application required with each act of coitus	
Nonparous	18	9	hx/o Toxic Shock Syndrome (TSS) or recurrent urinary tract infections (UTI)		allergy or sensitivity to latex			
			known or suspected cervical/uterine malignancy		vaginal or urinary tract infections		should not be used during menses	
			abnormal pap					
			vaginal or cervical infection					
			recent delivery or spontaneous/induced abortion					

Table continues . . .

TABLE 7-2: CONTRACEPTIVE METHODS (continued)

METHOD	FAILURE RATES % PREGNANCIES IN FIRST YEAR OF TYPICAL AND PERFECT USE		CONTRAINDICATIONS	BENEFITS	POTENTIAL SIDE EFFECTS	CONVENIENCE	DISADVANTAGES	COST (PUBLIC PROVIDER-MANAGED CARE SETTING)
	TYPICAL	PERFECT						
Diaphragm	18	6	latex allergy abnormal vaginal anatomy hx/o TSS or recurrent UTIs	limited STD protection reduces risk of PID	same as above	woman controlled can be inserted up to 6 hrs before intercourse	same as above, except may be used during menses	$15.00–$18.00 q 3 years + office visit & spermicide
Spermicides	21	6	allergy to nonoxynol-9	protection against some STDs, significant against gonorrhea/chlamydia *in vitro* activity against HIV	vaginal irritation allergy vaginal and urinary tract infection	woman controlled does not require a prescription easily available and inexpensive	efficacy reduced when used without a barrier method	$8.75–$12.00

Table continues . . .

TABLE 7-2: CONTRACEPTIVE METHODS *(continued)*

METHOD	FAILURE RATES % PREGNANCIES IN FIRST YEAR OF TYPICAL AND PERFECT USE		CONTRAINDICATIONS	BENEFITS	POTENTIAL SIDE EFFECTS	CONVENIENCE	DISADVANTAGES	COST (PUBLIC PROVIDER-MANAGED CARE SETTING)
	TYPICAL	PERFECT						
IUD	.1–2.0 (dependent on type of IUD)	.1–1.5	recent (within 3 mo) or recurrent pelvic infection post partum, post-abortion endometritis active STD severely distorted uterine cavity HIV infection (see text)	none	menstrual cramping increased bleeding risk of PID and uterine perforation following insertion anemia	provides contraception from 1 (progestasert) to 8 years (Copper T — Paraguard) requires no ongoing user action	no STD protection increased risk of PID	Progesterone T $82.00 every yr Copper T $109.00– $184.00 q 5 y insertion $62.42–$207.00 removal $10.80–$70.00
Female Sterilization	.4	.4	desire for future fertility	possible decreased risk of ovarian cancer decreased risk of salpingitis	pain at surgical site subsequent regret increased risk of ectopic pregnancy if failure	provides permanent contraception requires no ongoing user action	permanent no STD protection	$1,190.00– $2,466.80

Table continues . . .

VII

Table 7-2: Contraceptive Methods (continued)

Method	Failure Rates % Pregnancies in First Year of Typical and Perfect Use		Contraindications	Benefits	Potential Side Effects	Convenience	Disadvantages	Cost (Public Provider-Managed Care Setting)
	Typical	Perfect						
Male sterilization	.15	.10	desire for future fertility	none known	pain at surgical site subsequent regret	provides permanent sterilization for the man	same as above, except sterility not immediate	$353.28–$755.70

* polyurethane and latex-free natural rubber male condom now available — good alternative for men and women with latex allergy or sensitivity Hatcher RA, et al (eds), Contraceptive Technology, 1998.

CVD — cardiovascular disease

LDL — low density lipoprotein

HDL — high density lipoprotein

PMS — premenstrual syndrome

STD — sexually transmitted disease

Source: Hatcher, RA, et al (eds), Contraceptive Technology, 1998.

been associated with increased cervical ectopy, which has also been linked with genital tract HIV shedding. Similarly, ectopy or other epithelial changes secondary to hormonal contraception or associated effects on immune response may increase susceptibility to HIV and animal studies have suggested a link between progesterone implants and vulnerability to simian immunodeficiency virus (SIV). (Plummer, 1998; Mostad, 1998) Data from epidemiologic studies are conflicting and inconclusive regarding the relationship of these methods of contraception and HIV transmission. (Martin, 1998; Stephenson, 1998) At the current time, given their effectiveness, overall safety, and ease of use, hormonal methods of contraception remain an appropriate option for HIV-infected or at-risk women. These women should be advised that these contraceptives do not protect against HIV transmission and consistent condom use should be emphasized.

Use of the IUD has been linked to increased susceptibility for HIV transmission (Gervasoni, 1992) and is associated with increased menstrual flow and duration, possibly contributing to transmission risk and anemia in HIV-positive women; furthermore, risk of pelvic inflammatory disease (PID) is increased in IUD users who are at increased risk for acquiring other STDs. For these reasons, the IUD should generally be avoided in the setting of HIV infection.

Spermicides have in vitro activity against HIV and significant activity against gonorrhea and chlamydia; however, a recent study of a standard spermicidal dose of nonoxynol-9 (N-9) daily for one week found an increase in irritation, colposcopic and histologic evidence of inflammation, and decreased numbers of vaginal lactobacilli in N-9 users, as compared to placebo recipients (Stafford, 1998); these findings raise concerns that regular use of spermicides may not only negate any protective effect, but may potentially increase risk of HIV transmission. A recent randomized, double-blind, placebo-controlled study of vaginal film containing N-9 in over 1200 HIV uninfected sex workers in Africa found no difference in rates of HIV infection between the two groups. (Roddy, 1998)

Condoms — used consistently — provide the best known protection against sexual transmission of HIV and should be emphasized for all HIV-infected and at-risk.women to decrease risk of HIV transmission/acquisition, as well as transmission/acquisition of other STDs. Other barrier contraceptive methods provide limited STD protection and have not been shown to offer significant protection against HIV transmission.

Since male and female condoms are used for both prevention of infection and prevention of pregnancy, these two separate issues should be distinguished when counseling patients. Condom use should be reinforced for HIV-positive or at-risk women when prevention of pregnancy is not a concern: postmenopausal women; during pregnancy; infertility; and with the use of other methods of contraception.

VII

V. PREGNANCY TESTING

Indications for pregnancy testing in currently or recently sexually active women:

- missed menses (unless on Norplant or DepoProvera)
- irregular bleeding (unless on Norplant or DepoProvera)
- new onset of irregular bleeding after prolonged amenorrhea on Norplant/DepoProvera
- new onset pelvic pain
- enlarged uterus or adnexal mass on exam
- consider prior to institution of new therapies

Pregnancy tests are performed on blood or urine and may be qualitative (positive/negative) or quantitative. Quantitative tests are useful in early pregnancy when ectopic pregnancy or abnormal intrauterine pregnancy (e.g., missed abortion) are suspected. Several qualitative urine pregnancy tests are available over the counter. Most pregnancy tests in current use are positive before the first missed menses with normal intrauterine pregnancy. Table 7-3 lists types of available pregnancy tests and sensitivity.

TABLE 7-3: PREGNANCY TESTS

	SENSITIVITY	COMMENTS
Radioimmunossay ■ blood	positive within 7 days of fertilization	quantitative or qualitative used to follow women with possible ectopic pregnancy
Enzyme immunoassay (EIA) ■ blood ■ urine	positive approximately 10 days after fertilization	available for home urine testing — positive results require confirmation
Antibody agglutination inhibition ■ urine	positive approximately 18-21 days after fertilization	false positives with hypothyroidism, renal failure, immunologic disorders, increased lutenizing hormone (LH)

VI. HIV AND FERTILITY

Recent studies in Africa, as well as in developed countries, have suggested that HIV may have an adverse effect on fertility in both symptomatic and asymptomatic women. (Desgrees, 1999; Lee, 1998; Zaba, 1998) A cross-sectional study from Uganda found likelihood of pregnancy lower in HIV-positive women as compared to HIV-negative women and lowest in women who were symptomatic from HIV or were coinfected with syphilis. A prospective study in the same population found that pregnancy rates were lower and pregnancy loss was more common in HIV-infected women. (Gray, 1998)

EFFECTS OF PREGNANCY ON HIV INFECTION

A. CD4 COUNT AND HIV-RNA LEVELS IN PREGNANCY

In both HIV-positive and HIV-negative women there is a decline in absolute
CD4 cell counts in pregnancy, which is thought secondary to hemodilution; on
the other hand, percentage of CD4 cells remains relatively stable. Therefore,
percentage, rather than absolute number, may be a more accurate measure of
immune function for HIV-infected pregnant women. (Miotti, 1992; Brettle,
1995; European Collaborative Study and the Swiss HIV Pregnancy Cohort,
1997) When comparing changes in CD4 count/percentage over time, there is
no difference between HIV-positive pregnant and nonpregnant women (O'Sullivan, 1995), suggesting that pregnancy does not accelerate decline in CD4
cells. HIV-RNA levels (viral load) remain relatively stable throughout pregnancy in the absence of treatment (Burns, 1998).

B. CLINICAL COURSE OF HIV IN PREGNANCY

Most studies to date examining the impact of pregnancy on HIV disease have
been small but have not shown significant differences in HIV progression or
survival between pregnant women and nonpregnant women with HIV infection. A recent meta-analysis of seven prospective cohort studies found no
overall significant differences in death, HIV disease progression, progression
to an AIDS-defining illness, or fall in CD4 count to below $200/mm^3$ between
cases and controls. (French, 1998) A subsequently reported prospective study
of 331 women with known dates of seroconversion were followed for a
median of 5.5 years; during this time 69 women were pregnant. There were no
differences in progression between those who were and were not pregnant
during follow-up. (Alliegro, 1997)

VII. EFFECT OF HIV ON PREGNANCY COURSE AND OUTCOME

Adverse pregnancy outcomes may occur secondary to underlying disease
processes (or their treatment), as well as for unknown reasons. Approximately
10% of US pregnancies end prematurely and preterm birth is the leading
cause of perinatal morbidity and mortality. Data has accumulated that HIV,
especially when more advanced, may result in increases in certain pregnancy
complications. Furthermore, concerns have been raised that antiretroviral
treatment itself may increase some adverse outcomes in pregnancy. Table 7-4
summarizes the relationship between common pregnancy related complications and HIV. (Brocklehurst, 1998)

Both HIV and pregnancy may affect the natural history, presentation, treatment, or significance of certain infections, and these, in turn, may be associated with pregnancy complications or perinatal infection.

Table 7-4: Adverse Pregnancy Outcomes and Relationship to HIV Infection

Adverse Pregnancy Outcome	Relationship to HIV Infection
Spontaneous Abortion	Limited data, but evidence of possible increased risk
Stillbirth	No association noted in developed countries; evidence of increased risk in developing countries
Perinatal mortality	No association noted in developed countries, but data limited; evidence of increased risk in developing countries
Infant mortality	Limited data in developed countries; evidence of increased risk in developing countries
IUGR	Evidence of possible increased risk
LBW (< 2500g)	Evidence of possible increased risk
Preterm delivery	Evidence of possible increased risk, especially with more advanced disease
Pre-eclampsia	No data
Gestational diabetes	No data
Chorioamnionitis	Limited data; more recent studies do not suggest an increased risk; some earlier studies found increased histologic placental inflammation, particularly in those with preterm deliveries
Oligohydramnios	Minimal data
Fetal malformation	No evidence risk of increased risk

A. VULVOVAGINAL CANDIDIASIS

Pregnancy is associated with both increased rates of colonization and increase in symptomatic infections with species of Candida. HIV infection is also associated with increase in colonization and possible increased infection rates, especially with declining immune function. (Cu-Uvin, 1999; Schuman,1998; Duerr, 1997; Spinillo, 1994; Burns, 1997) Therefore, pregnant women with HIV infection may be particularly susceptible to yeast infections. Only topical azole agents should be used during pregnancy and should be given for at least 7 days. Prophylactic topical therapy should be considered during courses of systemic, especially broad spectrum, antibiotics are given.

B. BACTERIAL VAGINOSIS (BV)

Bacterial vaginosis has been associated with several adverse pregnancy outcomes, including preterm labor and birth, premature rupture of membranes, low birth weight infants, chorioamnionitis and amniotic fluid infection, postpartum and postabortal endometritis, and perinatal HIV transmission. If BV is diagnosed during pregnancy, preferred therapies are metronidazole 250 mg po tid x 7 days or clindamycin 300 mg po bid x 7 days, since only oral agents have been shown to reduce preterm births in women with BV. (Morales, 1994; McGregor, 1995; Hauth, 1995) Since the majority of BV episodes are asymptomatic, screening for BV should be performed at intervals during pregnancy and infection treated if identified. A recent meta-analysis (Caro-Paton, 1997) found no relationship between metronidazole exposure during the first trimester of pregnancy and birth defects.

C. GENITAL HERPES SIMPLEX (HSV)

Primary HSV infection during pregnancy has been associated with spontaneous abortion and prematurity. Congenital or intrauterine infection is uncommon but maternal HSV shedding at delivery is associated with neonatal HSV
infection, which is almost always symptomatic (including skin, eye, central
nervous system involvement, or disseminated infection involving multiple
organ systems) and frequently lethal. The risk of neonatal herpes is greatest
with primary HSV, especially when acquired close to delivery (approximately
50%), whereas only 0–3% of neonates become infected with recurrent maternal disease at delivery; however, since recurrent HSV is more common than
primary disease, the majority of neonatal infections are associated with recurrent HSV. Two-thirds or more of mothers with infected infants are asymptomatic during pregnancy; only one-third have a prior history of HSV in
themselves or their sexual partner. Since most neonatal infection occurs during
vaginal delivery, if genital lesions or prodromal symptoms are present at the
time of labor or membrane rupture, Cesarean section should be performed.
Cesarean section is not indicated for recurrent HSV distant from the genital
tract (e.g., thigh, buttocks). (ACOG, 1999)

HIV infection, particularly with evolving immunecompromise, is associated
with increased viral shedding and more frequent, severe, and prolonged
episodes of genital or perianal herpes. (Augenbraun, 1995) Higher doses
and/or longer courses of antiviral agents may be required and suppressive
therapy is often beneficial in nonpregnant individuals. Infection with HSV-2 is
common among pregnant HIV-infected women and reactivation of herpes in
labor occurs more frequently in the setting of HIV infection. (Hitti, 1997)

During pregnancy a first clinical episode of genital herpes, especially in late
pregnancy, may be treated with antiviral therapy. The use of oral acyclovir pro-
phylactically in late pregnancy has been shown to significantly reduce symptomatic recurrences and decreased need for Cesarean section, though not with
statistical significance. (Brocklehurst, 1998) Suppressive therapy may be indicated in women with frequent, severe recurrences; antiviral therapy may also
be considered at 36 weeks and beyond in women at risk for recurrent HSV.

There is no current evidence of increased risk for major birth defects or
other adverse pregnancy outcomes with exposure to acyclovir. Glaxo-Well-
come, Inc., in cooperation with CDC, maintains a registry to assess effects of
acyclovir and valacyclovir use during pregnancy. Women who receive either of
these drugs in pregnancy should be reported to this registry (telephone (888)
825-5249, ext. 39441).

Prevention of neonatal herpes should also emphasize prevention of acquisition of herpes in susceptible women in pregnancy. If her sexual partner has
a history of oral or genital HSV infection, serologic evidence of HSV infection, or infection status is unknown, the pregnant woman should be counseled
to avoid unprotected genital and oral sexual contact during pregnancy.

VII

D. HUMAN PAPILLOMA VIRUS (HPV)

Genital warts often enlarge and become friable during pregnancy and in some cases may mechanically obstruct the vaginal canal in labor; perinatal exposure can result in laryngeal papillomatosis in infants and children, although a recent prospective study suggests that the risk of perinatal transmission of HPV is low. (Watts, 1998) Both HPV infection in general and genital warts are more common in HIV-infected individuals, correlated with level of immunesuppression. Imiquimod, podophyllin, and podofilox should not be used in pregnancy. In women with large volume or bulk of genital warts treatment in late pregnancy with laser, excision, or cavitronic ultrasonic aspiration (CUSA) may be considered. Cesarean section is not currently recommended to prevent neonatal exposure to HPV, although in rare instances C-section may be indicated when extensive lesions obstruct the vagina.

E. SYPHILIS

Syphilis is more prevalent in HIV-infected populations and HIV may affect clinical manifestations, serologic response, or response to treatment for syphilis. Pregnancy does not alter the clinical manifestations of syphilis but untreated primary or secondary syphilis during pregnancy affects essentially all fetuses, with 50% rate of prematurity, stillbirth, or neonatal death. (Radolf, 1999) Even with later stages of syphilis, there is a significant increase in adverse pregnancy outcomes, although the frequency and severity of fetal disease decreases with longer duration of untreated maternal infection. Manifestations of congenital syphilis in the newborn include mucocutaneous lesions, hepatosplenomegaly, osteochondritis/periostitis, jaundice, petechiae/purpura, and meningitis.

Congenital syphilis can generally be prevented by identification and appropriate treatment of syphilis during pregnancy. All pregnant women should have serologic testing for syphilis at the beginning of prenatal care and testing should be repeated at 28 weeks gestation and at delivery, particularly in women who remain at risk for infection. Any woman with stillbirth after 20 weeks gestation should be tested for syphilis. Development of neurologic symptoms mandates evaluation for possible neurosyphilis. Treatment of syphilis during pregnancy should be the penicillin regimen appropriate for the stage of syphilis, although some experts recommend additional weekly doses in women with primary, secondary or early latent syphilis who are HIV-infected or pregnant. HIV-positive women with late latent syphilis or syphilis of unknown duration should have CSF examination before treatment. (CDC, 1998)

Ultrasound evidence of hydrops or hepatosplenomegaly suggesting fetal syphilis increases risk for treatment failure and should be managed with expert consultation. Treatment in the second half of pregnancy is associated with the Jarisch-Herxheimer reaction in up to 40% of cases, with resulting premature labor and/or fetal distress (Myles, 1998); they should be advised to seek immediate attention after treatment if contractions or decrease in fetal movements occur. Pregnant women with a history of penicillin allergy should be skin tested and, if necessary, desensitized and treated with penicillin, as there are no proven effective alternatives to penicillin for treatment and prevention of congenital syphilis. Even with appropriate treatment of the pregnant woman with syphilis, fetal infection may still occur and neonates should be carefully evaluated for evidence of congenital infection.

Clinical and serologic follow-up should be performed at 3,6,9,12, and 24 months after treatment. Treatment failure should be managed with CSF examination and re-treatment.

F. CYTOMEGALOVIRUS (CMV)

Cytomegalovirus is the most common cause of congenital viral infection in the U.S. with 0.2–2.2% of liveborn infants acquiring this infection perinatally. (ACOG, 1993) Most maternal CMV infections are asymptomatic but may cause a mononucleosis-like illness. Transmission can occur sexually or with injection drug use, since CMV has been recovered from virtually all body fluids. Perinatal transmission can occur with both primary and recurrent infection, but frequency of transmission and severity of infection in the infant are greater with primary infection. Ninety percent of infected infants are asymptomatic at birth, but symptomatic infection is more likely with maternal infection acquired early in pregnancy. Even if asymptomatic, many infected infants subsequently develop deafness, mental retardation, or delayed psychomotor development. More severe clinical manifestations include symmetric growth restriction, hepatosplenomegaly, chorioretinitis, microphthalmia, hydrocephaly, microcephaly, and cerebral calcifications.

In the setting of HIV infection, mothers seropositive for CMV do not appear to be more likely to transmit CMV perinatally than HIV-negative mothers. Furthermore, the frequency of CMV infection at birth is similar between HIV-infected and –uninfected infants born to HIV seropositive mothers. There have been some reports that co-transmission of HIV and CMV may be related to more rapid HIV progression. (Kovacs, 1999; Mussi-Pinhata, 1998)

There is no effective therapy to prevent or treat perinatal CMV infection. Testing for antibody to CMV should be considered in pregnancy, especially if the CD4 count is < 100/mm³; however, seropositivity is common and does not preclude viral shedding during pregnancy and perinatal transmission. Methods to reduce risk of exposure to CMV include safer sexual practices; careful handwashing; and transmission of only CMV antibody-negative blood products. Primary prophylaxis is not routinely recommended; however, after CMV disease, chronic suppression is indicated in pregnancy and should be continued with expert consultation concerning choice of agents. (see below OI Prophylaxis).

G. TOXOPLASMOSIS

Approximately one-third of U.S. women have toxoplasma antibodies, reflecting prior infection. Primary infection occurs in approximately 0.1–0.5% of pregnancies and places the fetus at risk for congenital toxoplasmosis. Congenital infection is more common when infection in the mother occurs during the third trimester (59% in third trimester vs 9% in first trimester) but is generally more severe when occurring in the first trimester. Although the majority of infected infants are asymptomatic at birth, most will develop some sequelae of congenital toxoplasmosis; two-thirds of infants infected after maternal first trimester infection have severe manifestations and 5% are stillborn or die in the perinatal period. (ACOG, 1993)

Congenital toxoplasmosis may affect all systems, but the most common findings are chorioretinitis, microcephaly, hydrocephaly, and cerebral calcifications.

Transmission of toxoplasmosis from a mother with antibody evidence of prior infection can occur in the setting of HIV infection, but does not seem to be common, although there is limited data in more immunosuppressed mothers. (Minkoff, 1997; European Collaborative Study and Research Network in Congenital Toxoplasmosis, 1996)

Testing for IgG antibodies to toxoplasma is recommended for all HIV-infected individuals soon after the diagnosis of HIV is made and should be considered as part of prenatal testing in HIV-positive pregnant women. Primary prophylaxis and prophylaxis against recurrent disease in pregnancy are discussed below. Pregnant women with symptoms including fever, chills, malaise, lymphadenopathy, myalgias, headache should be evaluated serologically for possible primary toxoplasmic infection. Evidence of primary infection or active toxoplasmosis should be evaluated and managed with expert consultation. Infants born to women infected with HIV and seropositive for toxoplasma should be evaluated for evidence of congenital toxoplasmosis.

To prevent exposure to toxoplasmosis, pregnant women should be counseled to avoid raw or undercooked meat; wash hands after contact with raw meat or with soil; and wash fruits and vegetables well before eating them raw. Cats should preferably be kept inside and fed only canned or dried commercial food; litter boxes should be changed daily, preferable by someone who is not HIV-positive or pregnant.

H. HEPATITIS B (HBV)

Approximately 300,000 new cases of hepatitis B occur each year and more than one million Americans are chronic carriers. Most patients who become infected have complete resolution of infection and develop protective levels of antibody (anti-HBs). Chronic HBV infection develops in 1–6% of persons who are infected as adults; they are chronically HbsAg+ and are at risk of chronic liver disease, including cirrhosis and hepatocellular carcinoma. (CDC, 1991) The presence of HbeAg indicates active viral replication and increased infectivity. HBV is transmitted parenterally, sexually, perinatally, and through household or institutional contact. Approximately one-quarter of regular sexual contacts of infected individuals will become seropositive and sexual transmission accounts for 30–60% of new infections. Perinatal transmission, usually with intrapartum contact with maternal blood and genital secretions, occurs in 10–20% of women who are HbsAg+, but increases to approximately 90% if the mother is also HbeAg+. Chronic HBV infection develops in about 90% of infected newborns, who are at high risk of chronic liver disease. (ACOG, 1998)

All pregnant women should be screened for HbsAg. Infants born to women who are HbsAg+ should receive hepatitis B immune globuline (HBIG) and initiate HBV vaccination within 12 hours after birth. HBV vaccine can be safely administered during pregnancy and should be considered in women who are high risk (injection drug use, STDs, multiple sexual partners, household or sexual contact of HBV carrier) and are anti-HBs or anti-HBc negative, indicating susceptibility. Some experts argue for more liberal use of vaccination in HIVinfected individuals, since HBV infection in the setting of HIV infection increases risk for chronic HBV infection. HIV can impair response to HBV vaccine, and, therefore, testing for hepatitis B surface antibody is recommended 1–2 months after the third vaccine dose. Full revaccination should be considered for those who are nonresponders. (ACOG, 1998; Bartlett, 1999)

I. HEPATITIS C (HCV)

Hepatitis C infection is primarily transmitted by injection drug use, but may also be transmitted sexually. Approximately 50% of those with acute HCV infection develop biochemical evidence of chronic liver disease, and 20% or more ultimately have chronic active hepatitis or cirrhosis and are at risk for hepatocellular carcinoma. (CDC, 1998) Women newly diagnosed with HIV in pregnancy should have testing for antibody to HCV by enzyme immunoassay; positive results should be confirmed with recombinant immunoblot assay (RIBA) or HCV PCR and liver function abnormalities should be documented. Women coinfected with HIV and HCV should avoid alcohol, both during and after pregnancy, since alcohol use increases risk of cirrhosis. Vaccination against hepatitis A, if the woman is anti-HAV negative, is recommended because the risk for fulminant hepatitis associated with hepatitis A is increased in HCV-infected individuals; this vaccination may be safely given during pregnancy. (ACOG, 1998; Bartlett, 1999)

Perinatal transmission of HCV has been documented and may be more likely in HIV coinfected women or in HIV-infected infants born to dually infected mothers. (Thomas, 1998; Papaevangelou, 1998) Furthermore, maternal coinfection with HIV and HCV may also increase risk for perinatal HIV transmission. (Hershow, 1997) Risk of vertical HCV transmission is proportional to amount of HCV RNA present in maternal blood. (Thomas, 1998)

VIII. PERINATAL TRANSMISSION

The baseline rate of perinatal HIV transmission without prophylactic therapy is approximately 25%. The timing of transmission is a critical factor impacting on development of preventive interventions. There is evidence that transmission can occur during the course of pregnancy, around the time of labor and delivery, or postpartum through breastfeeding; however, $^2/_3$ to $^3/_4$ of transmission appears to occur during or close to the intrapartum period, particularly in non-breastfeeding populations. (Mofenson, 1997)

A. POTENTIAL VARIABLES IN TRANSMISSION

HIV-RELATED FACTORS

■ **HIV-RNA level** (Garcia, 1999; Mofenson, 1999; Shaffer, 1999): HIV-RNA levels correlate with risk of transmission in both antiretroviral-treated and untreated women. The risk of perinatal transmission appears to be extremely low in women with undetectable plasma viral loads, but transmission has been reported at all levels of maternal HIV-RNA. There is no upper limit of HIV-RNA above which perinatal transmission always occurs.

■ **Strain variation (genotype):** Each HIV-infected individual's viral pool is comprised of a variety of HIV quasispecies. One recent study found that in utero transmission was associated with transmission of major maternal viral variants, whereas intrapartum transmission was associate with transmission of minor maternal viral variants, suggesting that different selective pressures may be involved in determining the pattern of viral strain transmission depending on timing of transmission. (Dickover, 2000) HIV in vaginal secretions can be derived from local expression and may have significant genotypic differences from plasma virus, with possible implications for perinatal transmission. (Subbarao, 1998)

■ **Biologic growth characteristics (phenotype):** Fetal blood mononuclear cells may be more susceptible to macrophage-tropic, non-syncytium-inducing HIV phenotypes and this may influence mother-to-infant HIV transmission. (Reinhardt, 1995; Palasanthiran P, 1994)

■ **Plasma vs genital tract viral load:** There is general correlation between plasma and genital tract viral load but discordance has been reported and may help explain some cases of transmission with undetectable plasma HIV-RNA. In the Thai short-course ZDV clinical trial, both plasma and cervicovaginal HIV-RNA levels were suppressed by ZDV treatment and both were independently correlated with transmission. (Chuachoowong, 2000) The female genital tract can also be a reservoir for virus with a different drug resistance pattern than that observed in plasma. (Fang, 1998) Further studies are needed to assess suppression of genital tract virus with other antiretroviral agents and with HAART therapy, and the association of this suppression with perinatal transmission.

■ **Genotypic resistance:** Use of antiretroviral regimens (particularly single agents) for the purpose of perinatal prophylaxis has raised concerns about the induction of resistance mutations, possibly increasing the risk for vertical transmission or progression in infected infants. Studies to date of resistance mutations in the setting of ZDV monotherapy during pregnancy have shown increasing prevalence of these mutations over time and an association with length of drug exposure. (Palumbo, 1999; Eastman, 1998; Kully, 1999; Fiscus, 1999) Perinatal transmission of virus with known ZDV resistance mutations has been described (Colgrove, 1998) and one recent study found that maternal ZDV use was associated with rapid disease progression in infants who acquired HIV despite maternal ZDV use. (Pitt, 2000) Most concerning, a recent study from the Women and Infants Transmission Study (WITS) of women who received ZDV during pregnancy, found that 25% of 142 maternal isolates had at least one ZDV-associated resistance mutations; a lower CD4 % and higher plasma HIV-RNA level were associated with ZDV resistance mutations at delivery and, with multivariate analysis, the presence of resistance mutations was independently associated with vertical transmission. (Welles, 2000)

Eschleman et al found that a subset of Ugandan women developed a K103N nevirapine resistance mutation after receiving a single dose of nevirapine at the onset of labor for prevention of perinatal transmission; the implications of this finding for perinatal prophylaxis with nevirapine and the relevance to HIV subtypes more prevalent in other areas of the world are unknown. (Becker-Pergola, 2000)

■ **CD4 cell count:** Lower CD4 count or decreased CD4:CD8 ratio have been consistently associated with increased risk of transmission.

■ **Maternal immune response:** Studies have been inconsistent when evaluating the role of maternal antibodies, including anti-gp120, anti-gp41, and autologous neutralizing antibody titers. Beta-chemokine and cytokine responses may affect risk of transmission. (Rich, 1998)

B. MATERNAL/OBSTETRICAL FACTORS

■ **Clinical stage:** Maternal symptomatic disease or AIDS-defining illness are consistently associated with higher risk for transmission. Women with primary HIV infection in pregnancy, at which time plasma viremia is high, are also at increased risk for transmission. (Nesheim, 1996)

■ **STDs/other coinfections:** STDs have been shown to increase genital tract HIV shedding and also increase plasma viremia (Plummer, 1998), both of which may increase risk for perinatal transmission. STDs (Mandelbrot, 1996), syphilis (Lee, 1998), bacterial vaginosis (Taha, 1998), and placental malaria have been associated with increased risk for vertical transmission, as have increased levels of genital tract inflammatory cells. (Panther, 2000)

■ **Vitamin A deficiency:** Vitamin A deficiency has been associated with increased risk of perinatal HIV transmission and increased genital tract HIV shedding. (Nimmagadda, 1998) However, a recent randomized trial of vitamin A supplementation in South Africa found no overall reduction in mother-to-child transmission of HIV, although vitamin A recipients were less likely to have a preterm delivery and in deliveries which were preterm, those infants assigned to the vitamin A group were less likely to be infected. (Coutsoudis, 1999)

■ **Substance abuse:** Illicit drug use during pregnancy has been associated with increased risk for perinatal transmission. (Landesman, 1996; Rodriguez, 1996; Lyman, 1993)

■ **Cigarette smoking:** Cigarette smoking has been associated with an increased risk of perinatal transmission. (Burns, 1994; Turner, 1997)

■ **Antiretroviral agents:** ZDV (antepartum/intrapartum/neonatal), ZDV/3TC (intrapartum/neonatal), and nevirapine (intrapartum/neonatal) have all demonstrated effectiveness in reducing periantal HIV transmission in randomized clinical trials. In the PACTG 076 study, reduction in viral load accounted for only 17% of ZDV's effectiveness, suggesting pre-and/or post-exposure prophylaxis as other possible mechanisms of action. (Sperling, 1996) Although there are no clinical trials completed with HAART regimens, these regimens result in optimal reductions in viral load, which would be expected to lead to reductions in transmission. Very few perinatal HIV infections have been reported in infants exposed to HAART.

■ **Sexual behavior:** Unprotected sex with multiple partners has been associated with increased risk for perinatal transmission. (Bultreys, 1997)

■ **Gestational age:** Preterm delivery has been associated with increased risk for perinatal transmission. (Kuhn, 1999; Kuhn, 1997)

■ **Duration of membrane rupture:** A recent meta-analysis from 15 prospective cohort studies, including over 7500 deliveries, examined the role of duration of ruptured membranes in perinatal transmission. (Read, 2000) The likelihood of transmission increased linearly with increasing duration of ruptured membranes, with a 2% increase in risk for each hour increment. Women with clinical AIDS had the most pronounced increase in risk, with a 31% probability of vertical transmission after 24 hours of ruptured membranes.

■ **Placental disruption-abruption, chorioamnionitis:** Clinical and histologic chorioamnionitis (Goldenberg, 1998) has been associated with increased risk of transmission. Placental abruption causing disruption of fetal-placental barrier and possible increased exposure of the fetus to maternal blood, has also been suggested as a risk factor for transmission.

■ **Invasive fetal monitoring:** Use of fetal scalp electrodes or fetal scalp sampling increases exposure of the fetus to maternal blood and genital secretions and may increase risk of vertical transmission. Amnioscopy and amnio-centesis increased risk in the French Perinatal Cohort (Mandelbrot, 1996)

■ **Episiotomy, forceps:** Use of episiotomy or vacuum extraction or forceps may potentially increase risk of transmission by increasing exposure to maternal blood/genital secretions with trauma to maternal or neonatal tissue. On the other hand, judicious use of these techniques to shorten duration of labor or ruptured membranes with vaginal delivery may decrease likelihood of transmission.

■ **Vaginal versus cesarean delivery:** Several recent studies indicate that cesarean delivery performed prior to the onset of labor and rupture of membranes significantly reduces the risk of perinatal HIV transmission. (Mandelbrot, 1998; Kind, 1998; European Mode of Delivery Collaboration, 1999; The International Perinatal HIV Group, 1999) Rates of transmission were reduced to approximately 2% with scheduled C-section and receipt of ZDV (similar risk of 2% or less is seen among women with HIV-RNA levels less than 1000c/ml, in the absence of systematic use of cesarean section). Whether cesarean delivery offers any benefit when the mother is on HAART and/or if she has low or undetectable viral load is unknown.

C. FETAL/NEONATAL FACTORS

Fetal/neonatal factors, including an immature immune system (particularly in the premature infant) and genetic susceptibility, as expressed by HLA genotype (Just, 1992) or CCR-5 receptor (a co-receptor for macrophage-tropic strains of HIV; a homozygous deletion in this gene confers a high degree of natural resistance to HIV sexual transmission) mutations may play a role in perinatal transmission. (Weiser, 1998; Mangano, 2000; Kostrikis, 1999) A recent study from South Africa (Kuhn, 2000) found that early acquired cellular immune responses to HIV, presumably from in utero exposure, were present in over one-third of 86 uninfected infants born to HIV-infected mothers. These detectable immune responses appeared to provide complete protection against subsequent HIV transmission at delivery and through breastfeeding.

D. BREASTFEEDING

Breastfeeding plays a more significant role in perinatal HIV transmission than was once thought and was estimated to have accounted for up to 50% of newly infected children globally in 1998. (Fowler, 1999) Breastfeeding in the setting of established maternal infection has an estimated additional risk of 14% transmission, while the risk is 29% in the setting of acute maternal infection or recent seroconverson. (Dunn, 1992) HIV-DNA can be detected in over 50% of breast milk samples and is correlated with CD4 depletion and vitamin A deficiency. Risk of transmission is highest in the earliest months of breastfeeding but increased duration of breastfeeding increases risk. (Kreiss, 1997; Leroy, 1998) Other potential variables include the presence of cracked nipples or breast abscess, infant oral candidosis, and the use of exclusive breastfeeding vs mixed feeding. A recent randomized clinical trial of breast-feeding vs formula in Kenya (Nduati, 2000) found that formula feeding prevented 44% of infant infections and was associated with a significantly improved HIV-free survival.

STRATEGIES FOR PREVENTION OF PERINATAL TRANSMISSION:

Based on the potential factors impacting on perinatal HIV transmission discussed above, several basic approaches to prevention have been suggested. These include decreasing viral load, decreasing viral exposure, identification and treatment of modifiable risk factors, and ultimately, stimulation of the immune system, such as with passive or active immunization.

IX. GUIDELINES FOR CARE

A. ANTEPARTUM

HISTORY/PHYSICAL EXAMINATION

(See Chapter IV on Primary Medical Care.)

- **HIV history**: date of diagnosis; history of HIV-related symptoms or opportunistic infections or malignancies; lowest CD4 cell count; complete antiretroviral history, including specific drugs, side effects or toxicity, length of treatment, adherence and response to treatment

- **Pregnancy history**: previous pregnancies and outcomes; complications; mode of delivery; use of antiretroviral prophylaxis; and HIV status of other children

- **Signs or symptoms of HIV/AIDS**: The initial and follow-up evaluations of HIV-positive women during pregnancy should assess signs or symptoms suggestive of symptomatic HIV infection or AIDS(e.g., generalized lymphadenopathy, thrush, constitutional symptoms such as fever (38.5 degrees C) or diarrhea > 1 month, herpes zoster involving two episodes or > 1 dermatome, peripheral neuropathy, wasting, dysphagia, shortness of breath, persistent mucocutaneous herpetic ulcerations, cognitive dysfunction, etc).

- **Signs or symptoms of pregnancy-related complications**: elevated blood pressure, significant edema, severe headache, vaginal bleeding or leakage of fluid, intractable nausea and vomiting, dysuria, abnormal vaginal discharge, persistent abdominal or back pain or cramping, decrease in fetal movement, etc.

  Certain symptoms of HIV disease and normal or abnormal pregnancy may overlap, resulting in possible delay in appropriate diagnosis and management.

- Relevant family history of possible heritable diseases.

LABORATORY EXAMINATION BY TRIMESTER

(See Table 7-5)

TABLE 7-5: LABORATORY EVALUATION IN THE HIV-INFECTED PREGNANT WOMAN

TEST	COMMENT
ENTRY INTO PRENATAL CARE	
HIV serology	unconfirmed HIV infection; + test with other techniques
CD4 cell count/% HIV-RNA	repeat every 3-4 mo; at milestones for therapeutic decisions, re: ARV therapy/OI prophylaxis
CBC	repeat every 3-6 mo; more frequent testing if low or receiving marrow-toxic drugs (e.g. ZDV)
Serum chemistry panel	repeat as indicated with abnormal results or use of hepatotoxic/nephrotoxic drugs
Syphilis serology	
Hepatitis serology HbsAg, anti-HCV	order anti-HBs or anti-HBc to screen for vaccine candidates
Rubella Blood type and Rh Antibody screen Urine culture GC/chlamydia testing Pap smear	
PPD	+ skin test= ≥ 5mm induration; anergy testing not indicated
Hemoglobin electrophoresis, red blood cell indices	perform in women at increased risk for hemoglobinopathies .
G6PD	optional — may consider screening black women or those receiving oxidant drugs (e.g. dapsone, sulfonamides)
CMV IgG	consider especially with CD4 < 100 mm³ or in patients at low risk for CMV
Toxoplasmosis IgG	screen all patients with initial HIV diagnosis; repeat with CD4 < 100/mm³ and not on TMP-SMZ, or with symptoms suggestive of toxoplasmic encephalitis
Urine toxicology screen	as indicated
Serum screening for Tay Sachs disease	consider screening both partners if at increased risk (Ashkenazi Jews, French-Canadian or Cajun descent)
16–20 WEEKS	
Ultrasound	gestational dating, anomaly screen
Maternal serum alpha fetoprotein*	screening test for neural tube and abdominal wall defects voluntary; requires counseling; abnormal result (usually > 2.5 multiple of the median) requires further evaluation
Triple screen (hcg, unconjugated estriol, alpha-fetoprotein)**	voluntary; requires counseling; noninvasive test to determine risk of neural tube & abdominal wall defects, Down syndrome and trisomy 18

* accurate gestational age is essential for interpretation of both tests

** Oligohydramnios:Minimal data; Fetal malformation: No evidence risk of increased risk

Table continues . . .

VII

TABLE 7-5: LABORATORY EVALUATION IN THE HIV-INFECTED PREGNANT WOMAN *(continued)*

TEST	COMMENT
24–28 WEEKS	
CBC Syphilis serology Antibody screen	
Diabetes screen	glucose 1 hour after 50 gm glucola — 3 hr oral GTT if abnormal; may need additional glucose monitoring in women on protease inhibitors
Bacterial vaginosis screening	women at high risk for preterm labor
32–36 WEEKS	
GC/chlamydia testing	
Group Bstrep culture (35–37 wks)	optional; offer intra-partum chemoprophylaxis with IV PCN G (2.5 million units q 4 hr) if positive. Alternative is prophylaxis strategy based on presence of intrapartum risk factors (CDC, 1996)
CD4, HIV-RNA	results may influence decisions about mode of delivery
Syphilis serology	consider in high risk patients or populations
ARV- antiretroviral	
OI- opportunistic infections	

ANTEPARTUM FETAL SURVEILLANCE/TESTING (ACOG, 1999)

The general purpose of antepartum fetal testing and surveillance is to identify fetal abnormalities or compromise so that appropriate interventions can be undertaken to optimize fetal health and prevent fetal damage or death; or, in some instances, to aid in decisions regarding continuation of pregnancy.

■ **Fetal surveillance:** Indications include:

- maternal conditions in which risk of fetal death is increased. This includes (but is not limited to) hemoglobinopathies, chronic renal disease, systemic lupus erythematosus, hypertension, and diabetes.

- pregnancy-related conditions in which risk of fetal death is increased. This includes pregnancy-induced hypertension, decreased fetal movement, oligohydramnios, polyhydramnios, intrauterine growth retardation, post-term pregnancy, mild to moderate isoimmunization, previous fetal demise, and multiple gestation.

  There are no data specifically on the need for and use of fetal surveillance techniques in the HIV-infected woman during pregnancy, and HIV per se is not an indication for fetal testing. However, HIV-infected women who have co-existing medical conditions placing the fetus at increased risk should have fetal surveillance; furthermore, HIV infection, especially when more advanced or associated with substance abuse, may be associated with increased risk for poor fetal growth, which places the fetus at increased risk. Need for fetal surveillance in the HIV-positive pregnancy should be determined on an individual basis.

Fetal surveillance techniques include:

➤ fetal movement assessment: perception of 10 distinct movements in a period of up to 2 hours is reassuring

➤ nonstress test (NST): reactive or reassuring test is defined as two or more fetal heart rate accelerations (at least 15 beats per minute above baseline and lasting at least 15 seconds from baseline to baseline on fetal monitor) within a 20 minute period.

➤ contraction stress test (CST): negative or reassuring test is absence of late or significant variable fetal heart rate decelerations with at least three contractions (lasting at least 40 seconds) within 10 minutes

➤ biophysical profile: consists of a NST combined with observations of fetal breathing, fetal movements, fetal tone, and amniotic fluid volume by real-time ultrasonography. Each component is given a score of 2(normal or present) or 0 (abnormal or absent); a composite score of 8 or 10 is normal.

➤ Modified biophysical profile: combines NST and amniotic fluid index (AFI), which is the sum of measurements of the deepest amniotic fluid pocket in each abdominal quadrant; normal AFI is > 5 cm. This test combines a short-term indicator of fetal acid-base status (NST) and an indicator of long-term placental function (AFI); placental dysfunction often leads to poor fetal growth and oligohydramnios.

➤ Umbilical artery doppler velocimetry: evaluation of flow velocity wave forms in the umbilical artery; in the normally growing fetus, characterized by high velocity diastolic flow; of benefit only in pregnancies complicated by intrauterine growth restriction.

Although data from randomized clinical trials are missing, antepartum fetal surveillance has been consistently associated with lower rates of fetal death than in untested pregnancies from the same institution or than historic controls with similar complicating factors. Testing should be initiated at 32–34 weeks gestation, but may be started as early as 26–28 weeks in pregnancies at very high risk. When the condition prompting testing persists, testing should be repeated periodically (weekly or, in some cases, biweekly) until delivery. Fetal reevaluation should also be repeated with significant deterioration in maternal medical condition or acute decrease in fetal movement, regardless of the time elapsed since the previous test.

NST, CST, biophysical profile and modified biophysical profile are the most commonly used forms of testing and have a negative predictive value > 99%. However, they are not predictive of acute events, such as placental abruption or umbilical cord accidents. On the other

VII

hand, the positive predictive value of an abnormal test can be quite low and the response to an abnormal result should be dictated by the individual clinical situation. Any abnormal test result requires further evaluation or action. Maternal perception of decreased fetal movements should be evaluated by NST, CST, biophysical profile or modified biophysical profile. If normal the mother can be reassured that the fetus is in no immediate danger. A nonreactive NST or abnormal modified biophysical profile is usually followed by additional testing with a CST or full biophysical profile. Management will be based on results of these tests, gestational age, degree of oligohydramnios (if assessed), and maternal condition. Oligohydramnios should prompt evaluation for membrane rupture. Depending on the degree of oligohydramnios, the gestational age, and the maternal medical condition, oligohydramnios warrants either delivery or close maternal/fetal surveillance.

■ **Ultrasound.** Indications for obstetrical ultrasound are many. Some of the more common include (ACOG, 1993):

- pregnancy dating
- evaluation of fetal growth
- evaluation of vaginal bleeding during pregnancy
- determination of fetal presentation
- suspected multiple gestation
- significant uterine size/clinical dates discrepancy
- pelvic mass
- suspected ectopic pregnancy
- document fetal viability/rule out fetal death
- biophysical profile for antepartum fetal surveillance
- suspected polyhydramnios/oligohydramnios
- placental localization
- abnormal serum alpha-fetoprotein or triple screen
- evaluation for fetal anomalies
- evaluation of fetal condition in late registrants for prenatal care

With transvaginal ultrasound, an intrauterine gestational sac can be seen by five weeks after the last menstrual period and fetal heart activity can be detected by 6 weeks. First–trimester bleeding is the most common indication for early ultrasound, when the major differential diagnoses are threatened abortion (miscarriage) and ectopic pregnancy. Accurate pregnancy dating is best accomplished in the late first and second trimesters.

In the setting of HIV infection, an ultrasound should be considered in the second trimester for accurate dating, which is important later in gestation if scheduled cesarean section is planned to avoid premature delivery (see below). This will also allow survey of fetal anatomy and screening for anomalies. Depending on the individual situation, including stage of illness, therapeutic regimen, and presence of other maternal/pregnacy-related factors, ultrasonography may be useful in monitoring fetal growth.

■ **Amniocentesis/Chorionic villous sampling (CVS)/Percutaneous umbilical blood sampling (PUBS).** Because of concerns about increasing risk of perinatal transmission with these invasive techniques, they should generally be avoided in pregnancies complicated by HIV infection.

ANTIRETROVIRAL TREATMENT

(See Table 7-6 on the following page) Although there are special considerations in using antiretroviral drugs during pregnancy, the basic principle is that therapies of known or possible benefit to the woman should not be withheld during pregnancy unless there are known adverse effects for mother, fetus or infant which outweigh the potential benefits. (Minkoff, 1997) Pregnant women meeting the criteria outlined for other adults and adolescents should be offered standard combination antiretroviral therapy, usually including two nucleoside reverse transcriptase inhibitors (NRTI) and a protease inhibitor (PI). (See Chapter IV on Primary Medical Care)

Nevertheless, there are additional issues to consider with treatment in pregnancy:

■ **Pharmacokinetics:** There are potential changes in dosing secondary to the physiologic changes during pregnancy; at the current time, pharmacokinetic information on existing antiretroviral agents during pregnancy is limited, but has not suggested need for dose adjustment.

■ **Perinatal transmission:** The effect of different drugs and drug combinations on vertical transmission. Current information on the use of antiretroviral agents during the antepartum period and perinatal transmission are summarized below:

• PACTG 076: ZDV given antepartum, intrapartum, and to the neonate for 6 weeks of life reduced risk of vertical transmission by 66%, from 22.6% in placebo recipients to 7.6% in ZDV recipients. (Sperling, 1996) All women participating in this trial had CD4 counts > 200/mm³ and were antiretroviral naïve. Subsequent studies, including women with more advanced disease and with prior ZDV exposure, confirm the effectiveness of this regimen with transmission rates as low as 3–4%.

• short-course ZDV: ZDV 300 mg twice daily beginning at 36 weeks gestation and 300 mg every 3 hours orally in labor reduced transmission by approximately 50% (19% placebo vs 9% ZDV) compared to placebo in a nonbreastfeeding population in Thailand. (Shaffer, 1999)

• ZDV/3TC: (PETRA trial) ZDV/3TC twice daily beginning at 36 weeks gestation and orally in labor (ZDV 600 mg and 3TC 150 mg orally at onset of labor, then ZDV 300 mg orally every 3 hours and

TABLE 7-6: PRECLINICAL AND CLINICAL DATA RELEVANT TO USE OF ANTIRETROVIRALS IN PREGNANCY

ANTIRETROVIRAL DRUG	FDA PREGNANCY CATEGORY[1]	PLACENTAL PASSAGE [NEWBORN:MATERNAL DRUG RATIO]	LONG-TERM ANIMAL CARCINOGENICITY STUDIES	RODENT TERATOGEN
zidovudine[2]	C	Yes (human) [0.85]	Positive (rodent, vaginal tumors)	Positive (near lethal dose)
zalcitabine	C	Yes (rhesus) [0.30–0.50]	Positive (rodent, thymic lymphomas)	Positive (hydrocephalus at high dose)
didanosine	B	Yes (human) [0.5]	Negative (no tumors, lifetime rodent study)	Negative
stavudine	C	Yes (rhesus) [0.76]	Not completed	Negative (but sternal bone calcium decreases)
lamivudine	C	Yes (human) [~1.0]	Negative (no tumors, lifetime rodent study)	Negative
abacavir	C	Yes (rats)	Not completed	Positive (anasarca and skeletal malformations at 1000 mg/kg [35x human exposure] during organogenesis)
saquinavir	B	Unknown	Not completed	Negative
indinavir	C	Yes (rats) ("Significant" in rats, low in rabbits)	Not completed	Negative (but extra ribs in rats)

[1] FDA Pregnancy Categories are:
A — Adequate and well-controlled studies of pregnant women fail to demonstrate a risk to the fetus during the first trimester of pregnancy (and there is no evidence of risk during later trimesters);
B — Animal reproduction studies fail to demonstrate a risk to the fetus and adequate but well-controlled studies of pregnant women have not been conducted;
C — Safety in human pregnancy has not been determined, animal studies are either positive for fetal risk or have not been conducted, and the drug should not be used unless the potential benefit outweighs the potential risk to the fetus;
D — Positive evidence of human fetal risk based on adverse reaction data from investigational or marketing experiences, but the potential benefits from the use of the drug in pregnant women may be acceptable despite its potential risks;
X — Studies in animals or reports of adverse reactions have indicated that the risk associated with the use of the drug for pregnant women clearly outweighs any possible benefit.

[2] Despite certain animal data showing potential teratogenicity of ZDV when near-lethal doses are given to pregnant rodents, considerable human data are available to date indicating that the risk to the fetus, if any, is extremely small when given to the pregnant mother beyond 14 weeks gestation. Follow-up for up to 6 years of age for 734 infants born to HIV-infected women who had in utero exposure to ZDV has not demonstrated any tumor development (93). However, no data is available on longer follow-up for late effects.

Table continues . . .

TABLE 7-6: PRECLINICAL AND CLINICAL DATA RELEVANT TO USE OF ANTIRETROVIRALS IN PREGNANCY *(continued)*

ANTIRETROVIRAL DRUG	FDA PREGNANCY CATEGORY[1]	PLACENTAL PASSAGE [NEWBORN:MATERNAL DRUG RATIO]	LONG-TERM ANIMAL CARCINOGENICITY STUDIES	RODENT TERATOGEN
ritonavir	B	Yes (rats) [mid-term fetus, 1.15; late-term fetus, 0.15–0.64]	Not completed	Negative (but cryptorchidism in rats)[3]
nelfinavir	B	Unknown	Not completed	Negative
amprenavir	C	Unknown	Not completed	Positive (thymic elongation; incomplete ossification of bones; low body weight)
nevirapine	C	Yes (human) [~1.0]	Not completed	Negative
delavirdine	C	Yes (rats) [late-term fetus, blood, 0.15 Late-term fetus, liver 0.04]	Not completed	Ventricular septal defect
efavirenz	C	Yes (cynomolgus monkeys, rats, rabbits) [~1.0]	Not completed	Anencephaly; anophthalmia; microphthalmia (cynomalgus monkeys)

[3] These effects seen at only at maternally toxic doses.

VII

3TC 150 mg orally every 12 hours) and for one week postpartum to the infant and mother reduced transmission by approximately 50% (17% placebo vs 9% ZDV/3TC) compared to placebo at 6 weeks. The majority of infants in this study were breastfed. (Saba, 1999)

■ **Fetal/infant adverse effects:** Potential teratogenicity, carcinogenicity, mutagenicity, or fetal/neonatal side effects/toxicity from transplacentally transferred drugs. The potential for adverse effects may be related to several factors: the drug itself, dose, gestational age at exposure, duration of exposure, interactions with other drugs or agents to which the fetus is exposed, and the genetic make-up of mother and fetus.

Information about the safety of drugs in pregnancy comes from animal toxicity studies, anecdotal experience, registry data, and clinical trials. Preclinical data do not necessarily correlate with adverse effects in humans. There are approximately 1200 known animal teratogens, but only about 30 are known human teratogens. Of currently available drugs, zidovudine (ZDV) is the agent for which there is the most information, and information about the other antiretrovirals is limited. Some specific concerns have been raised and are addressed below; for more in depth discussion of each drug, see Chapter XIV on Pharmacology and the U.S. Public Health Service Task Force Recommendations for the Use of Antiretroviral Drugs in Pregnant Women Infected with HIV-1 for Maternal Health and for Reducing Perinatal HIV-1 Transmission in the United States, which is updated regularly on-line at **http://www.hivatis.org**.

● **safety of ZDV exposure:** In the PACTG 076 study the only side effect significantly different between ZDV and placebo recipients was the presence of anemia in ZDV-exposed infants; however, the anemia was mild and resolved spontaneously without need for transfusion. (Connor, 1994) There has been no evidence of increase in congenital abnormalities in infant exposed to ZDV in utero, compared with the general population. Uninfected children who were participants in the PACTG 076 study have now been followed for over 4 years with no evidence of impact of ZDV on growth, neurodevelopment, or immunologic status. (Culnane, 1999)

ZDV carcinogenicity: Two transplacental carcinogenicity studies in mice showed different results: in one study (Olivero, 1997) two very high doses (approximately 25x and 50x daily human therapeutic exposure) were associated with an increase in lung, liver, and female genital tract tumors; in the second study (Ayers, 1997), a much lower dose (approximately 3x human therapeutic exposure) was not associated with an increase in tumors. A consensus conference reviewed all available information and concluded that the known benefits of zidovudine far outweighed the theoretical risks, but recommended long-term follow-up of infants exposed in utero to zidovudine or other antiretrovirals. In a follow-up of over 700 infants with in utero exposure to ZDV, no malignancies were observed in up to 6 years of age. (Hanson, 1999)

- **Efavirenz**: In primate studies efavirenz was associated with anencepahaly, anopthalmia, microphthalmia, and cleft palate at doses comparable to human exposure, suggesting that this drug should be avoided during pregnancy, particularly early pregnancy, and in women at risk for pregnancy (trying to get pregnant or unsafe sexual practices). Pregnant women who have conceived while on efavirenz should be counseled about possible fetal risks. It is important to acknowledge that animal studies in primates have not been performed with any of the other antiretroviral agents.

- **Hydroxyurea**: Although hydroxyurea is not a true antiretroviral drug, it has been used in many antiretroviral regimens, particularly in ddI-containing regimens. There is limited human information on the use of hydroxyurea in pregnancy and there are reports of exposure during pregnancy without apparent adverse outcome; however, hydroxyurea has been referred to as a "universal teratogen" with evidence of teragenicity in every animal species studied and defects involving multiple organ systems. This agent should be avoided during pregnancy and in women at risk for pregnancy; pregnant women who have conceived while on a hydroxyurea-containing regimen should be counseled about possible fetal risks.

- **Indinavir**: Indinavir has been associated with indirect hyperbilirubinemia and increased risk for renal stones. Because of theoretical concerns about risk for renal stones in neonates who cannot voluntarily hydrate themselves adequately and possible complications associated with exacerbation of physiologic hyperbilirubinemia (especially in premature infants, who are at greater risk for neonatal jaundice and kernicterus), this drug should be avoided in late pregnancy. Because of its short half-life, these concerns may not apply to use of indinavir earlier in pregnancy.

- **Amprenavir:** Amprenavir oral solution contains high levels of propylene glycol (the capsule form does not contain propylene glycol). Pregnant women and infants and children under the age of 4 are unable to adequately metabolize and eliminate propylene glycol, leading to accumulation and potential serious adverse events, including hyperosmolarity, lactic acidosis, seizures, and respiratory depression. Amprenavir oral solution is contraindicated in pregnancy and in children under the age of 4 years.

- **Preterm delivery**: concerns about possible increased risk for preterm delivery were raised by a small retrospective series of pregnant women on combination antiretroviral therapy (Lorenzi, 1998); however, some studies have found increased preterm birth rates in women who were not on ARV therapy, especially with more advanced disease. (Martin, 1997; Leroy, 1998; Brocklehurst, 1998) Furthermore, other factors, such as substance abuse, nutritional status, smoking, and cocaine use, may also increase risk and be confounding variables. Preliminary analyses of multiple PACTG clinical trials do not show an increased rate of preterm birth in women on ARV therapy, with or without protease inhibitors.(Shapiro, 2000)

- **Mitochondrial toxicity:** a small series of uninfected infants exposed in utero to nucleoside analogue agents was reported with laboratory or clinical evidence of mitochondrial dysfunction; two developed severe neurologic disease and died. (Blanche, 1999) Subsequent studies have been reassuring. A review of 353 deaths in over 20,000 children (with and without ARV exposure) born to HIV-positive mothers followed prospectively in the U.S. found no evidence of mitochondrial toxicity as a contributing factor in the deaths. (Smith, 1999) Neurologic adverse events were reviewed in 1,798 infants exposed to ZDV/3TC or placebo in the PETRA study, an African perinatal prophylaxis trial; no increased risk of adverse neurologic events was observed in infants exposed to ZDV/3TC as compared to placebo. (Lange, 1999) Although these studies do not rule out the possibility of an association between mitochondrial dysfunction and ARV exposures in utero, the likelihood of severe or fatal manifestations appears to be extremely small.

Given the limited and relatively short-term experience with all antiretroviral agents in pregnancy, long-term follow-up of infants exposed to these medications in utero is important.

- ■ **Interaction of drugs with pregnancy-related side effects/physiologic changes:**

  - Drugs which cause GI upset may not be well tolerated in early pregnancy when morning sickness is common and may increase risk for nonadherence or inadequate blood levels from vomiting

  - Protease inhibitors and hyperglycemia: protease inhibitors have been associated with the development or worsening of existing hyperglycemia or diabetes and pregnancy also increases risk for glucose intolerance. It is unknown whether the use of PIs in pregnancy will exacerbate risk for development of gestational diabetes. Women receiving protease inhibitors in pregnancy should have their glucose levels monitored closely.

General Principles for Antiretroviral Treatment in Pregnancy (CDC, 2000)

- ■ Decisions regarding initiation or alteration of antiretroviral therapy should be the same in pregnant and nonpregnant women, with the additional considerations outlined above.

- ■ Monitor CD4 count/viral load according to guidelines for nonpregnant adults: in pregnancy, this should be done approximately each trimester, but may be needed more frequently with failing or altered therapy. CD4 percentage may be a more accurate reflection of immune status during pregnancy than absolute CD4 cell count, because of possible variation in absolute CD4 count secondary to dilutional effects associated with hemodynamic changes in pregnancy.

■ The three-part ZDV chemoprophylaxis regimen (Table 7-7) should be recommended for all HIV-infected pregnant women to reduce the risk of perinatal HIV transmission. Current clinical trial and epidemiologic data confirm the effectiveness of this regimen; furthermore, no other regimen studied to date in randomized clinical trials has shown superior results.

TABLE 7-7: ZIDOVUDINE PERINATAL TRANSMISSION PROPHYLAXIS REGIMEN

ANTEPARTUM	Initiation at 14–34 weeks gestation and continued throughout pregnancy A. PACTG 076 REGIMEN: ZDV 100 mg 5 times daily B. ACCEPTABLE ALTERNATIVE REGIMEN: ■ ZDV 200 mg 3 times daily or ■ ZDV 300 mg 2 times daily
INTRAPARTUM	During labor, ZDV 2 mg/kg intravenously over 1 hour, followed by a continuous infusion of 1 mg/kg intravenously until delivery.
POSTPARTUM	Oral administration of ZDV to the newborn (ZDV syrup, 2 mg/kg every 6 hours) for the first 6 weeks of life, beginning at 8 – 12 hours after birth.

In women already receiving antiretroviral therapy when they become pregnant and this regimen does not include zidovudine, ZDV should be added or substituted for another nucleoside analogue agent after 14 weeks' gestation. There is evidence that duration of prior ZDV therapy in women with more advanced disease may not reduce effectiveness of ZDV in decreasing perinatal transmission. (Stiehm, 1999) However, ZDV should not be substituted for another antiretroviral agent when this is likely to reduce the efficacy of this regimen in treatment of maternal disease, i.e., with previous clinical failure of ZDV or history of documented ZDV resistance.

In some circumstances ZDV cannot be used during the antepartum period (e.g., intolerance to ZDV). d4T and ZDV appear to be pharmacologically antagonistic and should not be used together; therefore, women on d4T-containing regimens with prior ZDV failure should be continued on the most effective regimen for their disease and ZDV should be excluded if d4T is maintained. ZDV administration is recommended during the intrapartum period and for the newborn regardless of the antepartum antiretroviral regimen.

Women who present in labor with no prior antepartum antiretroviral therapy may be treated with one of several effective regimens, described below (Intrapartum Management) and in Table 7-8.

TABLE 7-8: COMPARISON OF INTRAPARTUM/POSTPARTUM REGIMENS FOR HIV-INFECTED WOMEN IN LABOR WHO HAVE HAD NO PRIOR ANTIRETROVIRAL THERAPY (SCENARIO 3)

DRUG REGIMEN	SOURCE OF EVIDENCE	MATERNAL INTRAPARTUM	INFANT POSTPARTUM	DATA ON TRANSMISSION	ADVANTAGES	DISADVANTAGES
Nevirapine	Clinical trial, Africa; compared to oral ZDV given intrapartum and for 1 week to the infant	Single 200 mg oral dose at onset of labor	Single 2 mg/kg oral dose at age 48-72 hours* * If the mother received nevirapine less than 1 hour prior to delivery, the infant was given 2 mg/kg oral nevirapine as soon as possible after birth and again at 48-72 hours.	Transmission at 6 weeks 12% with nevirapine compared to 21% with ZDV, a 47% (95% CI, 20-64%) reduction	Inexpensive Oral regimen Simple; easy to administer Can give directly observed treatment	Unknown efficacy if mother has nevirapin-resistant virus
ZDV/3TC	Clinical trial, Africa; compared to placebo	ZDV 600 mg orally at onset of labor, followed by 300 mg orally every 3 hours until delivery AND 3TC 150 mg orally at onset of labor, followed by 150 mg orally every 12 hours until delivery	ZDV 4 mg/kg orally every 12 hours AND 3TC 2 mg/kg orally every 12 hours for 7 days	Transmission at 6 weeks 10% with ZDV/3TC compared to 17% with placebo, a 38% reduction	Oral regimen Compliance easier than 6 weeks of ZDV alone as infant regimen is only 1 week	Potential toxicity of multiple drug exposure

Table continues . . .

TABLE 7-8: COMPARISON OF INTRAPARTUM/POSTPARTUM REGIMENS FOR HIV-INFECTED WOMEN IN LABOR WHO HAVE HAD NO PRIOR ANTIRETROVIRAL THERAPY (SCENARIO 3) (continued)

DRUG REGIMEN	SOURCE OF EVIDENCE	MATERNAL INTRAPARTUM	INFANT POSTPARTUM	DATA ON TRANSMISSION	ADVANTAGES	DISADVANTAGES
ZDV	Epidemiologic data, U.S.; compared to no ZDV treatment	2 mg/kg intravenous bolus, followed by continuous infusion of 1 mg/kg/hr until delivery	2 mg/kg orally every 6 hours for 6 weeks	Transmission 10% with ZDV compared to 27% with no ZDV treatment, a 62% (95% CI, 19-82%) reduction	Has been standard recommendation based on clinical trial results	Requires intravenous administration and availability of ZDV intravenous formulation Compliance with 6 week infant regimen
ZDV and Nevirapine	Theoretical	ZDV 2 mg/kg intravenous bolus, followed by continuous infusion of 1 mg/kg/hr until delivery AND Nevirapine single 200 mg oral dose at onset of labor	ZDV 2 mg/kg orally every 6 hours for 6 weeks AND Nevirapine single 2 mg/kg oral dose at age 48-72 hours	No data	Potential benefit if maternal virus is resistant to either nevirapine or ZDV Synergistic inhibition of HIV replication with combination in vitro	Requires intravenous administration and availability of ZDV intravenous formulation Compliance with 6 week infant ZDV regimen Unknown efficacy and limited toxicity data

VII

■ Women with high CD4 counts and low or undetectable HIV-RNA levels, for whom initiation of antiretroviral therapy for the treatment of maternal infection would be considered optional, should be counseled about the potential benefits and risks of standard combination therapy and offered this therapy, along with the three-part ZDV perinatal prophylaxis regimen.

Using ZDV alone is an option in this situation. This has the advantage of limiting exposure to other drugs during pregnancy but there are theoretical concerns about the selection of ZDV-resistant viral variants and limitation of future maternal therapeutic options, as well as increasing the risk for transmission. A recent study in women with moderately advanced HIV, many of whom had been treated with ZDV before pregnancy, found that maternal ZDV resistance was predictive of transmission. (Welles, 2000) However, the development of resistance should be minimized by the relatively short duration of therapy and the more limited viral replication present in individuals with low HIV-RNA level and high CD4 count. Follow-up of women enrolled in the PACTG 076 study has shown no significant differences in immunologic status or progression of disease (median follow-up 4.2 years) in women who received ZDV compared to placebo recipients. (Bardeguez, 1999)

■ In antiretroviral naïve patients clinicians may consider delaying initiation of ARV therapy until after 10–12 weeks of gestation, based on considerations of the woman's health status, the potential risk of delaying therapy for several weeks, and the potential benefits of avoiding first trimester drug exposure for the fetus.

■ In antiretroviral-experienced patients, who become pregnant or are referred into prenatal care while on ARV therapy, therapy should be continued or modified, subject to the considerations outlined above. If pregnancy is recognized in the first trimester, some women and their clinicians may consider temporary discontinuation of therapy until after completion of the first trimester because of concerns about potential teratogenicity, or because of significant nausea and vomiting in early pregnancy leading to concerns about inadequate absorption of medications.

Current data are insufficient to either support or refute fetal risk with early exposure to antiretroviral agents. Discontinuation of therapy may lead to viral rebound, which could theoretically increase risk of intrauterine HIV transmission or have an adverse effect on maternal disease. The woman's clinical, immunologic, and virologic status should also be considered in decisions regarding continuation of therapy in the first trimester.

If the decision is made to stop therapy temporarily, all agents should be stopped simulataneously and restarted simultaneously in the second trimester to avoid development of drug resistance.

■ Decisions regarding use of ARV therapy during pregnancy should be made
by the woman after detailed discussion of benefits and potential risks of
therapy. This includes discussion of:

- Treatment recommendations for health of the HIV-infected woman
- Current information regarding effectiveness of antiretroviral therapy
  in reducing perinatal transmission
- Known or potential effects of antiretroviral drug exposure on the
  fetus/newborn
- The importance of adherence to any prescribed antiretroviral regimen

There continue to be missed opportunities in prevention of transmission
of HIV from mother to child. HIV has to first be identified in the woman; situations where counseling and testing have not been available or not utilized
because of lack of perception of risk on the part of the woman or her health
care provider have been associated with perinatal transmission in some cases.
Women who become infected or seroconvert during pregnancy may be missed
unless HIV testing is repeated later in pregnancy. Lack of prenatal care and
active substance abuse, which frequently co-exist, have also been linked to
potentially avoidable increased risk for transmission. (Bardeguez, 2000)

Antiretroviral Pregnancy Registry

The Antiretroviral Registry is a collaborative effort between pharmaceutical
companies, the Centers for Disease Control and Prevention, the National
Institutes of Health, and obstetrical and pediatric practitioners to collect
observational information on antiretroviral exposure during pregnancy in
order to assess potential fetal/infant anomalies after exposure to these agents.
Patient names are not used and information is confidential. Health care
providers who are treating HIV-infected pregnant women are strongly encouraged to report cases of prenatal exposure to antiretroviral drugs to the Registry: 1410 Commonwealth Drive, Wilmington, NC 28403; telephone (800)
258-4263; fax (800) 800-1052.

OPPORTUNISTIC INFECTION PROPHYLAXIS

Indications and recommendations for primary prophylaxis of opportunistic
infections in pregnancy are noted in Table 7-9. Once an individual has had the
following infections, prophylaxis to prevent recurrence is recommended as
standard of care for the life of the individual (see Chapter IV on Primary
Medical Care). First-choice regimens are outlined:

■ **Pneumocystis carinii pneumonia:** same regimen as for primary prophylaxis

■ **Toxoplasmic encephalitis:** sulfadiazine 500–1000 mg po q.i.d. **plus**
pyrimethamine 25–75 mg po q.d. **plus** leucovorin 10–25 mg po q.d.; counsel regarding concerns about potential teratogenicity of pyrimethamine and
benefits of life-long therapy

TABLE 7-9: OPPORTUNISTIC INFECTIONS AND PRIMARY PROPHYLAXIS IN PREGNANT WOMEN

STRONGLY RECOMMENDED

PATHOGEN	INDICATION	REGIMEN	ALTERNATIVES	COMMENTS
Pneumocystis carinii (PCP)	CD4< 200/mm^3 **or** oral thrush	TMP-SMZ DS 1 po qd TMP-SMZ SS 1 po qd	Dapsone 50mg po bid Dapsone 100mg po qd Aerosolized pentamidine (AP) 300mg q mo (via Respirgard II nebulizer) TMP-SMZ DS 1 po tiw	Some providers may prefer to use AP in first trimester because of lack of systemic absorption and fetal exposure, secondary to theoretical concerns about possible teratogenicity with systemic medications.
Mycobacterium tuberculosis (M.tb) INH[1] sensitive	TST reaction ≥5mm **or** prior positive TST without treatment **or** contact with active TB	INH 300mg po qd **plus** pyridoxine 50mg po qd x 9 mo INH 900mg po biw **plus** pyridoxine 100mg po biw x 9 mo	Rifampin 600mg po qd x 4 mo	Some providers may choose to initiate phrophylaxis after the 1st trimester, because of concerns about possible teratogenicity. Anecdotal experience with rifampin has not been associated with adverse pregnancy outcomes. Pyrazinamide should generally be avoided, particularly in the 1st trimester, because of lack of information concerning fetal effects.
INH resistant multi-drug resistant	same; high probability of exposure to resistant M.tb			Choice of drugs requires consultation with obstetrical experts and public health authorities

Table continues . . .

TABLE 7-9: OPPORTUNISTIC INFECTIONS AND PRIMARY PROPHYLAXIS IN PREGNANT WOMEN *(continued)*

STRONGLY RECOMMENDED

PATHOGEN	INDICATION	REGIMEN	ALTERNATIVES	COMMENTS
Toxoplasma gondii	IgG antibody to Toxoplasma *and* CD4 < 100/mm³	TMP-SMZ[2] DS 1 po qd	TMP-SMZ SS 1 po qd	If patient cannot tolerate TMP-SMZ, the recommended alternative is dapsone-pyrimethamine; however, because of the low incidence of TE[3] during pregnancy and possible fetal risk with pyrimethamine, chemoprophylaxis may reasonably be deferred until after pregnancy
Mycobacterium avium complex	CD4 < 50 mm³	Azithromycin 1200mg po qw	Rifabutin 300mg po qd	Some providers may prefer to defer prophylaxis until after the first trimester, because of general concerns about administering drugs in early pregnancy. Experience with rifabutin in pregnancy is limited.

[1] INH — isoniazid

[2] TMP-SMZ — trimethoprim-sulfamethoxazole

[3] TE- toxoplasmic encephalitis

Source: Adapted from 1999 USPHS/IDSA Guidelines for the Prevention of Opportunistic Infections in Persons Infected with Human Immunodeficiency Virus, *MMWR* 48 (RR-10):1-66, 1999.

VII

- **Disseminated MAC:** azithromycin 500 mg po q.d. **plus** ethambutol 15 mg/kg po q.d.

- **CMV:** choice of agents should be individualized in pregnancy after consultation with experts; discontinuation of maintenance therapy with history of CMV retinitis may be considered with sustained (> 3–6 months) elevation of CD4 count above 100–150/mm^3 and durable suppression of plasma HIV-RNA levels. Opthalmologic consultation is recommended if discontinuation of secondary prophylaxis is considered.

- **Histoplasmosis:** amphotericin B 1.0 mg/kg iv q.w.- may be preferred, particularly during the first trimester, because of occurrence of craniofacial and skeletal abnormalities in infants after prolonged in utero exposure to fluconazole.

- **Crytococcosis:** amphotericin B 0.6–1.0 mg/kg iv q.w.-t.i.w.- may be preferred, particularly during the first trimester, because of occurrence of craniofacial and skeletal abnormalities in infants after prolonged in utero exposure to fluconazole.

- **Coccidiomycosis:** same as for histoplasmosis

IMMUNIZATIONS (CDC, 1993; CDC, 1999; ACOG, 1991)

Immunization should be considered in pregnancy when the risk for exposure is high, risk of infection for mother or fetus is high, and the vaccine is thought unlikely to cause harm. HIV-infected individuals should avoid live virus or live bacteria vaccines. HIV-positive persons who are symptomatic or have low CD4 cell counts may have suboptimal responses to vaccination. Some, but not all, studies have shown a transient (< 4 weeks) increase in viral load after immunization. This is of some theoretical concern, given the association between viral load and perinatal transmission. This increase in viremia may be prevented with appropriate antiretroviral therapy. (Bartlett, 1999) For this reason, clinicians may consider deferring routine vaccination until after the patient is on an effective antiretroviral regimen and avoiding administration late in pregnancy, close to delivery, when most transmission is thought to occur.

Current immunization recommendations for HIV-positive pregnant women are:

- **pneumococcal vaccine** — "generally recommended"
- **influenza vaccine** — "generally recommended"; administer before flu season
- **tetanus-diphtheria (Td) vaccine** — booster dose every ten years after completion of primary series
- **hepatitis B vaccine** — "generally recommended" for all susceptible (anti-HBc-negative) patients; three doses at 0,1,6 months
- **hepatitis A vaccine** — "generally recommended" for all susceptible (anti-HAV-negative) patients with chronic hepatitis C ; also indicated

prior to travel to endemic areas, in injection drug users, and with community outbreaks; two doses at 0,6 months

■ **enhanced potency inactivated polio vaccine** — use if not previously immunized and traveling to areas where risk for exposure is high; oral polio vaccine is a live virus vaccine and is contraindicated in HIV-positive persons

■ **immune globulins**

● immune globulin recommended for measles exposure in symptomatic HIV-positive persons and hepatitis A with exposure to HAV in close contact/sex partner or travel to underdeveloped country (especially in patient with advanced HIV, who have have poor antibody response to vaccine)

● hyperimmune globulins recommended:

➤ varicella-zoster immune globulin (VZIG)-susceptible adult (undetectable antibodies to VZV) after significant contact (household, hospital room, close indoor contact > 1 hour, prolonged face-to-face contact) to chickenpox or zoster; give within 96 hours of exposure

➤ hepatitis B immune globulin (HBIG)-needlestick or sexual contact with HbsAg+ person in susceptible individual (anti-HBc-negative); HBIG and HBV vaccine series should be started within 14 days of last exposure

REDUCTION OF SECONDARY RISK FACTORS

Treatment of STDs or other co-infections; encouragement of safer sexual practices during pregnancy; discouragement of smoking and drug use; and substance abuse treatment should be employed as measures which may decrease risk of perinatal transmission.

FREQUENCY OF VISITS

Determined on an individual basis, based on gestational age, health of the mother, presence of pregnancy-related complications, antiretroviral regimen and response, and psychosocial needs. In uncomplicated pregnancies visits generally are scheduled monthly in early pregnancy and every 1–2 weeks from 28–30 weeks of gestation until delivery.

COUNSELING AND SUPPORT

■ **Support systems:** At the initial visit the health care provider should assess the patient's support system — who knows her HIV status, problems encountered with disclosure, family and/or friends to whom she turns for ongoing support, barriers to disclosure to sexual or needle-sharing partners. These issues should be readdressed at intervals throughout pregnancy as needed. The use of peer counselors may be especially helpful.

■ **Contraception use postpartum**: Discussion about postpartum contraceptive plans should be initiated in early to mid-pregnancy to allow comprehensive education and counseling about available options and adequate time for informed decision making.

■ **Condom use during pregnancy**: Sexual activity should be reviewed at each visit and condom use reinforced.

■ **Drug use/treatment**: History of and/or ongoing substance abuse, including tobacco and alcohol, as well as illicit drugs, should be assessed at the initial visit and at intervals during prenatal care, if indicated. Type of substance(s), amount of use, route of administration, and prior drug or alcohol treatment should be documented. The patient should be counseled about specific risks associated with substance abuse in pregnancy (See Chapter X on Substance Abuse) and drug or alcohol treatment during pregnancy should be encouraged and facilitated for active problems.

■ **Adherence**: Each patient should be educated and counseled about the importance of adherence to prescribed medications, particularly antiretroviral drugs, before they are initiated and medication adherence should be assessed and reinforced at each visit. (see Chapter V on Adherence)

■ **Clinical trials**: Pregnant HIV-positive women should be informed about the availability of and offered participation in clinical trials to which they are eligible.

■ **Advance directives**: The issue of advance directives for care in the event of sudden deterioration in the woman's health, as well as guardianship plans for children in the event of the mother's incapacitation or death should be discussed; legal assistance should be facilitated, if needed.

X. INTRAPARTUM

A. UNIVERSAL PRECAUTIONS

Gowns, gloves, and eye protection should be used in all deliveries and in examinations or procedures likely to generate splashing of blood or amniotic fluid. (See Chapter XIII on Occupational Exposure)

B. FETAL/MATERNAL MONITORING

External fetal monitoring should be employed but avoid use of fetal scalp electrodes or fetal scalp sampling. Avoid artificial rupture of membranes if possible.

C. MODE OF DELIVERY

Based on data showing a reduction in perinatal HIV transmission (in addition to that seen with ZDV prophylaxis alone) with scheduled C-section (see above), all HIV-infected pregnant women should be counseled about the possible benefit versus risk of scheduled C-section and the limitations of current studies. Infants born to mothers with high plasma viral loads benefit most from planned Cesarean delivery. Data are insufficient to demonstrate benefit in women with very low or undetectable viral loads and/or women on HAART therapy. There is no evidence that performing C-section after onset of labor or ruptured membranes reduces transmission rate; this needs further study given the recent data about duration of ruptured membranes and increasing risk of transmission. Women should be informed that there is no therapy or combination of therapies which can guarantee an uninfected infant.

Ultimate decisions about the route of delivery must be individualized and the woman's autonomy must be respected. If scheduled C-section is planned, best clinical estimates of gestational age should be used and scheduling is recommended at 38 completed weeks of gestation to minimize the likelihood of labor and membrane rupture. (ACOG, 1999)

D. INTRAPARTUM ARV PROPHYLAXIS

Women who have been on an appropriate antiretroviral regimen during the course of pregnancy should receive ZDV in labor: 2mg/kg ZDV in a one-hour IV loading dose, followed by 1 mg/kg/hr by IV infusion. If scheduled cesarean section is planned, ZDV infusion should be begun 3 hours preoperatively to achieve adequate blood levels.

For women who present in labor with no prior antiretroviral therapy, there are several effective regimens available. (Guay, 1999; Saba, 1999; Wade, 1998; Perinatal HIV Guidelines Working Group, 2000) These are outlined in Table 7-8.

Women of unknown HIV status who present in labor with no prenatal care may be offered rapid HIV testing, after careful counseling and with informed consent. Positive results should be confirmed by standard serologic testing but enable the initiation of an appropriate antiretroviral regimen to reduce the risk of perinatal transmission.

E. ANTIBIOTIC PROPHYLAXIS:

Data are limited on the relationship between HIV infection and incidence of peripartum (e.g., chorioamnionitis, postpartum endometritis) infections. Results of histologic placental studies are conflicting but more recent studies do not suggest an increased risk of chorioamnionitis in HIV-positive pregnancies. (Hofman, 1998; Ladner, 1998) Several earlier studies (Gichangi, 1993) found an increase in histologic chorioamnionitis in HIV-positive pregnancies, particularly in those with preterm deliveries. (Gichangi, 1993; Kumar, 1995) Maternal HIV infection has been associated with an increased risk of postpartum endometritis, particularly in more immunosuppressed women (Temmerman, 1994); furthermore, some studies have shown an increase in post-Cesarean section infectious morbidity in HIV-positive women, correlated

VII

with lower CD4 counts, (Maiques-Montesinos, 1999; Semprini, 1995) as compared to HIV-negative controls. A recent analysis of complications according to mode of delivery among HIV-positive women with CD4 < 500/mm³ found peripartum infectious complications were common and were seen more frequently in women delivered by C-section compared to vaginal delivery; however, rates of complications were not significantly different from those found in similar HIV-uninfected women; in this study peripartum antibiotic prophylaxis was given in approximately three-quarters of patients undergoing C-section and in approximately one-third of those with vaginal delivery. (Watts, 1999) Increased rates of infectious complications may be related to confounding factors, such as poor nutritional status, substance abuse, or prevalence of genital tract infections, rather than to the presence of HIV infection. (Hanna, 1997)

There are currently no data on the role of prophylactic peripartum antibiotics in reducing risk of infectious morbidity for HIV-positive women. However, because of the concerns about possible increased risk of post-Cesarean infections in HIV-positive patients, prophylactic antibiotics are recommended at the time of scheduled C-section.

F. VAGINAL CLEANSING

A promising potential intervention to reduce transmission at the time of vaginal delivery is vaginal cleansing to decrease neonatal exposure to maternal blood and genital secretions. A clinical trial of 0.25% chlorhexidine manual vaginal cleansing on admission and every 4 hours until delivery had no significant impact on HIV transmission, except when membranes had been ruptured for more than 4 hours before delivery. (Biggar, 1996) Further study is needed.

XI. POSTPARTUM

A. INFANT FEEDING

When safe alternatives are available, breastfeeding is discouraged because of documented risk for transmission from mother to infant.

B. ASSESS HEALING

Assess healing of wound sites, uterine involution, and appropriate cessation of postpartum bleeding

C. CARE FOR MOTHER AND INFANT

HIV-infected mothers may neglect their own care while trying to provide appropriate care for their infant and other children or family members. It is essential that she be linked with comprehensive medical and supportive care services, including HIV specialty care; primary medical and gynecologic care;

mental health or substance abuse treatment services; and assistance with food, housing, transportation and legal/advocacy services, if needed.

Women who have received ZDV monotherapy during pregnancy should be re-evaluated in the postpartum period with clinical assessment, CD4 count and HIV-RNA level to determine need for ongoing antiretroviral therapy. It is essential that access to and continuity of antiretroviral treatment as needed for maternal health be ensured.

Similarly, the HIV-exposed infant should be linked into ongoing pediatric care, with HIV diagnostic tests as described below and appropriate HIV specialty care if HIV-infected.

D. CONTRACEPTION/CONDOM USE

Discussions about contraception and condom use should be continuous throughout pregnancy and reviewed and reinforced at the time of the postpartum visit.

E. LONG-TERM FOLLOW-UP OF MOTHER AND INFANT

All HIV-positive mothers and infants exposed to ZDV and/or other antiretroviral drugs or combinations during pregnancy should have long-term follow-up to assess possible late effects of these therapies on HIV progression in the mother or neoplasia or organ-system toxicity in exposed children.

XII. CARE OF THE HIV-EXPOSED INFANT (CDC, 2000)

A. DIAGNOSIS OF HIV

The standard for diagnosis of HIV infection in exposed infants is the use of viral assays (HIV-DNA PCR (preferred), HIV-RNA PCR, or viral culture) obtained within 48 hours of birth, at 1–2 months, and 3–6 months. HIV can be excluded with two or more negative tests, two of which are performed at age > or = 1 month, and one performed at age > or = 4 months. HIV IgG antibody tests will generally be positive in exposed infants up to 18 months of age because of transplacental passage; two negative tests performed at > or = 6 months and at least 1 month apart will also exclude infection in infants without clinical evidence of infection. P 24 antigen testing is less sensitive than other virologic tests and has a high frequency of false positive results in infants < 1 month of age.

HIV-DNA PCR is the preferred virologic assay for diagnosis with 93% (90% CI=76%–97%) sensitivity by age 14 days. Data on use of HIV-RNA PCR is more limited. HIV culture is sensitive for early diagnosis but is more complex, expensive, and has a longer turnaround time for results. Using these tests approximately 40% of infected infants can be identified by age 48 hours and are considered to have early or intrauterine infection; infants with initial negative testing during the first week of life and subsequent positive tests are considered to have intrapartum infection. Almost all infected infants can now be diagnosed by the age of 6 months. ZDV monotherapy for perinatal prophylaxis has not been shown to delay detection of HIV or decrease sensitivity or predictive value of virologic assays (Connor, 1994; Kovacs, 1995), although performance of these tests when the mother has received more intensive combination antiretroviral therapies has not been studied.

B. ARV TREATMENT

All HIV-exposed infants should receive ZDV prophylaxis (2 mg/kg/dose every 6 hours) for the first six weeks of life as part of the three-part zidovudine regimen to prevent perinatal HIV transmission. If the mother has received no antepartum or intrapartum ZDV, the newborn regimen should be started as soon as possible after delivery, preferably with 12–24 hours of birth. Initiation of ZDV prophylaxis for the neonate within 48 hours of birth resulted in an approximately 50% decrease in infection compared to no therapy. (Wade, 1998) When the mother has received no therapy, it is unknown whether combining newborn ZDV with administration of a single dose of nevirapine (2 mg/kg) to the infant as soon as possible after birth, or the use of nevirapine alone (particularly when there are concerns about the infant care provider's ability or willingness to administer ZDV for 6 weeks) will be as effective or more effective than zidovudine only. This approach has some theoretical attractiveness, since nevirapine can decrease plasma HIV-1-RNA concentration by over 1 log by 7 days after a single dose, is active immediately against both intracellular and extracellular virus, and has prolonged elimination in infants. Another theoretical benefit with combining ZDV and nevirapine includes potential efficacy in the presence of virus that is resistant to either drug.

Once infection is documented, more intensive combination antiretroviral therapy is recommended with clinical symptoms of HIV infection or evidence of immunesuppression (immune categories 2 or 3 — Table 7-10) regardless of age or viral load. Some experts recommend initiating potent ART as soon as the diagnosis is confirmed, regardless of clinical or immunologic status or viral load since HIV-infected infants under the age of 12 months are considered to be at high risk for disease progression and the prognostic value of standard virologic or immunologic parameters is less than that for older children. Once HIV infection is confirmed, decisions about antiretroviral therapy should be made in consultation with a specialist in the treatment of pediatric HIV infection.

C. PCP PROPHYLAXIS

All HIV-exposed infants should receive PCP prophylaxis with trimethoprim-sulfamethoxazole ($150/750$ mg/m^2/d in two divided doses po t.i.w. on consecutive days) beginning at 4–6 weeks and extending for the first year of life or until HIV infection is excluded. Dapsone or atovaquone are alternatives.

TABLE 7-10: 1994 REVISED HUMAN IMMUNODEFICIENCY VIRUS PEDIATRIC CLASSIFICATION SYSTEM: IMMUNE CATEGORIES BASED ON AGE-SPECIFIC CD4+T-LYMPHOCYTE COUNT AND PERCENTAGE*

IMMUNE CATEGORY	< 12 MONTHS		1–5 YEARS		6–12 YEARS	
	No./µL	(%)	No./µL	(%)	No./µL	(%)
Category 1: no suppression	≥ 1,500	(≥ 25%)	≥ 1,000	(≥ 25%)	≥ 500	(≥ 25%)
Category 2: moderate suppression	750–1,499	(15%–24%)	500–999	(15%–24%)	200–499	(15%–24%)
Category 3: severe suppression	< 750	(< 15%)	< 500	(< 15%)	< 200	(< 15%)

Source: Adapted from CDC. 1994 Revised classification system for human immunodeficiency virus infection in children less than 13 years of age. MMWR 1994; 43 (No. RR-12): 1–10.

REFERENCES

ACOG. Antepartum fetal surveillance. ACOG Practice Bulletin # 9, October, 1999.

ACOG. Management of herpes in pregnancy. ACOG Practice Bulletin 8, Oct 1999.

ACOG Committee Opinion # 219, August 1999. ACOG. Scheduled Cesarean delivery and the prevention of vertical transmission of HIV infection.

ACOG. Viral hepatitis in pregnancy. ACOG Educational Bulletin #248, July 1998.

ACOG. Ultasonography in pregnancy. ACOG Technical Bulletin # 187, December 1993.

ACOG. Perinatal viral and parasitic infections. ACOG Technical Bulletin #177, February, 1993.

ACOG. Immunization during pregnancy. ACOG Technical Bulletin # 160, October 1991.

Alliegro MB, Dorrucci M, Phillips AN, et al. Incidence and consequences of pregnancy in women with known duration of HIV infection. Italian Seroconversion Study Group. *Arch Intern Med* 157: 2585–2590, 1997.

Augenbraun M, Feldman J, Chirgwin K, et al. Increased genital shedding of herpes simplex virus type 2 in HIV-seropositive women. *Ann Intern Med* 123:845–847, 1995.

Ayers KM, Torrey CE, Reynolds DJ. A transplacental carcinogenicity bioassay in CD-1 mice with zidovudine. *Fundam Appl Toxicol* 38:195–198, 1997.

Bardeguez A, Mofenson LM, Fowler M, et al. Lack of clinical or immunologic disease progression with transient use of zidovudine (ZDV) to reduce perinatal HIV transmission in PACTG 076. 12th World AIDS Conference. Geneva, Switzerland, June 28–July 3, 1998 (abstract 12233).

Bardeguez A, Pompeo L, Bettica L, Holland B, Swerdlow J. Perinatal HIV transmission among women with no prenatal care. 7th Conf Retroviruses Opportunistic Infect (abst 711), Jan 30–Feb 2, 2000.

Bartlett JG. *1999 Medical Management of HIV Infection.* Baltimore, MD: Johns Hopkins University; 1999

Becker-Pergola G, Guay L, Mmiro F, et al. Selection of the K103N nevirapine (NVP) resistance mutation in Ugandan women receiving NVP prophylaxis to prevent HIV-1 vertical transmission (HIV-NET-006). 7th Conf Retroviruses Opportunistic Infect (abst # 658), Jan 30–Feb 2, 2000.

Biggar RJ, Miotti PG, Taha TE, et al. Perinatal intervention trial in Africa: effect of a birth canal cleansing intervention to prevent HIV transmission. *Lancet* 347:1647–1650, 1996.

Blanche S, Tardieu M, Rustin P et al. Persistent mitochondrial dysfunction and perinatal exposure to antiretroviral nucleoside analogues. *Lancet* 354:1084–1089, 1999.

Brettle RP,Raab GM, Ross A, Fielding KL, Gore SM, Bird AG. HIV infection in women:immunological markers and the influence of pregnancy. *AIDS* 9(10): 1177–1184, 1995.

Brocklehurst P, French R. The association between maternal HIV infection and perinatal outcome: a systematic review of the literature and meta-analysis. *Br J Obstet Gynaecol* 105: 836–848, 1998.

Brocklehurst P, Kinghorn G, Carney O, et al. A randomised placebo controlled trial of suppressive acyclovir in late pregnancy in women with recurrent genital herpes infection. *Br J Obstet Gynaecol* 105:275–280, 1998.

Bulterys M, Landesman S, Burns DN, Rubinstein A, Goedert J. Sexual behavior and injection drug use during pregnancy and vertical transmission of HIV-1. *J Acquir Immune Defic Syndr Hum Retrovirol* 15:76–82, 1997.

Burns DN, Landesman S, Muenz LR, et al. Cigarette smoking, premature rupture of membranes and vertical transmission of HIV-1 among women with low CD4 levels. *J Acquir Immune Defic Syndr Hum Retrovirol* 7:718–726, 1994.

Burns DN, Landesman S, Minkoff H, Wright DJ, Waters D, Mitchell RM, et al. The influence of pregnancy on human immunodeficiency virus type-1 infection: antepartum and postpartum changes in human immunodeficiency virus type-1 viral load. *Am J Obstet Gynecol* 178: 355–359, 1998.

Burns DN, Tuomala R, Chang BH, et al. Vaginal colonization or infection with Candida albicans in human immunodeficiency virus-infected women during pregnancy and during the postpartum period. Women and Infants Transmission Study Group. *Clin Infect Dis* 24 (2):201–210, 1997.

CaroPaton T, Carvajal A, Martin de Diego I, Martin_arias LH, Alvarez Requejo A, Rodriguez Pinilla E. Is metronidazole teratogenic? A meta-analysis. *Br J Clin Pharmacol* 44:179–182, 1997.

CDC. 1999 USPHS/IDSA guidelines for the prevention of opportunistic infections with persons infected with human immunodeficiency virus. *MMWR* 48 (RR-10): 1–66, 1999.

CDC. 1998 guidelines for treatment of sexually transmitted diseases. *MMWR* 47 (RR-1): 1–116, 1998.

CDC. Guidelines for the use of antiretroviral agents in HIV-infected adults and adolescents. *MMWR* 47(RR-5):39–82, 1998 (and updates **http://www.hivatis.org**).

CDC. Recommendations for prevention and control of hepatitis C virus (HCV) infection and HCV-related chronic disease. *MMWR* 47(RR-19), 1998.

CDC. Recommendations of the Advisory Committee on Immunization Practices (ACIP): Use of vaccines and immune globulins in persons with altered immunocompetence. *MMWR* 42 (RR-04): 1993.

CDC. Guidelines for the use of antiretroviral agents in pediatric HIV infection.(text and updates: **http://www.hivatis.org**.)

CDC. Hepatitis B virus: a comprehensive strategy for eliminating transmission in the United States through universal childhood vaccination: recommendations of the immunization practices advisory committee (ACIP). *MMWR* 40 (RR-13), 1991.

CDC. U.S. Public Health Service task force recommendations for the use of antiretroviral drugs in pregnant women infected with HIV-1 for maternal health and for reducing perinatal HIV-1 transmission in the United States. (**http://www.hivatis.org**)

Chuachoowong R, Shaffer N, Siriwasin W, et al. Short-course antenatal zidovudine reduces both cervicovaginal human immunodeficiency virus type 1 levels and risk of perinatal transmission. *J Infect Dis* 181:99–106, 2000.

Clarke JR, Braganza R, Mirza A, et al. Rapid development of genotypic resistance to lamivudine when combined with zidovudine in pregnancy. *J Med Virol* 59(3):364–368, 1999.

Colgrove RC, Pitt J, Chung PH, Welles SL, Japour AJ. Selective vertical transmission of HIV-1 antiretroviral resistance mutations. *AIDS* 12:2281–2288, 1998.

Connor EM, Sperling RS, Gelber R et al. Reduction of maternal-infant transmission of human immunodeficiency virus type 1 with zidovudine treatment. *N Engl J Med* 331: 1173–1180,1994.

Coutsoudis A, Pillay K, Spooner E, Kuhn L, Coovadia HM. Randomized trial testing the effect of vitamin A supplementation on pregnancy outcoomes and early mother-to-child HIV-1 transmission in Durban, South Africa. South African Vitamin A Study Group. *AIDS* 13:1517–1524, 1999.

Culnane M, Fowler MG, Lee SS, et al. Lack of long-term effects of in utero exposure to zidovudine among uninfected children born to HIV-infected women. *JAMA* 281:151–157, 1999.

Cu-Uvin S, Hogan JW, Warren D et al. Prevalence of lower genital tract infections among human immunodeficiency virus (HIV)-seropositive and high risk HIV-seronegative women. HIV Epidemiology Research Study Group. *Clin Infect Dis* 29:1145–1150, 1999.

Davis SF, Rosen DH, Steinberg S, Wortley PM, Karon JM, Gwinn M. Trends in HIV prevalence among childbearing women in the United States, 1989–1994. *J Acquir Immune Defic Syndr Hum Retrovirol* 19:158–164, 1998.

Desgrees du L A, Msellati P, Yao A, et al. Impaired fertility in HIV-1 infected pregnant women: a clinic-based survey in Abidjan, Cote d'Ivoire, 1997. *AIDS* 13:517–521, 1999

Dickover R, Garratty E, Plaeger S, Bryson Y. Perinatal transmission of major, minor, and multiple HIV-1 strains in utero and intrapartum. 7th Conf on Retroviruses and Opportunistic Infections (abst 181), Jan 30–Feb 2, 2000.

Duerr A, Sierra MF, Feldman J, Clarke LM, Ehrlich I, DeHovitz J. Immune compromise and prevalence of Candida vulvovaginitis in human immunodeficiency virus-infected women.. *Obstet Gynecol* 90:252–256, 1997.

Dunn DT, Newell ML, Ades AE, Peckham CS. Risk of human immunodeficiency virus type 1 transmission through breastfeeding. *Lancet* 340:585–588, 1992.

Eastman PS, Shapiro DE, Coombs RW, et al. Maternal viral genotypic resistance and infrequent failure of zidovudine therapy to prevent perinatal transmission of human immunodeficiency virus type 1 in Pediatric AIDS Clinical Trial Group Protocol 076. *J Infect Dis* 177:557–564, 1998.

European Collaborative Study and Research Network on Congenital Toxoplasmosis. Low incidence of congenital toxoplasmoswis in children born to women infected with human immunodeficiency virus. *Eur J Obstet Gynecol Reprod Biol* 68:93–96, 1996.

European Collaborative Study and the Swiss HIV Pregnancy Cohort. Immunological markers in HIV-infected pregnant women. *AIDS* 11(15): 1859–1865, 1997.

Fang G, Burger H, Anastos K, et al. Sequence analysis of the complete HIV-1 pol gene from virions in plasma and genital tract of women: genital tract reservoir and differential drug resistance. HIV Pathog Treat Conf (abst #4025), Mar 13–19, 1998.

Fiscus SA, Adimora AA, Schoenbach VJ, et al. Trends in human immunodeficiency virus (HIV) counseling, testing, and antiretroviral treatment of HIV-infected women and perinatal transmission in North Carolina. *J Infect Dis* 180:99–105, 1999.

Fowler MG, Bertolli J, Nieburg P. When is breastfeeding not best? The dilemma facing HIV-infected women in resource-poor settings. *JAMA* 282:781–783, 1999.

French R and Brocklehurst P. The effect of pregnancy on survival in women infected with HIV: a systematic review of the literature and meta-analysis. *Br J Obstet Gynaecol* 105: 827–835, 1998.

Garcia PM, Kalish LA, Pitt J, et al. Maternal levels of plasma human immunodeficiency virus type-1 RNA and the risk of perinatal transmission. *N Engl J Med* 341:394–402, 1999.

Gervasoni C, Lazzarin A, Musicco M, Saracco A, Nicolosi A. Contraceptive practices and man-to-woman HIV sexual transmission. The Italian Partner Study. Int Conf AIDS 8(2):C351 (abst PoC 4651) July 19–24, 1992.

Gichangi PB, Nyongo AO, Temmerman M. Pregnancy outcome and placental weight: their relationship to HIV-1 infection. *East Afr Med J* 70:85–9, 1993.

Goldenberg RL, Vermund SH, Goepfert AR, Andrews WW. Choriodecidual inflammation: a potentially preventable cause of perinatal HIV-1 transmission? *Lancet* 352:1927–1930, 1998.

Gray RH, Wawer MJ, Serwadda D, et al. Population-based study of fertility in women with HIV-1 infection in Uganda. *Lancet* 351(9096):98–103, 1998.

Greco P, Vimercati A, Fiore JR, et al. Reproductive choice in individuals HIV-1 infected in southeastern Italy. *J Perinat Med* 27:173–177, 1999.

Guay LA, Musoke P, Fleming T, et al. Intrapartum and neonatal single-dose nevirapine compared with zidovudine for prevention of mother-to-child transmission of HIV-1 in Kampala, Uganda. HIVNET 012 randomised trial. *Lancet* 354:795–802, 1999.

Hanna G, Hueppchen N, Kriebs J, Moore R, Anderson J, Pressman E. Post-cesarean febrile morbidity in HIV-infected patients. *Am J Obstet Gynecol* 176 (1 pt 2):59, 1997.

Hanson IC, Antonelli TA, Sperling RS et al. Lack of tumors in infants with perinatal HIV-1 exposure and fetal/neonatal exposure to zidovudine. *J Acquir Immune Defic Syndr* 20:463–467, 1999.

Hatcher RA, Trusell J, Stewart F, et al. *Contraceptive Technology,* 17th edition. Ardent Media, Inc, New York, 1998.

Hauth JC, Goldenberg RL, Andrews WW, DuBard MB, Copper RL. Reduced incidence of preterm delivery with metronidazole and erythromycin in women with bacterial vaginosis. *N Engl J Med* 333:1732–1736, 1995.

Hershow RC, Riester KA, Lew J, et al. Increased vertical transmission of human immunodeficiency virus from hepatitis C virus-coinfected mothers. Women and Infants Transmission Study. *J Infect Dis* 176 (2):414–420, 1997.

Hitti J, Watts DH, Burchett SK, et al. Herpes simplex virus seropositivity and reactivation at delivery among pregnant women infected with human immunodeficiency virus-1. *Am J Obstet Gynecol* 177(2):450–454, 1997.

Hofman V, Ladner J, Tran AT, et al. Placental infection in Rwanda: comparison an HIV infected population and a control population. *Ann Pathol* 18:466–472, 1998.

Just J, Louie L, Abrams E, et al. HLA genotype and risk of vertical transmission of HIV. Int Conf AIDS 8:C282 (abst PoC 4225), July19–24, 1992.

Kind C, Rudin C, Siegrist CA, et al. Prevention of vertical HIV transmission: additive protective effect of elective Caesarean section and zidovudine prophylaxis. *AIDS* 12: 205–210, 1998.

Kostrikis LG, Neumann AU, Thomson B, et al. A polymorphism in the regulatory region of the CC-chemokine receptor 5 gene influences perinatal transmission of human immunodeficiency virus type 1 to African-American infants. *J Virol* 73:10264–10271, 1999.

Kovacs A, Schluchter M, Easley K, et al. Cytomegalovirus infection and HIV-1 disease progression in infants born to HIV-1 infected women. Pediatric Pulmonary and Cardiovascular Complications of Vertically Transmitted HIV Infection Study Group. *N Engl J Med* 341 (2):77–84, 1999.

Kovacs A, Xu J Rasheed S, et al. Comparison of a rapid nonisotopic polymerase chain reaction assay with four commonly used methods for the early diagnosis of human immunodeficiency virus type 1 infection I neonates and children. *Pediatr Infect Dis J* 14:948–954, 1995.

VII

Kreiss J. Breasfeeding and vertical transmission of HIV-1. *Acta Paediatr* Suppl 421:113–117, 1997.

Kuhn L, Abrams EJ, Matheson PB, et al. Timing of maternal-infant HIV transmission: associations between intrapartum factors and early polymerase chain reaction results. New York City Perinatal HIV Transmission Collaborative Study Group. *AIDS* 11:429–435, 1997.

Kuhn L, Coutsoudis A, Moodley D, et al. HIV-1 specific T-helper cell responses detected at birth: protection against intrapartum and breast feeding-associated transmission of HIV-1. 7th Conf Retroviruses Opportunistic Infect (abst 702), Jan 30–Feb2, 2000.

Kuhn L, Steketee RW, Weedon J, et al. Distinct risk factors for intrauterine and intra-partum human immunodeficiency virus transmission and consequences for disease progression in infected children. Perinatal AIDS Collaborative Transmission Study. *J Infect Dis* 179:52–58, 1999.

Kully C, Yerly S, Erb P, et al. Codon 215 mutations in human immunodeficiency virus-infected pregnant women. Swiss Collaborative HIV and Pregnancy Study. *J Infect Dis* 179:705–708, 1999.

Kumar RM, Uduman SA, Khurranna AK. Impact of maternal HIV-1 infection on peri-natal outcome. *Int J Gynaecol Obstet* 49:137–143, 1995.

Ladner J, Lerooy V, Hoffman P, et al. Chorioamnionits and pregnancy outcome in HIV-infected African women. *J Acquir Immune Defic Syndr Hum Retrovirol* 18: 293–298, 1998.

Landesman SH, Kalish LA, Burns DN, et al. Obstetrical factors and the transmission of human immunodeficiency virus type 1 from mother to child. The Women and Infants Transmission Study. *N Engl J Med* 334:1617–1623, 1996.

Lange J, Stellato R, Brinkman K et al. Review of neurological adverse events in relation to mitochondrial dysfunction in the prevention of mother to child transmission of HIV: PETRA study. 2nd Conference on Global Strategies for the Prevention of HIV Transmission from Mothers to Infants. September 1–6, 1999, Montreal, Canada (Abstract 250).

Lee LM, Wortley PM, Gray RH, Fleming PL. Reduced fertility and duration of HIV-1 infection in American women. Int Conf AIDS 12: 479–480, 1998 (Abstract 24198)

Lee MJ, Hallmark RJ, Frenkel LM, Del Priore G. Maternal syphilis and vertical transmis-sion of human immunodeficiency virus type-1 infection. *Int J Gynaecol Obstet* 63:247–252, 1998.

Leroy V, Ladner J, Nyiraziraje M et al. Effect of HIV-1 infection on pregnancy outcome in women in Kigali, Rwanda, 1992–1994. Pregnancy and HIV Study Group. *AIDS* 12: 643–650, 1998.

Leroy V, Newell ML, Dabis F, et al. International multicentre pooled analysis of late postnatal mother-to-child transmission of HIV-1 infection. Ghent International Working Group on Mother-to-Child Transmission of HIV. *Lancet* 352:597–600, 1998.

Lindsay MK, Grant J, Peterson HB, Willis S, Nelson P, Klein L. The impact of knowl-edge of human immunodeficiency virus serostatus on contraceptive choice and repeat pregnancy. *Obstet Gynecol* 85:675–679, 1995.

Lorenzi P, Spicher VM, Laubreau B et al. Antiretrovrial therapies in pregnancy: maternal, fetal, and neonatal effects. Swiss HIV Cohort Study, the Swiss Collaborative HIV and Pregnancy Study, and the Swiss Neonatal HIV Study. *AIDS* 12:F241–247, 1998.

Lyman WD. Perinatal AIDS: drugs of abuse and transplacental infection. *Adv Exp Med Biol* 335:211–217, 1993.

Maiques-Montesinos V, Cervera-Sanchez J, Bellver-Pradas J, Abad-Carrascosa A, Serra-Serra V. Post-cesarean section morbidity in HIV-positive women. Acta *Obstet Gynecol* Scand 78:789–792, 1999.

Mandelbrot L, Le Chenadec J, Berrebi A, et al. Perinatal HIV-1 transmission: interaction between zidovudine prophylaxis and mode of delivery in the French perinatal cohort. *JAMA* 280:55–60, 1998.

Mandelbrot L, Mayaux MJ, Bongain A, et al. Obstetric factors and mother-to-child transmission of human immunodeficiency virus type 1: the French perinatal cohorts. SEROGEST French Pediatric HIV Infection Study Group. *Am J Obstet Gynecol* 175:661–667, 1996.

Mangano A, Gonzalez E, Catano G, et al. CCR5 haplotypes asscoaited with enhanced or reduced transmission of HIV-1 from mother to child. 7th Conf Retroviruses Opportunistic Infect (abst 448), Jan 30–Feb2, 2000.

Martin HL, Nyange PM, Richardson BA, et al. Hormonal contraception, sexually transmitted diseases, and risk of heterosexual transmission of human immunodeficiency virus type 1. *J Infect Dis* 178:10053–1059, 1998.

Martin R, Boyer P, Hammill H et al. Incidence of premature birth and neonatal respiratory disease in infants of HIV-positive mothers. The Pediatric Pulmonary and Cardiovascular Complications of Vertically Transmitted Huuman Immunodeficiency Virus Infection Study Group. *J Pediatr* 131:851–856, 1997.

McGregor JA, French JI, Parker R, et al. Prevention of premature birth by screening and treatment for common genital tract infections: results of a prospective controlled evaluation. *Am J Obstet Gynecol* 173:157–167, 1995.

McSherry GD, Shapiro DE, Coombs RW, et al. The effects of zidovudine in the subset of infants infected with human immunodefiency virus type-1 (Pediatric AIDS Clinical Trials Group 076). *J Pediatr* 134 (6):717–724, 1999.

Minkoff H, Augenbraun M. Antiretroviral therapy for pregnant women. *Am J Obstet Gynecol* 176:478–489, 1997.

Minkoff H, Remington JS, Holman S, Ramirez R, Goodwin S, Landesman S. Vertical transmission of toxoplasma by human immunodeficiency virus-infected women. *Am J Obstet Gynecol* 176(3):555–559, 1997.

Miotti P, Liomba G, Dallabetta GA, Hoover DR, Chiphangwi JD, Saah AJ. T lymphocyte subsets during and after pregnancy: analysis in human immunodeficiency virus type-1 infected and –uninfected Malawian mothers. *J Infect Dis* 165(6):1116–1119, 1992.

Mofenson LM, Lambert JS, Stiehm ER, et al. Risk factors for perinatal transmission of human immunodeficiency virus type 1 in women treated with zidovudine. *N Engl J Med* 341: 385–393, 1999.

Mofenson LM. Interaction between timing of perinatal human immunodeficiency virus infection and the design of preventive and therapeutic interventions. *Acta Paediatr* Suppl 491:1–9, 1997.

Morales WJ, Schorr S, Albritton J. Effect of metronidazole in patients with preterm birth in preceding pregnancy and bacterial vaginosis: a placebo-controlled, double-blind study. *Am J Obstet Gynecol* 171:345–347, 1994.

Mostad SB. Prevalence and correlates of HIV type 1 shedding in the female genital tract. *AIDS Res Hum Retroviruses.* 14 (suppl 1):S11–S15, 1998.

VII

Mussi-Pinhata MM, Yamamoto AY, Figueiredo LT, Cervi MC, Duarte G. Congenital and perinatal cytomegalovirus infection in infants to mothers infected with human immunodeficiency virus. *J Pediatr* 132 (2):285–290, 1998.

Myles TD, Elam G, Park-Hwang E, Nguyen T. The Jarisch-Herxheimer reaction and fetal monitoring changes in pregnant women treated for syphilis. *Obstet Gynecol* 92(5):859–864, 1998.

Nduati R, John G, Mbori-Ngacha D, et al. Breastmilk transmission of HIV-1. 7th Conf Retroviruses Opportunistic Infect (abst S-13), Jan 30–Feb 2, 2000.

Nesheim SR, Sawyer M, Meadows L, Grimes V, Nahmias A, Lindsay M. Perinatal HIV transmission among women with primary infection during pregnancy. Int Conf AIDS 11:369 (abst # Tu.C.2600), 1996.

Nimmagadda A, O'Brien WA, Goetz MB. The significance of vitamin A and carotenoid status in persons infected by the human immunodeficiency virus. *Clin Infect Dis* 26:711–718, 1998.

O'Sullivan MJ, Lai S, Yasin S, Helfgott A. The effect of pregnancy on lymphocyte counts in HIV infected women. HIV Infect Women Conf S20: Feb 22–24, 1995.

Olivero OA, Anderson LM, Diwan BA, et al. Transplacental effects of 3'-azido-2'3'-dideoxythymidine (AZT): tumorigenicity in mice and genotoxicity in mice and monkeys. *J Natl Cancer Inst* 89: 1602–1608, 1997.

Palasanthiran P, Ziegler JB, Dwyer DE, Robertson P, Leigh D, Cunningham AL. Early detection of human immunodeficiency virus type 1 infection in Australian infants at risk of perinatal infection and factors affecting transmission. *Pediatr Infect Dis J* 13: 1083–1090, 1994.

Palumbo P, Dobbs T, Holland B, et al. Antiretroviral (ARV) resistance mutations among pregnant HIV-infected women: frequency and clinical correlates. 2nd Conf on Global Strategies for the Prevention of HIV Transmission from Mothers to Infants. (abst #098), Sept 1–6, 1999.

Panther LA, Tucker L, Xu C, Tuomala RE, Mullins JI, Anderson DJ. Genital tract human immunodeficiency virus type 1 (HIV-1) shedding and inflammation and HIV-1 env diversity in perinatal HIV-1 transmission. *J Infect Dis* 181:555–563, 2000.

Papaevangelou V, Pollack H, Rochford G, et al. Increased transmission of vertical hepatitis C virus (HCV) infection to human immunodeficiency virus (HIV)-infected infants of HIV-and HCV-coinfected women. *J Infect Dis* 178(4):1047–1052, 1998.

Perinatal HIV Guidelines Working Group. USPHS task force recommendations for the use of antiretroviral drugs in pregnant women infected with HIV-1 for maternal health and for reducing perinatal HIV-1 transmission in the United States. (and updates) **http://www.hivatis.org**.

Pitt J, Colgrove R, Thompson B, Japour AJ, Welles S. Association of maternal ZDV use during pregnancy and infant ZDV genotypic resistance with rapid disease progression among infants in the WITS. 7th Conf Retroviruses Opportunistic Infect (abst# 709), Jan 30–Feb 2, 2000.

Plummer FA. Heterosexual transmission of human immunodeficiency virus type 1 (HIV): interactions of conventional sexually transmitted diseases, hormonal contraception and HIV-1. *AIDS Res Hum Retroviruses* 14 (suppl 1): S5–S10, 1998.

Radolf JD, Sanchez PJ, Schulz KF, and Murphy FK. Congenital syphilis. In *Sexually Transmitted Diseases* 3rd Edition. (Holmes, Sparling, Mardh, et al. Eds) NY: McGrawHill, 1999.

Read J for the Intl Perinatal HIV Group. Duration of ruptured membranes and vertical transmission of HIV-1: a meta-analysis from fifteen prospective cohort studies. 7th Conf Retroviruses Opportunistic Infect (abst # 659), Jan 30–Feb 2, 2000.

Reinhardt PP, Reinhardt B, Lathey JL, Spector SA. Human cord blood mononuclear cells are preferentially infected by non-syncytium-inducing, macrophage-tropic human immunodeficiency virus type 1 isolates. *J Clin Microbiol* 33:292–297, 1995.

Rich KC, Siegel JN, Leurgans SE, Landay AL. Induced beta-chemokine and cytokine response in pregnant HIV-1 infected women and risk of perinatal transmission. Int Conf AIDS 12:397 (abst #23279), 1998.

Roddy RE, Zekeng L, Ryan KA, Tamoufe U, Weir SS, Wong EL. A controlled trial of nonoxynol 9 film to reduce male-to-female transmission of sexually transmitted diseases. *N Engl J Med* 339:504–510, 1998.

Rodriguez EM, Mofenson LM, Chang BH, et al. Association of maternal drug use during pregnancy with maternal HIV culture positivity and perinatal HIV transmission. *AIDS* 10:273–282, 1996.

Saba J on behalf of the PETRA Trial Study Team. Interim analysis of early efficacy of three shot ZDV/3TC combination regimens to prevent mother-to-child transmission of HIV-1. The PETRA trial. 6th Conf Retroviruses Opportunistic Infect (abst S-7), January 1999.

Schuman P, Sobel JD, Ohmit SE, et al. Mucosal candidal colonization and candidiasis in women with or at risk for human immunodeficiency virus infection. HIV Epidemiology Research Study (HERS) Group. *Clin Infect Dis* 27:1161–1167, 1998.

Semprini AE, Castagna C, Ravizza M, et al. The incidence of complications after cesarean section in 156 HIV-positive women. *AIDS* 9:913–917, 1995.

Shaffer N, Chuachoowong R, Mock PA, et al. Short-course zidovudine for perinatal HIV-1 transmission in Bangkok, Thailand: a randomized controlled trial. *Lancet* 353:773-780, 1999.

Shapiro D, Tuomala R, Samelson R, et al. Antepartum antiretroviral therapy and pregnancy outcome in 462 HIV-infected women in 1998-1999 (PACTG 367). 7th Conf Retroviruses Opportunistic Infect (abst 664), Jan 30–Feb 2, 2000.

Smith ME and the U.S. Nucleoside Safety Review Working Group. Ongoing nucleoside safety review of HIV-exposed children in U.S. studies. 2nd Conference on Global Strategies for the Prevention of HIV Transmission from Mothers to Infants. September 1–6, 1999, Montreal, Canada (Abstract 096).

Smits AK, Goergen CA, Delaney JA, Williamson C, Mundy LM, Fraser VJ. Contraceptive use and pregnancy decision making among women with HIV. *AIDS Patient Care STDS* 12:739–746, 1999.

Sperling RS, Shapiro DE, Coombs RW et al. Maternal viral load, zidovudine treatment, and the risk of transmission of human immunodeficiency virus type 1 from mother to infant. *N Engl J Med* 335:1621–1629, 1996.

Spinillo A, Michelone G, Cavanna C, Colonna L, Capuzzo E, Nicola S. Clinical and microbiological characteristics of symptomatic vulvovaginal candidiasis in HIV-seropositive women. *Genitourin Med* 70:268–272, 1994.

St. Louis ME, Kamenga M, Brown C et al. Risk for peinatal HIV-1 transmission according to maternal immunologic, virologic, and placental factors. *JAMA* 269:2853–2859, 1993.

Stafford MK, Ward H, Flanagan A, et al. Safety study of nononynol 9 as a vaginal microbicide: evidence of adverse effects. *J Acquir Immune Defic Syndr Hum Retrovirol* 17:327–331, 1998.

Stephenson JM. Systematic review of hormonal contraception and risk of HIV transmission: when to resist meta-analysis. *AIDS* 12: 545–553, 1998.

VII

Stiehm ER, Lambert JS, Mofenson LM, et al. Efficacy of zidovudine and hyperimmune HIV immunoglobulin for reducing perinatal HIV transmission from HIV-infected women with advanced disease: results of Pediatric AIDS Clinical Trials Group Protocol 185. *J Infect Dis* 179:567–575, 1999.

Subbarao S, Wright T, Ellerbrock T, Lennox JL, Hart C. Genotypic evidence of local HIV expression in the female genital tract. 5th Conf Retroviruses Opportunistic Infect (abst 708), Feb 1–5, 1998.

Taha T, Kumwenda N, Liomba G, et al. Heterosexual and perinatal transmission of HIV-1: associations with bacterial vaginosis (BV). Int Conf AIDS 12:410–411 (abst # 527/23347), 1998.

Temmerman M, Chomba EN, Ndinya-Achola J, Plummer FA, Coppens M, Piot P. Maternal human immunoedeficiency virus-1 infection and pregnancy outcome. *Obstet Gynecol* 83:495–501, 1994.

The European Mode of Delivery Collaboration. Elective caesarean-section versus vaginal delivery in prevention of vertical HIV-1 transmission: a randomised clinical trial. *Lancet* 353:1035–1039, 1999.

The International Perinatal HIV Group. The mode of delivery and the risk of vertical transmission of human immunodeficiency virus type 1. *N Engl J Med* 340 (13):977–987, 1999.

The International Perinatal HIV Group. The mode of delivery and the risk of vertical transmission of human immunodeficiency virus type 1. *N Engl J Med* 340:977–987, 1999.

Thomas DL, Villano SA, Reister KA, et alo. Perinatal transmission of hepatits C virus from human immunodeficiency virus type-1-infected mothers. Womens and Infants Transmission Study. *J Infect Dis* 177(6):1480–1488, 1998.

Turner BJ, Hauck WW, Fanning R, Markson LE. Cigarette smoking and maternal-child HIV transmission. *J Acquir Immune Defic Syndr Hum Retrovirol* 14:327–337, 1997.

Wade NA, Birkhead GS, Warren BL et al. Abbreviated regimens of zidovudine prophylaxis and perinatal transmission of the human immunodeficiency virus. *N Engl J Med* 339:1409–1414, 1998.

Watts DH, Koutsky LA, Holmes KK, et al. Low risk of perinatal transmission of human papillomavirus: results from a prospective cohort study. *Am J Obstet Gynecol* 178 (2):365–373, 1998.

Watts DH, Mofenson L, Whitehouse J, et al. Complications according to mode of delivery among HIV-positive women with CD4 counts < 500. 6th Conf on Retroviruses and Opportunistic Infections (abst 684), Jan 31–Feb 4, 1999.

Watts DH, Spino C, Zaborski L, Katzenstein D, Hammer S, Benson C. Comaprison of gynecologic history and laboratory results in HIV-positive women with CD4+ lymphocyte counts between 200 and 500 cells/microl and below 100 cells/microl. *J Acquire Immune Defic Syndr Hum Retrovirol* 20:455–462, 1999.

Weiser B, Burger H, Charbonneau T, et al. CCR-5 genotype and resistance to mother-to-child transmission of HIV-1. HIV Pathog Treat Conf 79 (abst 3081), Mar 13–19, 1998.

Welles SL, Pitt J, Colgrove R, et al. HIV-1 genotypic zidovudine drug resistance and the risk of maternal-infant transmission in the women and infants transmission study. The Women and Infants Transmission Study Group. *AIDS* 14:263–271, 2000.

Wilson T, Barkan S, Gurtman A et al. The sexual and contraceptive behavior of women infected with HIV. Int Conf AIDS 11(2):434 (abst Th.D.5196), July 7–12, 1996.

Zaba B, Gregson S. Measuring the impact of HIV on fertility in Africa. *AIDS* 12 (suppl 1):S41–50, 1998.

VIII: Psychosocial and Cultural Considerations

Barbara Aranda-Naranjo PhD, RN and Rachel Davis RN

I. INTRODUCTION

Minority women are disproportionately affected by the HIV/AIDS epidemic.
The incidence of HIV is 19 times higher for African-American women and
seven times higher for Latina/Hispanic women, as compared to the incidence
in Caucasian women. Among women of color age 25 and older, 73% of
those with AIDS and 90% of those with HIV infection are African American. (CDC, 1998) Furthermore, the majority of the women diagnosed with
HIV infection are women of childbearing age between the ages of 16–44
years. These women must make a series of complex decisions concerning
contraception, pregnancy, and abortion. Although little is known about how
women living with HIV/AIDS make such decisions, the decision to have a
baby is likely influenced by the interrelationship of intrapersonal factors,
family influences and social pressures. (Sowell, 1993; Moneyham, 1997;
Aranda-Naranjo, 1999)

Growing rates of HIV infection among minority women have created a
burden on often already impoverished families. Numerous psychosocial and
economic obstacles may prevent these women from seeking health care. (Met-
calfe, 1998) When women in HIV clinics in a mid-south city were given an
opportunity to identify their concerns they listed 349 needs: 32% psychosocial,
14% physical, 13% service and maintenance, and 11% financial and legal.
(Bunting, 1999)

This chapter will identify the psychosocial issues for women living
with HIV infection: economic concerns, human relationship issues,
psychological issues, and cultural considerations. Interventions will be
introduced to address the challenges of working with women and their
families and to maintain cultural sensitivity. These interventions will
facilitate the treatment and care of Latina/Hispanic and African-American
women living with HIV. Providers may find it helpful to establish a broad
sociocultural program that can assess and address the women's lifestyle
issues. The inclusion of the socio-cultural aspects of a woman's life will
allow a program to be more holistic in the provision of care for the woman
and her family.

II. ECONOMIC ISSUES

A. DISCUSSION

The majority of women living with HIV infection live in poverty and struggle with complex economic issues as a result of homelessness, substance abuse, immigration status, mental health disorders, and violent relationships. They often lack health insurance. Those women who do have health insurance usually obtain it during their pregnancy and lose it after the baby is born. Most of their energy is spent meeting basic needs such as food, housing, and employment for themselves and their families, which take priority over any health problems, including HIV infection. Furthermore, because of past experiences, many minority women tend not to trust the medical system or the entire health and human service infrastructure. These factors combine to make health care less accessible and less of a priority in the lives of many HIV-infected women.

Strategies that utilize a linkage approach within the community have been effective in addressing basic economic needs. (Anderson, 1999) A number of resources are funded specifically for HIV infected individuals and there are community-based organizations that provide assistance with food, housing, and other basic needs. An important aspect of linkage development is to assign a case coordinator or case manager for the woman and her family. This individual can facilitate the development of a care plan and advocate for the family. Because the woman is usually the primary caregiver in the family, she will often be overwhelmed, especially in the first few months after learning of her diagnosis, with all the medical and social service appointments she will be asked to keep. The case coordinator or case manager can decrease anxiety for the woman by facilitating the appointments and serving as the broker in linking her to needed services.

B. INTERVENTIONS

- Assign a case manager/case coordinator to link the woman to social services which can meet her basic needs

- Teach the woman about the structure of the health and human services system in her community

- Establish peer interventions so that women are able to talk with other women about negotiating life with HIV disease

III. HUMAN RELATIONSHIP ISSUES

A. DISCUSSION

Women with HIV have many significant relationships-with their family, particularly their children, their partner/significant other, friends, members of the health care team, and with themselves. Each of these relationships may affect the others and each can have a profound impact on how the woman deals with her HIV infection and other comorbidities.

HIV infection in women is clearly a family issue, imposing social, psychological, and economic burdens on women who care for family members while they are ill. Many women see themselves as they relate to their children and significant others and to the roles they take in their family structure.

When multiple family members are also infected with HIV, a systems approach, which looks at the whole in order to understand the parts, is needed to assist the woman in managing her own care and that of her entire family. The well-being and the return of normalcy for a family depend on the care-seeking ability of the woman and the sensitivity of health care providers in facilitating the process of seeking care. Women often defer their needs to those of their children and significant others. In a recent study of inner-city HIV-positive women and their infants, the large majority of women studied were likely to secure medical care for their infants, while only 46% reported ever seeking HIV-related health care for themselves. (Butz, 1993)

Many women have low self-esteem and have trouble negotiating safe sexual practices with their partners. The implementation of an empowerment program for Latina immigrant women demonstrated that targeting broader socio-cultural issues may increase the skills necessary for these women to avoid transmission of HIV infection by their sexual partners.(Gomez, 1999) The women in this study showed significant increases in comfort with sexual communication, were less likely to maintain traditional sexual gender norms, and reported changes in decision-making power (N=74).

Because many women with HIV live with other conditions, such as substance abuse and/or mental illness, in addition to poverty and domestic violence as a part of their lives, they have had to rely on the government public health and social service system for help and health care. Many have experienced difficult moments in asking for help and have suffered humiliation on behalf of their families in trying to get what they need. Because of issues of stigma and poverty, women are vulnerable to a decreased ability to meet their needs such as housing, food, and work as well as decreased access to health care services, and/or delayed health-care seeking for themselves. (Amaro, 1990; Mays, 1987) Women with dependent children and those who are pregnant may be even more reluctant to seek care, due partly to a fear of having their children taken from them. Issues of substance abuse or prostitution may make the decision to seek health care more complex. (Pivnicka, 1991)

A case manager or coordinator can help establish trust by participating in the initial overall assessment (if possible, in the home), giving straightforward explanations, and having a working knowledge of the structure and roles the woman plays within her defined family. Medical providers should also make extra time for the initial visit in order to begin the process of developing trust with the patient.

Within the African-American population, one can find various arrangements that constitute a family. Some women may have "play sisters" or "play moms" who are not biological family members but who provide great support for the women in times of crisis. (Asante, 1995) Many Hispanic women have madrinas (godmothers) and comadres (friends related by marriage or baptism) who are great sources of support for them during times of crisis. Understanding the family dynamics is important for providers to facilitate trust and understanding. Before giving the initial HIV test results and discussing disclosure issues, it is essential to have an understanding of the communication dynamics in the family, especially with the "significant other" of the woman.

B. INTERVENTIONS

■ Don't rush the first visit; trust takes time

■ Initial assessment by the case manager in the home may give additional insights into the family structure and the roles the woman plays within her family

■ Give simple straightforward explanations

■ Family dynamics needs to be understood before recommending disclosure actions

■ Develop or link with empowerment programs targeting sexual communication, negotiation and self-esteem

■ Understand each woman's priorities and develop strategies to meet those needs she considers most important

IV. PSYCHOLOGICAL ISSUES

A. DISCUSSION

Women face an array of psychological issues, not only related to possible coexisting substance abuse, mental illness, domestic violence, and poverty, but also related to the stresses of living with HIV disease and being the primary care provider for the family. Most HIV/AIDS-infected minority women are stigmatized even before HIV, infected by drug use, race and poverty. (Wofsy, 1987) The majority of these women are single heads of households with young dependent children, and, in general, lack a community of support such as that seen among gay men. (Weiner, 1991) This situation affects the actual and perceived availability of supportive resources to respond to varied manifestations of HIV disease. Limited financial and emotional resources affect HIV-infected women's access to both psychological and medical services. Low self-esteem is the rule rather than the exception and plays a major role in ability to access and adhere to care.

Many women experience a variety of emotions related to infecting their child and/or the mode of transmission for themselves. They may feel anger at a partner who infected them sexually or guilt with a partner to whom they have been unable to disclose. Some of the emotional issues can be categorized by the time of the encounter with the woman. At the initial visit with the medical provider the women is most vulnerable to a number of emotions such as shock, disbelief, guilt, anger, sadness and even suicidal ideation. At intermediate visits, which may be with various members of the multidisciplinary team (social worker, nurse, psychologist, counselor, nurse practitioner or physician), many of the same emotions are still present, although some may be more attenuated while others may have greater prominence. The importance of intermediate visits is to continue emotional assessments in order to provide effective interventions and help establish trust. Regular visits are those visits established for routine follow-up and for optimal health maintenance. Typically, women maintain the regular visit schedule for all members of the family. Therefore, it is important to take time to address the emotional needs of the women at these regular visits. The most difficult visits are those occurring for crisis reasons. Crisis visits often occur frequently until the woman and her family stabilize their lives and the medical conditions of all family members. Reasons for crisis range from HIV issues to domestic violence to medical deterioration of one or more family members. It is not unusual for a women to be hospitalized at the same time as her child. These scenarios call for all team members to work together and provide anticipatory guidance – that is, devise a plan or procedure that will address the issues and problems that may arise. A debriefing session by the care coordinator/social worker with the woman after the crisis has been resolved is important to prevent potential future crises.

Despite this complex picture and against all odds, many of these women have strong coping abilities and profound survival instincts. Some studies have suggest that interventions to support attempts to use active coping strategies as physical symptoms increase may be effective in promoting positive adaptation to HIV disease. (Moneyham, 1998)

B. INTERVENTIONS

- The initial visit is often filled with shock, disbelief, guilt, anger, sadness, or even suicidal ideation. Take time to deal with these reactions, assess possible suicidal thoughts, and give information in "small bites" over several closely spaced visits

- During intermediate visits, work on the establishment of trust between the woman and her provider/health care team

- During regular visits, inquire about the health status of all members of the family, especially the children; continue to assess the emotional status of the woman

■ At times of crisis address the situation at hand, consider the possible value of peer counselors; after resolution, revisit it and develop plans to prevent reoccurrence of similar situations when possible

V. CULTURAL ISSUES

A. DISCUSSION

Since the majority of women living with HIV infection come from two primary groups, African and Hispanic Americans, this section will focus on the cultural beliefs of these two groups. Culture functions as a guiding framework that assists individuals, families and communities to interpret and respond to internal and external stimuli. "Culture describes learned behavior affected by home, religion, ethnic group, language, neighborhood, school and age-group." (Cruickshank, 1989)

B. HISPANIC CULTURE

DISCUSSION

In Hispanic populations, one complex facet of cultural sensitivity and competency lies in the diversity of the subgroups that make up this population in the United States. The subgroups and their representation are: Mexican American, 62 percent; Puerto Rican, 13 percent; Cuban, 5 percent; Central and South American, 12 percent; other Hispanic (Spanish/Mexican/Native American population in the Southwest), 8 percent. (U.S. Bureau of Census, 1990) Each of these subgroups has their distinct culture, as well as various levels of assimilation into the general population.

Providers need to address these distinctions in developing intervention and prevention programs for HIV/AIDS and other health issues. Amidst the diversity among Hispanic Americans, social scientists have identified cultural values that are shared by most Hispanics regardless of country of origin. The identified core values are (Marin, 1989):

■ **Familismo** — the importance of the family to the individual

■ **Colectivismo** — the importance of friends and extended family members such as godmothers (madrinas) and godfathers (padrinos)

■ Simpatía — the act of being polite; respectful not confrontational

■ **Personalismo** — the preference to be with other persons of the same ethnic group

■ **Respeto** — the act of upholding one's own integrity without damaging another person

For Hispanics, HIV/AIDS is not an individual issue, but one that affects the family structure and the unity within the community. In many Hispanic families the husband makes the decisions for all members of the family, including his wife. The extended family in the Hispanic culture may also play a major role in the making of decisions. Clinicians need to assess the role of the woman within her culture and her adherence to strict cultural beliefs.

Interventions

■ Identify the woman's ethnic subgroup of origin

■ Provide a bilingual provider on the health care team (do not use the children or the custodian to translate; this demonstrates a lack of respect)

■ Diagram the family structure and discuss the role of each member

■ Review the role of women in her family

■ Link the woman to appropriate social service providers

Case Study: Hispanic

Name: DE
Age: 35 years
Ethnicity: Mexican American

DE came into our program on 11/4/93 – her first visit with the physician was the day she learned of her HIV status. She was 27 weeks pregnant with her second child. She had a 14 month-old daughter who was followed by a specialist because of urological problems. Her risk factors included two heterosexual partners and history of a blood transfusion after her first pregnancy in 1992 secondary to hemorrhage. She stated she was tested because of the blood transfusion.

We performed HIV testing on her daughter, and explained the risk to her unborn child because of her HIV status; the plan of care for the child after birth was reviewed.

At the time of diagnosis DE received a classification of AIDS due to a CD4 count of 178. Despite these obstacles, she maintained her health during her pregnancy, continued to care for her daughter, and began getting care for her own HIV disease. DE tested in the lower ranges for verbal intelligence and conceptual processing with psychological evaluation.

DE's support system included her mother (who initially did not know DE's status), and her common-law husband, who was not the father of her oldest child, but was the father of the child she was carrying. The HIV test results for her daughter and husband were negative. DE experienced an variety of emotions, including fear, anxiety, and depression, and needed much support from the entire staff to assist her in understanding more fully not only what HIV was or how it affected her and her family, but also in obtaining financial support.

As with most new clients, DE was distrustful of staff initially, but with care, concern and perseverance, our entire team (physicians, nurses, social workers, psychologist, foster granny volunteers, etc.) developed a trusting relationship with her. DE was empowered to take control of her own life and that of her children. Her second child was a boy, and within

1–2 months of life it was obvious he was infected and he had a very low CD4 count. She never missed a clinical appointment for him, and in fact, was always there even before clinic began. DE provided excellent care to her son, learned to give him his medications, and had good relationships with the medical staff, so that she would call with any problems he was having.

By 1996 her own health had deteriorated significantly and her care was transferred to another physician, but she continued to bring her son to our program for care. She was linked with hospice services and almost died several

Case Study continues . . .

CASE STUDY: HISPANIC *(continued)*

times, but each time improved to the point where she was ultimately taken off the hospice list. Her determination to personally care for her son was a strong motivating factor in her ability to not only stay alive, but to actually improve her health status.

DE was able to make the choice as to how and where her son would spend his last days, and was at his bedside when his short life ended. She let balloons loose into the sky at his burial to signify that her son had gone to heaven.

DE continues to live, and both she and her husband have dropped in to the clinic occasionally to visit and to show us photos of the family trip to Disneyworld, pictures of her son in his last hours, etc. DE has also become involved with the Pediatric AIDS quilt project, started by one of our program nurses.

C. AFRICAN-AMERICAN CULTURE

DISCUSSION

As in other minorities, African Americans experience high rates of unemployment and overall poverty. Any discussion of core values must be evaluated in the context of these sociodemographics characteristics. According to Gibbs, even though family conflict is reported in all races and socioeconomic groups, minorities have a higher rate because they are more vulnerable to detection and arrest by the police and referral to public agencies. (Gibbs, 1990) These problems may be more appropriately viewed as community problems rather than problems of the black family. Amidst the complexity of life for African-American individuals and their families they are sustained by their core values which have historical roots in Africa.

The core values that most African Americans embrace have been described by Sudarkasa. (Sudarkasa, 1996) They are the seven "R's": respect, responsibility, reciprocity, restraint, reverence, reason and reconciliation. The core values defined are:

- **Respect** — the respect of others from parents and relatives to elders or leaders in the community
- **Responsibility** — being accountable for self and for those less fortunate in one's own extended family and even one's community
- **Reciprocity** — giving back to family and community in return for what has been given to one (mutual assistance)
- **Restraint** — giving due consideration to the family or community/group when making decisions
- **Reverence** – deep awe and respect firstly toward God, the ancestors as well as for many things in nature
- **Reason** — taking a reasoned approach to the settling of disputes within the family or the community

■ **Reconciliation** — the art of settling differences; that is, putting a matter to rest between two parties

Two of these values, respect and responsibility, were major guiding principles for behaviors within families from Africa which have been carried over to African-American families today. "Restraint" is related to the notion of "sacrifice." Parents exercise restraint over their own destinies in order to provide for their children, who in turn repay the "sacrifice" by putting their parent's needs before their own in many instances. (Sudarkasa, 1988)

Spirituality is a strong cultural value among both African- and Hispanic-American women. Historically, the church in the African-American community has been the single most important organization advocating for public policies to influence improvements in health, education and financial quality of life. (Poole, 1996) From this perspective there is a continuum between religion and one's quality of life. "As the center for the extended family, reinforcing the sense of self and self-esteem within the culture, the church offers opportunities for the whole family's development." (Butler, 1992) Churches in the African-American community have created and mobilized leaders and increased hope. (Neeleman, 1998; DHHS,1998) In order to provide comprehensive health care to these populations, programs should include the spiritual dimension and beliefs in all aspects of care.

Many African Americans share a distrust of the health care system related to historical experiences such as the Tuskegee experiment. Airhihenbuwa, (1990) suggests that African Americans operate in a society where rules and social systems appear to be adversarial. "The degree to which they perceive the odds against them as manageable or overwhelming will depend to a significant degree on the transactional competency and success of their parents, the competence of the role models in their primary community, and the availability and accessibility of resources and support to help them in their coping efforts." (Meyers, 1983)

INTERVENTIONS

■ Trust is a continuous, dynamic process requiring open and ongoing communication between women and their health care providers/team

■ Educate team members about the values of African Americans

■ Show respect for spiritual beliefs and how they affect advanced directives and other decisions the woman may make

■ Recognize extended family members as key supports for the patient

■ An essential role for the case manager/coordinator is to help the woman negotiate multiple parts of the health care/social services system and to serve as a broker and advocate for her specific needs

---

CASE STUDY: AFRICAN AMERICAN

NAME: BA
AGE: 43
ETHNICITY: AFRICAN AMERICAN

BA was referred to the program after delivering a baby boy 7½ weeks prematurely; he was born withdrawing from drugs and was found to be HIV infected. After the referral was made at 5 p.m. on a Friday, two nurse-case managers went to the hospital to meet with BA and to initiate the process of caring for her child. While there, local law enforcement officers came into the patient's room and informed her that they were removing her newborn son from her custody because of her drug use during pregnancy.

BA was 43 years old and had a history of injectable drug use since the age of 15 when she ran away from home. She was homeless at the time of delivery and was attempting to reunite with her family.

On initial assessment she was happy but nervous and apprehensive about the possibility that her child could be infected with HIV. She did not get prenatal care because doctors had told her that her uterus was so badly scarred from sexually transmitted diseases that she was unlikely to get pregnant. This pregnancy was a pleasant surprise for her and she saw this baby as a gift, a miracle from God.

She was admitted to an outpatient drug rehabilitation program and her baby was placed in foster care. With the help of her caseworker she reunited with her mother and sisters after revealing her HIV status. She also met with her spiritual counselor on a regular basis to discuss life and death issues.

She completed her 6-month drug rehabilitation program successfully and was able to petition the courts and get her son back. She was in the hospital when her son became very ill and was also hospitalized. She was able to talk with her pediatrician and sign advanced directives for her child. He died during their simultaneous hospitalization in his mother's arms. When the nurses and caseworker came to be with her at the hospital she shared the following story:

"I have done a lot of things wrong in my life and I didn't think I had a chance to get in the pearly gates. But you know I have loved my son and he knew that. I tried to be the best mother I could be for the short time I had him. So when I die and I go up and see St. Peter at the pearly gates he is just going to nod his head "no" . As I am just about to leave I hear someone running and I turn around to hear a little boy screaming: "St. Peter, that's my mom and she loved me and I love her. You have to let her in!"

BA remained clean for the entire year that her infant was alive, but relapsed back into drug addiction upon his death. This was the way she had always coped before. BA was distrustful of the system (all the team members), had been estranged from her family, and had an array of health problems. Early in her assessment she said, "I have come home to die." She did live two years, during which time she was back and forth between drug rehabilitation programs and hospitalizations for her HIV infection. A key factor in her care was the assignment of a case manager and the coordination with her drug rehabilitation team. She had constant contact with her spiritual counselor, with whom she had had a long-lasting relationship since her childhood. She was referred late in the stages of HIV infection. She was given medical information about herself and child in a straightforward manner, which she appreciated, commenting "tell it to me straight." She had a very close relationship with her child's pediatrician. She tended not to keep her own medical appointments and deferred most of her energy to her child's care. BA died one month after her son's death surrounded by her family, the staff and her spiritual counselor.

D. COMMUNITY

DISCUSSION

In addition to the major core values of a culture, other considerations are the "vital signs" of the community in which the woman lives. Community "vital signs" include, but are not limited to: prevailing cultural beliefs, pressing issues for the community, employment rate, the level of poverty, the definition of health espoused by most people in the community, access to health care, characteristics of the community leaders and their followers, support structures, and the level of trust in the health care system.

These factors can be described as a community's ecological system. (Meyer, 1988) Health care practitioners should be encouraged to view the people of the community in the context of their environment. The interrelatedness of individuals to their environment leads one to view people not as solitary subjects, but as integral parts of a whole community.

With both Hispanics and African Americans the community is vital to a good and healthy life. However, both of these populations experience a disproportionate level of displacement due to the requirements for economic survival. Health and human service providers who want to serve these populations with sensitivity and quality must understand the complexity of living with HIV disease in poverty. According to Mindy Fullilove (1996), psychological well-being depends on strong, nurturing places.

INTERVENTIONS

- Identify and have a working knowledge of the core values of the community you are serving

- Develop an alliance with key community based organizations

- Teach staff about the effect of community on the woman's decision making and belief system

- Identify women who have to leave their community for long periods of time for employment (e.g., migrant workers), and assist them in making connections for health care while away and in ensuring access to needed medications

VI. SUMMARY

Women living with HIV infection are living with a multitude of medical and social problems. They live not in isolation but as integral members of their communities and primary caregivers for their families. Although HIV infection is often not their primary concern, this does not mean they do not want help. To understand and assist women living with HIV, it is important to take a systems approach, to look at the whole in order to understand the parts, to think in loops rather than in straight lines. (O'Connor, 1997) High quality care for women living with HIV disease is best given by addressing not only her medical needs, but also her economic needs, her relationships, her emotional responses, and her culture and her community-all of the faces of a multifaceted life.

REFERENCES

Airhihenbuwa, C. Health Promotion Disease Prevention Strategies for African Americans: A Conceptual Model. In R. Braithwaite & S. Taylor (Eds.), *Health Issues In The Black Community.* (pp. 267–280). San Francisco: Jossey-Bass Publishers, 1990.

Amaro, H. Love, sex, and power: Considering women's realities in HIV prevention. *American Psychologist,* 50 (6), 437–447, 1995.

Anderson, M.D.., Smereck, G.A., Hockman, E.M., Ross, D.J., & Ground, K.J. Nurses decrease barriers to health care by "Hyperlinking" multiple diagnosed women living with HIV/AIDS into care. *Journal of the Association of Nurses in AIDS Care* 10(2): 55–65, 1999.

Asante, M.K. *African-American History: A Journey of Liberation.* Maywood, NJ: Peoples Publishing Group, 1995.

Bunting, S.M., Bevier, D.J., Baker, S.K. Poor women living with HIV: Self-Identified needs. *Journal of Community Health Nursing,* 16, 41–52, 1999.

Butler, J.P. Of kindred minds: The ties that bind. In Orlandi, M.A. (ed). *Cultural competence for evaluation: A guide for alcohol and other drug abuse prevention practitioners working with ethnic/racial communities.* Rockville, Maryland: U.S. Department of Health and Human Services, 1992.

Butz, A.M., Hutton, N., Joyner,M.,Vogelhut, J., Greenberg-Friedman, D., Schreibeis, D., & Anderson, J.R. HIV-infected women and infants: Social and health factors impeding utilization of Health Care. *Journal of Nurse-Midwifery.* 38 (2), 103–109, 1993.

Centers for Disease Control and Prevention. *HIV/AIDS Weekly Surveillance Report,* 1998.

Cruickshank, J.K. & Beevers, D.G. *Ethnic Factors in Health and Disease.* Wright Butterworth & Co., 1989.

Fullilove, M.T. Psychiatric implications of displacement: Contributions from the psychology of place. *American Journal of Psychiatry,* 153, 1516–1523, 1996.

Gibbs, J.T. "Developing Intervention Models For Black Families: Linking Theory and Research." In Harold E. Cheatham & James B. Stewart (Ed.), *Black Families. Interdisciplinary Perspectives.* New Jersey: Transaction Publishers, 1990.

Gomez, C.A., Hernandez, M. & Faigeles, B. Sex in the New World: AN empowerment model for HIV prevention in Latina immigrant women. *Health Education & Behavior,* 26, 200–212, 1999.

Marin, G. AIDS prevention among Hispanic needs, risk behaviors and cultural values. *Public Health Reports,* 104, 411–415, 1989

Mays, V.M., & Cochran, S.D. Acquired immnodeficiency syndrome and Black-Americans: Special psychological issues. *Public Health Reports,* 102, 224–231, 1987.

Metcalf, K.A., Langstaff, J.E., Evans, S.J., Paterson, H.M.& Reid, J.L. Meeting the needs of women living with HIV. *Public Health Nursing,* 15, 30–34, 1998.

Meyer, C.H. "The eco-system perspective." In R. A. Dorfman (Ed.), *Paradigms of Clinical Social Work.* New York: Brunner Mazel, 1988.

Moneyham, L., Hennessy, M., Sowell, R., Demi, A., Seals, B. & Mizuno, Y. The effectiveness of coping strategies used by HIV-seropositive women. *Research in Nursing & Health,* 21, 351–362, 1997.

Myers, H.F., & King, L. M. "Mental Health Issues in the Development of the Black American Child." In E.G. Powel (Ed.), *The Psychosocial Development of Minority Group Children.* New York: Bruner/Mazel, 1983.

Neeleman, J.,Wessely, S., & Lewis, G. Suicide acceptability in African and white Americans: The role of religion. *Journal of Nervous and Mental Disease*, 186, 12–16, 1998.

O'Connor, J., & McDermott, I. *The Art of Systems Thinking:: Essential Skills for Creativity and Problem Solving.*. San Francisco: Harper Collins Pub., 1997.

Pivnicka. Reproductive decisions among HIV-positive drug using women: The importance of mother/child co-residence. International Conference on AIDS, 7 (2), 352, 1991.

Poole, Thomas G., Black Families and the Black Church: A Sociohistorical Perspective. In H.E. Cheatham & James B. Stewart (Ed.), *Black Families. Interdisciplinary Perspectives.* New Jersey: Transaction Publishers, 1990.

Sowell, R., Moneyham, L. & Aranda-Naranjo, B. The care of women with AIDS: Special Needs and Considerations. *Nursing Clinics of North America* 34(1): 179–99, 1999.

Sudarkasa, N., African and Afro-American family structure. In Cole, J.B. (ed.). *Anthropology for the Nineties*. Collier Macmillan, Inc.: New York, 1988.

Sudarkasa, N. *The Strength of Our Mothers. African & African American Women & Families: Essays and Speeches.* New Jersey: Africa World Press, Inc., 1996.

U.S. Bureau of Census. *Department of Statistical Information,* Washington, D.C., 1990.

U.S. Department of Health and Human Services. Cultural Competence working with African-American communities: Theory and Practice. *CSAP Cultural Competence Series* 7, 1998.

Weiner, D.C. Health Issues at the U.S. Mexican Border. *Journal of the American Medical Association*, 265 (2), 242–247, 1991.

Wofsy, C.B. Human Immunodeficiency Virus infection in women. *Journal of the American Medical Association*, 257 (15), 2074–2076, 1987.

VIII

This *Guide* is a PRELIMINARY EDITION.

We need YOUR HELP to make the NEXT EDITION as useful as possible!

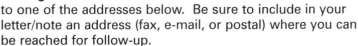

Please send your
comments
criticisms
corrections
suggested changes, and
other guidance
to one of the addresses below. Be sure to include in your
letter/note an address (fax, e-mail, or postal) where you can
be reached for follow-up.

Translation Partners Needed

Write to us if you can help us find partners to help us have
this *Guide* translated into your native language. For
instance, provide us with a contact who works with translation in your country's Ministry of Health, or tell us about a
group at a medical school that translates medical texts.

Send Us Your Comments

E-mail: womencare@hrsa.gov

Fax to the attention of "Womencare": 301-443-0791 (USA)

Postal address: Womencare
Parklawn Building, Room 11A-33
5600 Fishers Lane
Rockville, Maryland 20857
USA

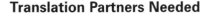

Note that this and subsequent editions of
A Guide to the Clinical Care of Women with HIV
will be available online.

Go to the HIV/AIDS Bureau Web site
and click on the publication *Women's Guide*:
http://www.hrsa.gov/hab

IX: PSYCHIATRIC ISSUES
Joyce Kobayashi, MD

I. OVERVIEW

The experience of being a woman who is HIV-positive must be examined from several perspectives: A) from the perspective of the individual seropositive woman as she makes the journey through the common emotional milestones of HIV; B) from the perspective of women as a group, because women, in contrast to men, tend to cope with HIV within the context of the relationships which are most important to their self-definition; and C) from the perspective of the contemporary context of most HIV-positive women who are, on average, African-American and Hispanic women living and needing to survive in poverty, in the midst of drugs and commonly with personal experiences of childhood sexual abuse or adult victimization through sexual or physical assault.

The experience of the woman living with HIV may be affected by the emotional dynamics described by any or all of these three perspectives. The healthcare provider who is mindful of all three may be able to provide care with deeper understanding and more precise appreciation of her daily struggles with this disease.

Even the asymptomatic phase of being seropositive should be managed and understood in these psychological dimensions. In fact, the experience of the asymptomatic phase of HIV is entirely emotional and psychological, rather than a disease characterized by physical symptoms. It can be an intense experience ranging from individual fears of stigma and suffering, to common concerns about rejection and abandonment by a partner, to a deep feeling about HIV as further victimization in the context of daily concerns about survival.

Interventions by the healthcare provider during normal adjustment phases and common emotional transitions include skilled emotional support, education and empathy, while maintaining awareness of the provider's own reactions to the HIV-positive woman, her experiences and her ways of coping .

Accurate assessment might also indicate the need for referral to a substance treatment program or psychiatric evaluation, in addition to referral to programs of social support, housing, case management and concrete services, depending on the needs of the individual. Care providers who focus on medication adherence without a comprehensive treatment plan addressing harm reduction and treatment for illicit drug use, psychiatric treatment for comorbid psychiatric conditions, and a full range of support services are likely to fail, leaving the HIV-positive woman with the feeling that her real sources of pain and suffering have been left unrecognized.

When normal adjustment issues give way to formal psychiatric disorders, accurate diagnosis is essential as well as knowledge of appropriate treatment and awareness of potential drug-drug interactions, complemented by thorough assessment of suicide risk.

This chapter will address this range of psychiatric issues relating to HIV disease in women and will make specific recommendations for provider and program response, evaluation and management.

II. THREE PERSPECTIVES ON THE EXPERIENCE OF BEING A WOMAN WITH HIV

A. EMOTIONAL MILESTONES: THE EXPERIENCE OF THE INDIVIDUAL HIV-POSITIVE WOMAN

Emotional adjustment to the experience of learning that one is HIV-positive, coping with the demands of being HIV-positive in daily function, and becoming a patient for HIV care commonly follow a natural course of progression through stages. The milestones which mark the transition from one stage to another are often powerful emotional experiences and should be understood as important opportunities for clinical intervention. (See Table 9-1) Knowledge of these milestones will enable the healthcare provider to provide appropriate emotional support, education and empathy.

Reproductive decisionmaking has not been included in Table 9-1, as discussion of this complex decision must be individually tailored to the current circumstances, both social and clinical, of the particular woman considering the variety of options now available. The decision to get pregnant is an important and emotional one and the healthcare provider should be ready to explore a variety of feelings with the patient within the emotionally intensified circumstances of seropositivity without a sense of pressure, before launching into current percentage rates of vertical transmission. (See Chapter VII: HIV and Reproduction)

B. COPING WITH HIV: THE EXPERIENCE OF HIV-POSITIVE WOMEN IN THE CONTEXT OF THEIR RELATIONSHIPS

Contemporary psychiatric research about the developmental psychology of women suggests fundamental differences in the way women and men think about themselves (Gilligan, 1990), with significant implications for clinical practice. While it may be speculative as to whether these differences are more evolutionary and transcultural or locally socialized and economic, an understanding of this perspective is likely to amplify sensitivity in working with HIV

TABLE 9-1: PROVIDING HIV CARE AT EMOTIONAL MILESTONES

PATIENT MILESTONES	HEALTHCARE PROVIDER SKILLS REQUIRED AT THESE TRANSITIONS	EDUCATION ABOUT:	EMPATHY AROUND:
HIV prevention	ease with discussing high risk behaviors ease with discussing prevention measures (e.g. condoms, safe sex, clean needles)	HIV, HIV disease HIV transmission negotiating safe behaviors	denial lack of interest high risk behaviors
Deciding to get HIV tested	ease with details of sexual histories identify high risk behaviors preparation for results anticipate emotional impact	HIV antibody testing	denial ambivalence fear
Accepting, Understanding HIV positive serostatus	ability to tell bad news with empathy anticipate common concerns encourage discussion assess emotional impact	HIV antibody testing HIV disease, prognosis HIV transmission behaviors CD4, viral load	denial, anger fears of rejection, stigma fears of death continuing high risk behaviors
Disclosure of HIV serostatus	discuss decisions about whom to tell discuss decisions about when to tell	anticipating reactions negotiating safe sex	conflicts re: disclosure rejection, fears of rejection
Accepting the "Patient Role"	establish rapport, trust, mutual respect encourage partnership, foster autonomy elicit concerns, encourage questions communicate clearly patient tasks	patient tasks patient responsibilities	ambivalence, distrust anger, rejection oppositional behavior testing limits
Initiating Positive Health Behaviors	identify harmful behaviors refer for substance, psychiatric treatment establish alliance around health	health promotion harm reduction lifestyle, behavior change	anger, grief difficulty changing behaviors resistance to treatment
Appointments, Adherence	forge treatment alliance understand barriers to treatment discuss risk/benefit decisionmaking anticipate side effects	importance of follow-up medications, side effects adherence skills viral resistance	anger, defiance, hostility burden of adherence demands fear of failure, self-blame missed appointments, doses

Table continues . . .

IX

TABLE 9-1: PROVIDING HIV CARE AT EMOTIONAL MILESTONES (continued)

Patient Milestones	Healthcare Provider Skills Required at these Transitions	Education About:	Empathy Around:
Coping with Physical Symptoms	identify symptoms, provide relief; encourage accurate description of symptoms; emotional support, compassion for distress	etiology of symptoms; limitations of treatment; risks/benefits of treatment	discomfort, distress; breakthrough of denial; anger, impatience; fear of progression of illness
Confronting Serious Illness	diagnose, treat, diminish suffering; ability to tell bad news with empathy; compassion, recognize emotional impact; provide emotional support	illness, treatment specifics; prognosis; opportunities for change in behaviors; "lessons"	anger, blaming self, provider; fear of dying; suffering; dependency needs
Improvement in Health Status	consolidate lessons learned from illness; encourage health promotion behaviors	realistic expectations; reassessing work limitations	unrealistic expectations; return of denial
Transition to Disability	ease in initiating discussion re: disability; accurate assessment of legal disability; provide emotional support	realistic goals, expectations; advance care directives; disability entitlements; permanency planning	grief, demoralization; anger, denial; loss of self esteem
Confronting Death	balance hope, discuss common fears; accurate prognosis, allow time to prepare; palliative care, communication with "family"	prognosis, likely course; palliative measures	denial, anger, blame; fear, grief

seropositive women, whatever the ethnicity or racial background.

While acknowledging that any generalization about gender is often wrong in the individual case, two overarching propositions derived from this research may help health care providers understand the ways HIV-positive women often differ from men in their adjustment to being seropositive or having AIDS. First, women more frequently define themselves in the context of their relationships to others. Second, while men may fear intimacy, women more often fear separation. (Surrey, 1982)

For example, it is not uncommon to hear HIV-positive men express fears about becoming dependent on others in the course of their illness, while HIV-positive women often tend to worry more about those who are dependent on them as their illness progresses. Of course, everyone fears being abandoned and left alone when they are dying. While these differences may sound simple or obvious, in clinical practice the differences are striking.

Men often lose self-esteem if they are not able to continue working, or feel anger and may wish to distance themselves from others whom they feel obligated to support, while women more frequently lose self-esteem if they are unable to continue taking care of others. Many HIV-positive women are single mothers and feel deep shame if they are unable to take care of their children or provide for them as they feel they should.

Women may also accept being the target of anger or even abuse, or suppress their own anger, in order to avoid finding themselves alone. They may be more likely to end up in an abusive relationship if they have been abused in their childhood. (See Section C)

There are subtleties in these differences which can guide the care provider in recognizing the adaptive and maladaptive aspects of these concerns for their female patients, and should inform their clinical approaches to seropositive women as they struggle with emotional adjustment to the vicissitudes of HIV-related illness.

On the positive side, women who are coping with HIV/AIDS may be motivated to take care of others to the extent that they can undertake major changes in their own behavior, such as giving up longstanding drug dependencies during pregnancy, or engaging in discussions about permanency planning which frighten them or that they would rather avoid. Other HIV-positive women may take on the responsibility of bringing their children or partners into medical care despite great distance or significant barriers (including their own fatigue or ill health). They may also demonstrate remarkable resourcefulness in seeking out additional avenues of support for others.

The clinician who understands that the strength of this motivation often derives from a deeper level of self-definition and not simply a conventional wish to "do good" will realize the importance of pausing to show respect for the degree of caring the woman demonstrates in making this effort. These are clinical opportunities to build trust and strengthen an alliance around common concerns.

The maladaptive side of similar situations for an HIV-positive woman may include starting or continuing to use drugs simply out of fear of losing a substance using partner; staying in a dysfunctional or even abusive relationship because of anxiety about the loss of the relationship; feeling guilty about taking time away from responsibilities for others to address her own needs; or simply not being able to self-motivate and establish good self-care independently when "no one" will benefit from these efforts except herself.

Women who have lived in poverty or have in multiple additional ways experienced powerlessness about their lives are even less convinced about self efficacy; or at a deeper level, that they are "worth it."

IX

Astute care providers understand that affirming or even "giving permission" for the seropositive woman to attend to her own needs may over time be more important than instructions about what specific health behaviors to follow. In certain circumstances, such as in negotiating safe sex with an unreceptive partner, the provider may even be more directive, without implying criticism about past behaviors, and encourage a woman to develop the necessary skills to become more assertive about her own health concerns.

The practitioner who is able to establish a trusting relationship with the patient should also learn to feel comfortable with the fact that the strength of their relationship may help motivate the HIV-positive woman as much as lectures about viral load. Another provider may convey frustration or disappointment about a patient's nonadherence to medication or some other medical recommendation, only to find that the patient does not return because she has personalized this as a rejection within the context of their relationship.

The woman with AIDS who may feel guilty about taking any time for herself will feel much more supported by a healthcare provider who first acknowledges the importance of her concerns for taking care of others and then builds on that concern by gently reminding her she will not be able to continue unless she takes care of her own health first. This is most effectively done within the context of a relationship where the seropositive woman has felt her values have been respected, and where sufficient trust has been established that maladaptive behavior may be confronted by the provider, and yet be experienced as caring and supportive, rather than as rejection or criticism by the patient.

C: SURVIVING WITH HIV: CONTEMPORARY HIV-POSITIVE WOMEN IN THEIR CONTEXT OF POVERTY, SEXUAL ABUSE AND DRUGS

POVERTY

"The majority of women with AIDS in the United States are unemployed, and 83% live in households with incomes less than $10,000 per year. Only 14% are currently married, compared to 50% of all women in the United States, aged 15–44 years. Twenty-three (23%) of HIV-infected women live alone, 2% live in various facilities, and 1% are homeless. Approximately 50% have at least one child less than the age of 15 years. Similar to other population groups with AIDS in the United States, the majority of women with AIDS are from minority racial and ethnic groups, with African Americans comprising 57% of women with AIDS in the U.S., Latinas comprising 20% and Caucasians comprising 23%." (CDC, 1997; Barkan 1998)

The clinician should be as mindful of the devastating impact of poverty and intermittent homelessness on the person and personality, as the physical sequelae of HIV. For many women who are working the streets, are constantly on the move in transient residences, or are feeling overwhelmed by the needs of their children, illicit drugs are sometimes the most available antidote. It is hard to make the medical treatment needs for HIV relevant unless the woman feels her provider recognizes and has some understanding of her daily struggles for survival. There are many concrete services such as transportation, childcare, food programs and housing that can increase the ability of these HIV-positive women to participate in their healthcare, amplified by the knowledge that their treatment team wants to address all issues which are fundamental to her survival and longevity.

In the book, *Women, Poverty and AIDS* (Farmer, 1996), which contains a comprehensive discussion of these issues, Shayne and Kaplan state that "safe sex is an economic compromise for many poor women who rely on sex as a source of employment, as a means to establish ownership or proprietary rights in relationships, or as a means of getting tanglible supports, generally short in supply." (Shayne, 1991)

Most women with AIDS in the United States are unemployed minority women living in poverty, often as single mothers, and frequently without easy access to medical care. Poverty and the related experiences of racism, sexism and stigmatization are the predominant themes in their lives. This may leave these women with the feeling that their medical teams are simply adding to their burdens by admonishing them to adhere to complicated medical recommendations such as antiretroviral medications. In one study investigating ways to improve healthcare utilization by inquiring about needs for services, a sample of two groups of HIV-positive women, from a Needle Exchange Program and a correctional facility, all indicated that "shelter and food/clothing ranked first among unmet needs for services." (Thompson, 1995)

While a source of income is not traditionally conceptualized as within the realm of medical treatment, it certainly becomes a major factor in medical illness and cannot be ignored. Many women who have substance abuse disorders with psychiatric comorbidity may qualify for entitlement programs which

IX

TABLE 9-2: A DEMOGRAPHIC COMPARISON OF HIV-POSITIVE WOMEN AND MEN

	WOMEN	MEN	LEVEL OF SIGNIFICANCE
African American	54%	27%	< .001
Unemployed	76%	59%	NA
Incomes < $5,000/year	30%	17%	< .001
Without medical insurance	85%	63%	< .001
< 35 years old	44%	31%	< .001

Analysis based on 1996 figures of men versus women living with HIV/AIDS;

Women were 26% of 231,4000 reported cases

Source: Bozzette, 1998.

they have not explored. Vocational rehabilitation programs often entail medical or psychiatric referrals. While housing is not traditionally considered part of medical care, it is also a major factor in medical illness and should be considered. For example, residential programs which require substance abuse treatment contracts should be made available when feasible. Treatment teams should consider this dimension of care in making a comprehensive plan to encourage antiretroviral medication adherence.

CHILDHOOD SEXUAL ABUSE AND ADULT VICTIMIZATION

Sexual abuse, sexual assault and domestic violence are experienced within the lifetimes of a significant portion of American women regardless of their economic status or ethnicity. When childhood sexual abuse is defined as physical contact of a sexual nature to children under 14 years of age, estimates range from 28% to 36%. (Wyatt, 1986) Childhood abuse research is limited by the methodology of self-report, sampling and definitional issues, but shows remarkably consistent high lifetime prevalence rates for women who are HIV-positive or at risk for HIV, for both childhood sexual abuse and adult sexual assault. In turn, these are associated with multiple HIV transmission and risk behaviors.

In a study of 186 HIV-positive or at risk individuals, 28% of the women (and 15% of the men) had been sexually abused during childhood. The female survivors of sexual abuse were significantly more likely to work as prostitutes, become pregnant during teenage years, abuse alcohol or tranquilizers, and were less likely to finish high school. (Zierler, 1991)

A recent study of 1645 subjects enrolled in the Women's Interagency HIV Study (Cohen, 2000) found that among both HIV-positive and seronegative-at-risk women 2 out of every 3 women (67%, 66%) had experienced domestic violence during their lifetimes, and almost one out of three (31% and 27%) had been sexually abused as children. There was no significant difference in prevalence associated with race, ethnicity, education level or marital status, although domestic violence was more frequently reported among older, unmarried, unemployed women.

Early sexual abuse was strongly associated with increased HIV risk behaviors:

- using drugs
- having more than 10 male sexual partners
- having male partners at risk for HIV infection
- exchanging sex for drugs, money or shelter

Sexual assault for adult women has been estimated to be two to four times as likely in women who were survivors of childhood sexual abuse. In a study of 327 women with or at risk for HIV, Zierler (1996) found that35%of women with HIV were sexually assaulted as adults. Forty-five percent of women who reported rape as adults had been sexually abused during childhood or as teenagers. Among women with HIV, adult rape experiences were associated with:

■ more sexual partners

■ unprotected sex involving drugs

■ earlier age of injection drug use

■ teen pregnancy

■ sexually transmitted diseases

■ gynecologic surgery

Similar results were found in a study of street-recruited women from three different major urban sites, with demographics similar to a large portion of the female HIV-positive population: 114/918 women (12%) reported they had been sexually assaulted in the previous 12 months. In comparison to those who were not sexually assaulted, this study (Wong, 1993) found that rape was associated with:

■ higher rates of sex for drug exchanges (79% vs 37%)

■ reporting more than 100 lifetime sex partners (55% vs 18%)

■ smoking crack (86% vs 55%)

■ twice the likelihood of being infected with HIV and syphilis

In another study, of 40 HIV-positive women seeking medical care in one survey, a trauma history was reported by 95%: 63% reported sexual abuse and 70% reported physical abuse. (Nelson, 1996)

In addition, multiple studies have established a relationship between childhood sexual abuse in women and adult-onset depression. (Weiss, 1999) Of interest is that HIV-positive and HIV-at risk women both have higher rates of depression than the general population, although depression increases with physical symptoms. There is also evidence that a range of psychiatric disorders are more prevalent in women and are associated with childhood sexual abuse:

■ Bulimia nervosa

■ Panic disorder with agoraphobia

■ Generalized anxiety disorder

■ Borderline personality disorder

■ Adult-onset depression

There are major implications from these findings for medical care, psychiatric and substance treatment as well as for HIV prevention efforts. A significant segment of the HIV-positive and at risk female population have experienced childhood sexual abuse and/or sexual assault as an adult and their feelings about their disease, their likelihood of continuing high risk transmission behaviors, their methods of coping, such as the use of substances, and their relationship to the healthcare system are seen through the prism of those experiences.

IX

Medical care and treatment targeting women should be conceptualized with attention to the important impact of violence and trauma in the lives of these women. When individuals whom these women were supposed to be able to trust have victimized them, it is not surprising that healthcare providers will have to very consciously earn their trust. Lack of trust, low self-esteem and feelings of powerlessness are frequently experienced by these women and supportive measures such as: having a female healthcare provider, participation in women's support groups, getting supportive therapy or treatment with psychiatric medications, providing social resources or vocational rehabilitation can increase trust, self-esteem and ultimately empower them. Education about prevention should also be a part of medical treatment when there is high risk for continuing transmission behaviors.

It is also important to be aware that women with a history of childhood sexual abuse may be susceptible to a variety of misperceptions. A directive style of recommending medical treatment, for example, may be perceived as coercive by women sensitized through past experiences. A treatment with major side effects or a surgical procedure may be experienced as abusive intrusions in their lives or bodies. A friendly relationship with a healthcare provider may take on unwarranted sexual overtones. Efforts at health education may not be heard when the individual is suddenly lost in thought or actually dissociating because of suddenly being overwhelmed by memories of abuse. Pain may be amplified because of experiences of physical abuse and might be dismissed as drug-seeking.

Clinicians, in turn, may have particular responses to these women and should understand their vulnerability to unproductive "countertransferential" reactions such as either being provoked into being the anticipated abusive figure, or feeling compelled to rescue the individual. Responses of the clinician are more specifically addressed later in this chapter.

Finally, it must be noted, that the clinician must ask in order to know. A simple and direct question may be used, such as, "Would you mind if I ask if you have ever been the victim of physical or sexual abuse?" or "Has anyone ever hurt you physically or abused you sexually?" This should routinely be asked as a pertinent part of the medical history. If there is a positive response, the details need not be explored. If there is a negative response, the possibility of an abuse history should nevertheless be kept in mind. With regard to the possibility of domestic violence, the clinician can ask, "Is there anyone in your life right now who makes you feel unsafe?" If there is a positive response, the details should be explored.

ILLICIT DRUG USE

Women with HIV who are impoverished and struggling with sequelae of childhood abuse and adult victimization are also frequently struggling under the burden of significant substance use which is often further complicated by psychiatric comorbidity. Whether or not they are etiologically related, each factor can exacerbate the other and relapses, in turn, are often associated with increased medical morbidity. Medical providers who consider a substance using HIV-positive woman an inappropriate candidate for multiple drug anti-retroviral medication should consider clinical efforts to assure that she is enrolled in substance abuse treatment as a specific part of the treatment plan.

While it is beyond the scope of this chapter to explore the range of studies addressing substance use among HIV-positive women, a few have been selected for discussion. (Also see Chapter X on Substance Abuse)

■ **There is a high rate of psychiatric comorbidity among HIV-positive women who use substances:**

In a study of a population of HIV-positive individuals on methadone, 79% were found to have a current DSM-III-R Axis I psychiatric disorder and nearly two thirds had two or more concurrent disorders. (Batki, 1996) If psychiatric and substance use treatment are not offered at the same time, a relapse in one condition can often destabilize the other, such as with crack use and bipolar disorder, or with intravenous drug use and post-traumatic stress disorder. Investigators using a National Survey of Veterans found that the combination of substance abuse and PTSD increased the rate of HIV infection by almost 12 times, as compared those without either disorder. (Hoff, 1997) Psychiatric evaluation and treatment should accompany substance treatment when there is comorbidity, and has been shown to be effective. (Lyketsos, 1997)

■ **As many as one-third of HIV-infected women exposed to HIV through heterosexual contact use noninjection drugs and engage in high risk behaviors:**

Analysis of data from 2270 questionnaires administered to HIV-infected women from 12 state or local health departments over five years focussed on the 488 (21%) who used noninjection drugs only.

● 36% of crack users, 11% of primarily marijuana users and 7% of primarily cocaine users had received money for sex in the past five years;

● 66% of crack users, 37% of marijuana only and cocaine primarily users had had an STD. (Kacanek, 1996)

■ **Crack cocaine use results in increased HIV exposure and HIV-positive status in multiple ways:**

Comparing a national sample of 796 high-frequency (daily during the previous month) and 855 low-frequency (1–10 days during the previous month) crack using women, high fequency users were more likely to be infected with HIV (14.2% vs 5.8%), had six times the number of sex partners (13 vs 2.4), were more than three-fold as likely to have sex while high, were nine times more likely to trade sex for drugs or money, and were about 50% more likely to have had unprotected oral sex, as compared to low-frequency users. (Klein, 1997)

It is likely that one of the most important interventions for preventing further HIV transmission in the seropositive woman who continues to use crack is substance abuse treatment and needed psychiatric and other concrete services.

■ **Women IDUs frequently borrow injection works or follow as a second user with shared needles, increasing the risk of HIV transmission:**

- New York neighborhood with high HIV seroprevalence: Among 286 women IDUs who had been injecting drugs an average of 14 years and on an average had injected 55 times/month during the past 12 months, 48% reported having borrowed used injection works. Being African American and having more than one injecting male sex partner in an average month during the past year was significantly (p< .05) associated with borrowing used needles. (Abdul-Quader, 1993)

- San Francisco Needle Exchange Programs: Among 150 female IDUs, younger women (< 30 years) were more likely to be Caucasian, have an IDU parent, start injecting at an early age and more likely to share needles and inject second when sharing with a main partner (74% vs 38%). (Lum, 1998) Needle exchange programs have been found to be effective in preventing HIV exposure and reducing transmission of HIV among injection drug users.

■ **HIV-positive women with substance abuse problems have high utilization of emergency services, low utilization of health services, and HIV-positive women in general tend to have lower rates of utilization of antiretrovirals and OI prophylaxis.**

Seropositive individuals who use drugs are more likely to be without a primary care provider and use emergency medical services than people with AIDS who do not use drugs. (Mauskopf, 1994) Injection drug users either tend to delay initiation of treatment (Broers, 1994), or have less access to antiretroviral medications as a group. (Shapiro, 1999) In women with < 200 CD4/mm³, at a baseline visit, utilization of antiretroviral medication was only 49%, and prophylaxis for opportunistic infections, 58%. (Solomon, 1996) People who use injection drugs are often not diagnosed as HIV-positive until they are symptomatic. (Hu, 1994)

III. NEED FOR MULTISERVICE CLINICAL PROGRAMS

As the above discussions indicate, many HIV-positive women have multiple diagnoses, and require a variety of services to be adequately supported through this illness. Many HIV-positive women are living in poverty or as sex workers, often while still addicted to drugs. A large percentage of seropositive women are also struggling with the multiple sequelae of childhood sexual abuse and may have formal psychiatric disorders.

The varied needs of these HIV-positive women will generally require specific multiservice program components and care provider training as listed below for good comprehensive care. Common clinical issues for these diverse subpopulations of HIV-positive women with complex histories and comorbidities can be managed best through such programs, which are responsive to both their clinical and concrete needs. Some of these services may be available through community-based AIDS service organizations and require close coordination with medical care.

Optimally, treatment for formal psychiatric and substance use disorders, which will be discussed below, would be available on site (Kobayashi, in press) and be integrated with primary medical care. Savings from emergency room visits and hospitalizations prevented help offset the labor intensive costs of these multiservice programs; if a broad array of services is not provided for these populations with such a complex layering of needs, routine medical care will generally be complicated by intermittent follow-up, medication non-adherence or frequent presentations in crisis in emergency room settings.

TABLE 9-3: MULTISERVICE CLINICAL PROGRAM COMPONENTS

COMMON CLINICAL ISSUES FOR HIV-POSITIVE WOMEN	CLINICAL PROGRAM RESPONSE
lack of trust; fears of abandonment	continuity of care; non judgmental attitude; patience; female providers
chronic low self-esteem	respect, acceptance, listening, time
complex personal situations	multiservice coordination: housing; transportation; vocational rehabilitation and education; linkage to entitlement programs
responsibility for children and others in household	childcare, respite programs; integrated pediatric and women's care; permanency planning and advance directives assistance
stigmatization	awareness of care provider reactions; social support groups
continuing high risk behaviors	prevention education via the primary healthcare provider
feelings of powerlessness; lack of assertiveness and skills	case management; outreach support; patient education; new skills training
domestic violence; exploitive relationships	women's shelters; domestic violence counseling; legal aid; psychotherapy
substance use and psychiatric comorbidities	psychiatric and substance tx programs integrated with medical care

IV. PSYCHIATRIC DISORDERS

There are a number of formal psychiatric disorders among women with HIV infection which require diagnosis and treatment. Women with HIV as well as women at risk for HIV have higher lifetime prevalence of major depressive disorder, PTSD and borderline personality disorder than the general population. If women with these disorders do not receive appropriate treatment, their participation in medical follow-up or their ability to adhere to complicated medication regimes can be compromised.

Seropositive women with untreated psychiatric disorders which are associated with impulsive or self-destructive tendencies may also engage in high risk transmission behaviors, potentially infecting others or being exposed to other STDs themselves. Abuse histories frequently leave them susceptible to feelings of learned helplessness or powerlessness in sexual situations which may result in high risk behaviors, inability to negotiate safe sex, or engaging in sex for drug exchanges. (Fullilove, 1992)

Women across cultures and around the world have lifetime incident rates of major depressive disorders twice that of men. In the United States, the incidence of major depression in the general population is approximately 10–15%. (DSM-IV, 1994) Among a sample of 234 African-American men who have sex with men (159 HIV-positive and 75 HIV-) and African-American women (100 HIV-positive and 35 HIV-), there was a high prevalence of anxiety spectrum disorders (38%) and mood disorders (23%) in both samples, and signifcant rates of PTSD (50%) among the women. (Myers, 1999)

Major depressive disorders may be missed as care providers project their own feelings and think "I'd be depressed too, under those circumstances." Once diagnosed, these disorders are often undermedicated with doses of antidepressant medication which are too low to insure a clinical response. Substance disorders are sometimes missed as contributors to the depression, and bipolar disorder is often not recognized when depression is the presenting symptom.

There are a number of specific psychiatric issues for the clinician who is treating HIV-positive to consider. Women who are incarcerated have a higher prevalence of psychiatric disorders and substance use disorders than women in the general population or even men who are incarcerated . The chronically mentally ill have higher rates of HIV than the general population in high seroprevalence areas. (Cournos, 1991) Psychotic symptoms also need to be differentiated from delirium in any HIV-positive individual. Central nervous system causes of change in mood and mental status should be ruled out. (The differential diagnoses of minor cognitive motor disorder, HIV-associated dementia, and other CNS diseases such as cryptococcus, syphilis, herpes, CNS lymphoma, progressive multifocal leukoencephalopathy, toxoplasmosis and other conditions are beyond the scope of this chapter.) Although initial rates of suicide were much higher than in the general population in the early days of the epidemic, it is likely that these rates are decreasing. (Marzuk, 1997) Suicidal ideation may be used defensively, as a reminder that the individual still retains ultimate control over their illness; these cases should be differentiated from those individuals who are actively suicidal.

Some of the clinical misperceptions which get in the way of evaluating these disorders are listed below, along with reminders for the complete assessment. For the complete diagnostic criteria of each disorder, see the DSM-IV of the American Psychiatric Association. (DSM-IV, 1994)

TABLE 9-4: COMMON CLINICAL MISPERCEPTIONS REGARDING PSYCHIATRIC ISSUES

PSYCHIATRIC ISSUE/ DISORDER	CLINICAL MISPERCEPTIONS	REMEMBER TO ASK ABOUT
Major Depression	"Anyone would be depressed or grieving," forgetting biologic depression	**Vegetative symptoms** (early AM awakening, diurnal mood variation, appetite disturbance); anhedonia more than sadness
Bipolar Mood Disorder	"Depressed mood must mean depression," forgetting bipolar sx	**Hypomanic/Manic sx** (hx of racing thoughts, hyperactivity, no need for sleep, grandiose plans, irritability)
Psychosis	"The patient seems normal," forgetting hallucinations and paranoia	**Psychotic sx:** "Do you ever hear your name called, turn around and no one is there? or a phone ringing?" "Ever feel like people are talking about you walking down the street?"
Delirium	"The patient is clearly schizophrenic or psychotic" forgetting acute medical etiologies	**Distractibility, Disorientation, Dysarthric speech;** Inability to sustain, focus attention; misperceptions; mumbling or muttering
Sexual Abuse/ Assault Hx	"Too personal; may embarrass or offend"	"Were you ever sexually, physically abused in childhood? Assaulted as an adult?" **Do not ask details.**
Anxiety, Panic, Agoraphobia	"Must be drug-seeking"; "Anyone would be anxious"	Panic sx, sense of Doom, Tachycardia repeated episodes, **impairment of function;** avoids crowded places
Domestic Violence	"Seems like a nice person"	"Is there anyone in your life now or in the past who makes you feel unsafe?"
Suicidal Ideation	"May plant the thought in their mind, provoke it"	"Have you ever felt like hurting or killing yourself? **Have a plan?"** Have the means?

V. DIAGNOSIS OF MAJOR DEPRESSIVE DISORDER

The diagnosis of a major depressive disorder should focus on "anhedonia," or the loss of pleasure in all activities, rather than sadness alone. The sadness of grief, for example, can be as profound, but is often accompanied by moments of pleasure or even laughter as the most acute grief subsides. Sadness from other sources, such as major disappointments, is also responsive to environmental change such as an enjoyable activity, and the mood would be quickly reversed if the source of the disappointment were to change. This is not the case in a major depressive episode, where the world has no joy regardless of the activity or turn of events, where the outlook is gloom and doom regardless of the likelihood of positive events, and where there can be obsessive rumination on past wrongs or regrets which are impossible to balance with any feelings of accomplishment or hope. The mood is often worst in the morning, whereas the sadness of adjusting to difficult or stressful events tends to worsen over the course of the day and the new day is often filled with more hope. Hopelessness indicates severe depression and is the most consistent predictor of completed suicides; suicidal ideation is associated with both depressive and bipolar mood disorders.

In addition to depressed mood and anhedonia, often with a sense of hopelessness, there are a variety of vegetative or biologic symptoms which should be explored: low energy and psychomotor retardation; sleep disturbance (hypersomnia or insomnia), frequently with early morning awakening around 2:00 AM to 4:00 AM; appetite disturbance (hyperphagia or hypophagia) usually accompanied by loss of appetite and enjoyment of food regardless of the amount actually consumed; constipation may occur. Finally, there may be cognitive changes such as decreased attention and concentration (see Table 9-5); social withdrawal and tendency toward isolative behavior; preoccupation with guilt or regrets; obsessive rumination; diminished range of affect; uncharacteristic irritability; and increased use of substances of abuse. A family history of mood disorders is often present. In the most severe cases, psychotic symptoms such as delusions and hallucinations can be present. The fact that there

TABLE 9-5: DIFFERENTIAL DIAGNOSIS OF MAJOR DEPRESSIVE DISORDER (MDD)

DISORDER	DIFFERENTIATED FROM MDD BY:
Bipolar Disorder	Racing thoughts, increased energy, decreased need for sleep irritability, hypersexuality (these may coexist with depressed mood in a mixed Bipolar state)
Grief	Onset associated with the loss; responsive to changes in the environment with less sadness or enjoyment; decreasing severity over time; preoccupation with deceased; "psychotic" symptoms related to deceased such as seeing, being visited by the deceased; rare suicidal intent although reunion fantasies may exist
Adjustment Disorder with Depressed Mood	Sadness is rarely as profound; little anhedonia; no vegetative symptoms; identifiable precipitant; responsive to environmental change; suicidal ideation and intent may still occur
Organic Mood Disorder	Identifiable agent linked by time; less anhedonia or hopelessness; test for specific medical conditions such as TSH, B12, VDRL CNS evaluation; no family history
Dementia	Less concern re: cognitive decline; more gradual changes; may respond with laughter; worse at night; specific neurological deficits; CT scan often abnormal
Delirium	Fluctuating mental status with altered level of consciousness; distractibility; inability to focus or sustain attention; dysarthric speech; agitation; medical etiology
Medication-Induced Substance-Induced Mood Disorders	Onset with use of: steroids, anticholinergics, sedative-hypnotics, anticonvulsants, antiparkinsonians, Beta-blockers, anti-TB meds; sympathomimetics; Azidothymidine, Stavudine; all illicit drugs; urine tox screen; medication history

is a constellation of depressive symptoms which develop together over a course of weeks or months helps differentiate major depressive disorders from similar disturbances related to medical illnesses.

VI. PSYCHOPHARMACOLOGY FOR THE HIV-POSITIVE WOMAN: GENERAL GUIDELINES

There have been numerous studies indicating that psychotropic medications are safe for HIV-positive individuals, and do not adversely affect the immune system. While specific medications and dosing will be discussed later, the following general guidelines should be kept in mind when approaching psychotropic medications with the seropositive woman:

■ **"Start Low, Go Slow":** Low dosing, slow upward titration as with geriatric patients.

■ **"Always expect the unexpected":** HIV-positive patients often experience unusual side effects; or common side effects at low doses; or complicated drug-drug interactions.

■ **"Dynamic Monitoring":** Changes in weight, metabolism, other medications, or medical illness episodes require frequent updating and reevaluating dosing ranges.

■ **"Interdisciplinary Coordination":** Psychiatrists should be in regular communication with primary healthcare providers, and vice versa, about clinical updates, dosing changes, major medical events.

■ **"Suspect Substances":** Depression may be complicated by alcohol, anxiety by withdrawal syndromes, mania by psychostimulants; patients often forget that, when their consumption has decreased, their CNS sensitivitiy to the effects of these substances increases over time.

■ **Amplify psychotropic medication adherence** with medication boxes, simple regimes, written instructions, coordination with antiretroviral therapies and patient education.

■ **The primary Cytochrome P450 systems at issue for psychiatric medications are Cyp2D6 and Cyp3A4.** The major Cytochrome P450 drug-drug interactions to keep in mind are: ritonavir may increase levels of benzodiazepines, desipramine and selective serotonin reuptake inhibitors (2D6), or nefazadone (3A4); venlafaxine (and St. John's Wort) may decrease indinavir concentration; nevirapine may decrease methadone levels; methadone increases zidovudine levels; valproate increases the level of zidovudine. (See Chapter Chapter XIV on Pharmacologic Considerations in HIV-infected Pregnant Patients for more information re: drug-drug interactions)

While a complete discussion of psychotropic medications (including complete side effect profiles) is beyond the scope of this chapter, the following medications are useful for the practitioner wishing to initiate psychotropic medications, with dosage ranges for common indications. (Modifed from Schatzberg, 1998)

Common potential side effects of all of the antidepressant medications include agitation, irritability, sedation, sexual dysfunction, weight gain, headache, gastrointestinal distress, dry mouth and potentiation of mania. Side effects of antipsychotics include cognitive slowing, the extrapyramidal symptoms of dystonia and akathisia with long-term risk of dyskinesia; with the newer "atypical" antipsychotics, hyperprolactinemia may occur and with olanzapine in particular, significant weight gain. There are discontinuation syn-

TABLE 9-6: COMMON PSYCHIATRIC MEDICATIONS

DISORDER	MEDICATION(S)
Major Depressive Disorder (with or without anxiety)	Sertraline (Zoloft) 25–200mg (SSRI) Fluoxetine (Prozac) 10–80mg (SSRI) Paroxetine (Paxil) 10–50mg (SSRI)\ Citalopram (Celexa) 10–40mg (SSRI) Venlafaxine (Effexor-XR) 37.5–225mg Buproprion (Wellbutrin-SR) 50–300mg ; in divided doses
HIV-related Depression/ fatigue (with or without Minor Cognitive Motor Disorder)	Methylphenidate 10–80mg in divided doses
Bipolar Mood Disorder	Valproate/Valproic Acid (Depakote) 500–2000mg, titrated by blood levels (50–100 micrograms/ml) Lithium Carbonate 600–1800mg titrated by blood levels (0.6–1.0mEq/L)
Psychotic Symptom (also severe PTSD)	Olanzapine (Zyprexa) 2.5–20mg Risperidone (Risperdal) 0.5–6mg Quetiapine (Seroquel) 50–600mg
Anxiety Disorders (also PTSD)	Buspirone (Buspar) 15–30mg in divided doses Lorazepam (Ativan) 1–6mg in divided doses Alprazolam (Xanax) 1–4mg in divided doses Clonazepam (Klonopin) 1–4mg in divided doses
Panic Attacks	Paroxetine (Paxil) 10–40mg Sertraline (Zoloft) 25–200mg Imipramine (Tofranil) 25–200mg Alprazolam (Xanax) 1.5–4mg in divided doses Lorazepam (Ativan) 3–6mg in divided doses
Insomnia	Lorazepam/Clonazepam at night dose Temazepam (Restoril) 15–60mg Zolpidem (Ambien) 5–10mg Trazadone (Desyrel) 25–100mg
Alcohol Dependence	Disulfiram (Antabuse) 250–500mg
Alcohol Withdrawal	Tranxene 15–30mg q2–6hrs
Opiate Dependence	Methadone 60–120mg
Opiate Withdrawal	Methadone 5–20mg in divided doses, tapered by 5 mg/day Clonidine 0.3mg in three divided doses; increase to 2mg/day in divided doses

dromes with paroxetine and venlafaxine; these drugs should be tapered. Sedation and cognitive effects; tolerance, dependence and withdrawal syndromes, including rebound anxiety, occur with the benzodiazepines (BZDZ), especially with alprazolam.

Patients who require multiple medications, have severe side effects, have multiple diagnoses, or are not responding routinely or at routine doses should be referred for psychiatric evaluation.

VII. EVALUATION OF SUICIDE RISK

Women are significantly more likely to attempt suicide than men, while men are significantly more likely to complete the suicide by a male:female ratio of at least 4:1. Caucasians commit suicide at twice the rate of African Americans and Hispanics. It is estimated that 90% of individuals have a psychiatric disorder at the time of suicide, 45–79% of whom have major depression. Fifteen percent of individuals with a mood disorder commit suicide. (Buzan, 1999)

Women more commonly attempt suicide by overdose, while men use more violent means such as firearms or hanging. Women who have few social supports, have been widowed or divorced, or who have a history of sexual abuse are at increased risk for suicide. Women with children attempt suicide less frequently. Any risk factor is increased by the presence of alcohol, psychosis or an organic mental syndrome.

As mentioned, it is likely that suicide rates are decreasing among HIV-positive individuals. This may be due to antiretroviral therapies which can improve organic mood disorders and cognitive function (Ferrando, 1998), as well as increase longevity and hope.

IX

TABLE 9-7: RISK FACTORS AND CONSIDERATIONS IN THE EVALUATION OF SUICIDALITY
■ Significant Suicidal Ideation*
■ Specific Intent or Plan*; available means
■ Hopelessness*
■ Previous Suicide Attempts*
■ Depressed Mood, Mood Disorders*
■ Family History of suicide or Mood Disorders*
■ Schizophrenia, Psychosis (not necessarily command hallucinations)*
■ Organic Mental Syndromes*
■ Intoxication with Alcohol*, other Substances
■ Recent Major Loss, particularly through suicide
■ Preoccupation with death
■ Fantasies of Reunion through death
■ Homocidal Rage
■ Caucasian Race*
* These factors have been documented as risk factors for suicidality.

In order to assess suicide risk, the clinician must inquire about it. This does not increase the likelihood an individual will attempt suicide. The clinician should practice a standard way of asking, such as "Have you ever had thoughts of hurting yourself?" or ". . . of ending your life?" or "Do you ever feel that life is not worth living?"

VIII. CARE PROVIDER ISSUES

One of the most important relationships the seropositive woman has is the relationship with her healthcare provider. The dynamics of this relationship can have significant impact on the experience of the individual HIV-positive woman, and the woman will be affected not only by what the clinician communicates about HIV disease and treatment, but by the way the information is communicated, and the manner in which the provider relates to the HIV-positive woman herself.

Whether or not it is conscious, healthcare providers may experience different reactions to HIV-positive women than with seropositive men. As previously discussed, it has been estimated that one out of every three women in the United States has experienced a sexual assault, from childhood sexual abuse to rape. This is even more common among women in poverty where the HIV epidemic increasingly resides.

Women who have been victims of abuse or assault may provoke a variety of reactions in care providers, the most common of which is frustration and disapproval of the substance use which many women use to distance themselves from their trauma. Male or female care providers may find it particularly difficult not to be angry or put off with the substance using woman who is pregnant or who has children.

Providers may also collude with the seropositive woman's feelings of powerlessness and try to take control over things she can actually handle with sufficient support; protective concerns and anger at an abusing partner may tempt the caring provider to cross professional boundaries and try to rescue the patient.

The provider may feel anger when the woman's sense of powerlessness, particularly in sexual situations, results in submitting repeatedly to unsafe sex. They may unknowingly continue the trail of abuse by not allowing her concerns to be heard or with inadequate pain control, often in response to provocative and insistent behavior on the part of the patient, which provokes the clinician to try to assert control. It is important to stop to consider the powerful drive for self preservation that leads women with few options to try to neutralize or forget painful memories with drugs or alcohol. Pregnancy and motherhood do not automatically erase these feelings.

As with other medical populations, nonadherence with medications or medical follow-up can be personalized by providers as lack of commitment, clinical failure or an affront to their good intentions, rather than adherence to different priorities. Appointments missed to take care of children or because of problems with transportation may be misinterpreted as not caring about medical follow-up.

Frank disregard or avoidance of medical treatment, on the other hand, may be mistakenly excused without exploring the real meaning of the behaviors. Careproviders often assume that a woman is missing visits because she is overwhelmed with the care of her children, when she is actually angry at a particular provider, or so frightened about the illness that she avoids treatment in order not to be confronted with it. Initiating multiple medications may be the point at which she is forced to break through the denial and confront her illness.

For the woman health care provider, the experience of taking care of HIV-positive women can be both more rewarding and more depleting than general medical or HIV care. Personal identification with the patient may work positively to increase empathy, or negatively to increase projection of one's own values and expectations on the individual. Female providers may also experience amplified grief, through personal identification, concern for orphaned children, or because of the death of a patient with whom they developed a genuine connection. Providers who are either prone to experience patient deaths as their own clinical failures, or who have deep compassion for the suffering of their patients, may be vulnerable to experiencing professional burn out, particularly if subjected to multiple, sequential losses.

IX

REFERENCES

Abdul-Quader AS, Tross S, Silvert HM, et al. Women who borrow: determinants of borrowing injection equipment in female injecting drug users in New York City. Int Conf AIDS (2):822, 1993.

American Psychiatric Association. *Diagnostic and Statistical Manual of Mental Disorders,* 4th Edition. Washington, DC, American Psychiatric Association, 1994.

Barkan SE, Melnick SL, Preston-Martin S, et al. The Women's Interagency HIV Study. The WIHS Collaborative Study Group. *Epidemiology* 9:117–125, 1998.

Batki SL, Ferrando SJ, Manfredi LB, et al. Psychiatric disorders, drug use, and medical status in injection drug users with HIV disease. *Am J Addictions* 5:249–258, 1996.

Boland RJ, Moore J, Schuman P. The Longitudinal Course of Depression in HIV-Infected Women. *Psychosomatics* 40(2):160, 1999.

Boland RJ, Moore J, Solomon L, et al. Depression and HIV in Women: Prevalence and Associations in a National Cohort. *Psychosomatics* 37(2):198, 1999.

Bozzette SA, Berry SH, Duan N, et al. The Care of HIV infected adults in the United States. *New England Journal of Medicine* 339:1897–1904, 1998.

Broers RP, Morabia A, Hirschel B. A cohort study of drug users' compliance with zidovudine treatment. *Arch Intern Med* 154:1121–1127, 1994.

Brown GR, Rundell JR, McManis SE, et al. Prevalence of Psychiatric Disorders in Early Stages of HIV Infection. *Psychosomatic Medicine* 54:588–601, 1992.

Buzan R. Assessment and management of the suicidal patient. In Jacobson JL, Jacobson AM.. *Psychiatric Secrets*. Philadelphia: Hanley & Belfus, Inc., 1996.

Centers for Disease Control. Estimated incidence of AIDS and deaths of persons with AIDS, adjusted for delays in reporting, by quarter year of diagnosis/death, United States, January 1985 through June 1987. *HIV/AIDS Surveillance Report* 9:1–43, 1997.

Centers for Disease Control. Estimated incidence of AIDS and deaths of persons with AIDS, adjusted for delays in reporting, by quarter year of diagnosis/death, United States, January 1985 through June 1987. *HIV/AIDS Surveillance Report* 9:1–43, 1997.

Cohen M, Deamant C, Barkan S, et al. Domestic violence and childhood sexual abuse in HIV-infected women and women at risk for HIV. *Am J Public Health* 90(4):560–565, 2000.

Farmer P, Connors M, Simmons J, eds. *Women, Poverty and AIDS*. Monroe, Maine: Common Courage Press, 1996.

Ferrando S, van Gorp W, McElhiney M, et al. Highly active antiretroviral treatment in HIV infection: benefits for neuropsychological function. *JAIDS* 12:F65–F70, 1998.

Gilligan, C. *In a Different Voice*. Cambridge: Harvard University Press, 1982.

Hoff RA, Beam-Goulet J, Rosenheck RA. Mental disorder as a risk factor for human immunodeficiency virus infection in a sample of veterans. *J Nerv Ment Dis* 185(9):556–560, 1997.

Hu DJ, Byers R Jr, Fleming PL, et al. Characteristics of persons with late AIDS diagnosis in the United States. *Am J Prev Med* 11:114–119, 1995.

Kacanek D, Diaz T, Ward JW. Noninjection drug use and sexual risk behaviors of women with HIV and AIDS — United States. Int Conf AIDS 11(1):252, 1996.

Klein H, Rodriguez-Crane SM, Hoffman JA, et al. HIV risk behavior involvement among low-frequency and high-frequency crack-using women. Natl Conf Women HIV 120, 1997.

Kobayashi and Standridge, in press.

Lyketsos CG, Fishman M, Hutton H, et al. The Effectiveness of Psychiatric Treatment for HIV-Infected Patients. *Psychosomatics* 38(5):423–432, 1997.

Lum PJ, Guydish JR, Brown E, Allen R. Younger female injection drug users report higher riskd for HIV and drug-related harm in San Francisco. Int Conf AIDS 12:382 (abst 23202), 1998.

Markowitz JC, Kocsis JH, Fishman B, et al. Treatment of Depressive Symptoms in Human Immunodeficiency Virus-Positive Patients. *Arch Gen Psych* 55:452–457, 1998.

Marzuk P, Tardiff K, Leon A, et al. HIV seroprevalence among suicide victims in New York City, 1991–1993. *Am J Psychiatry* 154: 1720–1725, 1997.

Mauskopf J, Turner BJ, Markson LE, et al. Patterns of ambulatory care for AIDS patients and association with emergency room use. *Health Serv Res* 29: 489–510, 1994.

Myers HF, Durvasula RS. Psychiatric disorders in African-American men and women living with HIV/AIDS. *Cultural Diversity and Ethnic Minority Psychology* 5(3):249–262, 1999.

Nelson WL, Ferrando SJ, Stanislawski DM, et al. Childhood trauma, substance abuse, and distress in HIV-infected women. Intl Conf AIDS ll(2):429, 1996.

Paone D, Caloir S, Shi Q, et al. Sex, drugs, and syringe exchange in New York City: women's experiences. *JAMA* 50(3–4):109–114, 1995.

Shapiro MF, Morton SC, McCaffrey DF et al. Variation sin the care of HIVinfected adults in the United States: results from the HIV Cost and Services Utilization Study. *JAMA* 281:2305–2315, 1999.

Schatzberg AF, Nemeroff CB. *Textbook of Psychopharmacology.* Washington DC: American Psychiatric Press, 1998.

Shayne VT, Kaplan BJ. Double Victims: Poor Women with AIDS. *Women and Health* 17(1):21–37, 1991.

Solomon L, Stein M, Flynn CP, et al. Service Utilization by HIV-1 infected women from four United States urban centers: the HERS study. Int Conf AIDS 11(2):20, 1996.

Surrey JL. The 'Self-in-Relation': A Theory of Women's Development. Work in Progress Series, The Stone Center, Wellesley College, 1982.

Thompson AS, Blankenship KM, Winfrey J, et al. Improving health care utilization and access for drug-using women with or at risk for HIV infection in a correctional facility and at needle exchange sites. HIV Infect Women Conf S19, 1995.

Weiss EL, Longhurst JG, Mazure CM. Childhood Sexual Abuse as a Risk Factor for Depression in Women: Psychosocial and Neurobiological Correlates. *Am J Psychiatry* 156 (6): 816–828, 1999.

Wong L, Irwin K, Edlin B, et al. Risk factors for rape and prevalence of HHIV and syphilis infection among the rape victims in 3 US cities. The Multicenter Crack Cocaine and HIV Study Team. Intl Conf AIDS 9(2):649, 1993.

Wyatt GE, Peters SD. Issues in the definition of child sexual abuse in prevalence research. *Child Abuse and Neglect* 10:231–240, 1986.

Zierler S, Feingold L, Laufer D, et al. Adult Survivors of Childhood Sexual Abuse and Subsequent Risk of HIV Infection. *Am J Public Health* 81:572–575, 1991.

IX

This *Guide* is a PRELIMINARY EDITION.

We need YOUR HELP to make the NEXT EDITION as useful as possible!

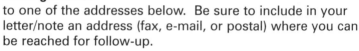

Please send your
comments
criticisms
corrections
suggested changes, and
other guidance
to one of the addresses below. Be sure to include in your letter/note an address (fax, e-mail, or postal) where you can be reached for follow-up.

Translation Partners Needed

Write to us if you can help us find partners to help us have this *Guide* translated into your native language. For instance, provide us with a contact who works with translation in your country's Ministry of Health, or tell us about a group at a medical school that translates medical texts.

Send Us Your Comments

E-mail: womencare@hrsa.gov

Fax to the attention of "Womencare": 301-443-0791 (USA)

Postal address: Womencare
Parklawn Building, Room 11A-33
5600 Fishers Lane
Rockville, Maryland 20857
USA

Note that this and subsequent editions of
A Guide to the Clinical Care of Women with HIV
will be available online.

Go to the HIV/AIDS Bureau Web site
and click on the publication *Women's Guide*:
http://www.hrsa.gov/hab

X: SUBSTANCE ABUSE

Henry L Francis, MD and Victoria A Cargill, MD, MSCE

I. SUBSTANCE ABUSE

Substance use is more prevalent in the United States than most persons realize. Statistics described in the 1998 National Household Survey on Drug Abuse (NHSDA) give the following picture on drug use in American men and women. (NHSDA, 1998) Approximately 53% of the American population will use an illegal drug in their lifetime. It is estimated from the NHSDA data that in the general population, 8.1% of males and 4.5% of women have used illegal drugs in the last month. Over the past year, 23.1 million persons Americans will have used an illegal drug. Only a fraction of drug using persons are truly drug addicted (also called drug dependent). It is estimated that at there are 4.1 million people who meet the definition of drug addiction, defined as compulsively continuing drug seeking and drug using behavior even in the face of negative health consequences.

The general rates of legal drug addiction dwarf the amount of illegal drug addiction. In 1998, 113 million persons reported consuming alcohol in the last 30 days and 64 million persons consumed cigarettes. At least 43 million of the alcohol consumers are dependant on alcohol through binge or very heavy drinking. The alcohol dependant individuals are more than twice as numerous as the number of illegal drug users combined. In contrast to illegal drug use rates where twice as many men use illegal drugs than women, alcohol consumption rates are nearly equal for men (59%) and women (45%) in the general population. However, women were much less likely to be binge drinkers. Regular use of cigarettes, nicotine dependence, was nearly equal for men and women, 29.7% vs. 25.7 % respectively.

Unfortunately, the majority of substance dependant women and men, who could benefit from substance abuse, and substance abuse related emotion/psychological and health treatment never receive any form of therapeutic intervention. In 1998, 846,000 substance dependent women needed clinical health care, 1.6 million women needed emotional/psychological treatment and more than1.7 million women needed substance abuse care. Yet only 390,000 of all three groups of women combined received any care at all.

This chapter will focus on addiction as a disease, discuss associations with a variety of comorbid conditions, review the epidemiology of substance abuse in the United States, and outline ways to identify and treat substance abuse in women.

II. EPIDEMIOLOGY OF SUBSTANCE ABUSE

The frequency and danger of drugs and behaviors of drug use are greatly underestimated by the American public and health care professionals. The two commonly used legal drugs, alcohol and tobacco, are more frequently consumed than all the illegal drugs combined (Table 10-1). Marijuana, and cocaine (including crack cocaine) are the most frequently used illegal drugs. Inhalants are used predominately by adolescents. A more recent trend in adolescents is to use club drugs like gamma-hydroxybutyrate (GHB), Ecstasy (MDMA), Rohypnol, Ketamine, methamphetamine and LSD at all night parties called "raves" or "trances". Surprisingly, heroin, which is viewed as a highly prevalent drug is actually one of the least favored drugs of preference in the U.S. population.

TABLE 10-1: PREVALENCE OF DRUG USE	
DRUG	CURRENT USERS ESTIMATE
■ Alcohol	113,000, 000
■ Tobacco	64,000,000
■ Marijuana	11,000,000
■ Cocaine	2,187,000
■ Hallucinogens	1,500,000
■ Inhalants	713,000
■ Stimulants	633,000
■ Opiates	180,000
Source: Adapted from Summary from the 1998 National Household Survey on Drug Abuse, DHHS, SAMSHA.	

The rates of illicit drugs used vary by slightly by ethnicity and in a major way by gender. Estimates for the gender specific drug use indicate that women are at least 50% less likely to use illicit drugs compared to males. The male to female illicit drug use rate relationship is consistent thorough out all ethnic groups (Table 10-2). However, African American males and females have higher rates of illicit drug use than White Americans and Hispanic Americans. Ethnic comparisons of drug used demonstrated that the highest rated of drug use occurs in the adolescents, aged 18–25. The males in all 3 ethnic groups are comparable though

TABLE 10-2: ILLICIT DRUG USE ESTIMATES BY AGE, GENDER, AND ETHNICITY IN THE U.S.			
	PERCENT U.S. POPULATION		
AGE	WHITE	HISPANIC	AFRICAN AMERICAN
12–17	10.3	9.9	9.9
18–25	13.6	11.1	17.1
26–34	7.1	5.4	9.4
> 35	3.2	3.5	4.8
Male	7.7	7.7	12.0
Female	4.5	4.5	5.2
Source: Adapted from Summary from the 1998 National Household Survey on Drug Abuse, DHHS, SAMSHA.			

African Americans are to be more likely to use drugs past the age of 26.

White American men and women have higher rates of alcohol use than African Americans or Hispanic Americans (Table 10-3). For all alcohol using groups, alcohol consumption is highest in adolescents. White Americans have a notably higher rate of chronic alcohol consumption after the age of 26 than Hispanic or African Americans.

TABLE 10-3: ALCOHOL USE ESTIMATES BY AGE, GENDER, AND ETHNICITY IN THE U.S.

AGE	PERCENT U.S. POPULATION		
	WHITE	HISPANIC	AFRICAN AMERICAN
12–17	20.9	18.9	13.1
18–25	65.0	50.8	50.3
26–34	65.2	53.1	54.8
> 35	56.2	47.7	38.3
Male	61.2	56.8	49.0
Female	49.2	33.6	32.3

III. CO-MORBIDITY RELATED TO SUBSTANCE ABUSE

Substance abuse is associated with a number of medical consequences, as well as co-morbid conditions. Some of these are listed in Table 10-4, and include the hepatitis's (A, B, C, D and G), sexually transmitted diseases (STD's), tuberculosis and trauma. These represent conditions associated directly and indirectly with substance use. Not only does the abuse of psychoactive substances cause a significant number of accidents, but excessive alcohol intake places users at risk for cirrhosis, malignant disease, neurological disorder, neuropathy and psychiatric disorders. Intravenous drug use is a major factor in transmission of certain infectious diseases. Smoking of drugs is the most common cause of bronchial carcinoma, other malignancies and airway diseases.

TABLE 10-4: MEDICAL CONDITIONS AND SEQUELAE ASSOCIATED WITH SUBSTANCE USE

▪ HIV	▪ Cellulitis
▪ STDs	▪ Thrombophlebitis
▪ Tuberculosis	▪ Poor nutrition
▪ Hepatitis (A, B, C, D, and G)	▪ Pneumonia
▪ Endocarditis	▪ Cutaneous abscesses
▪ Alcoholism	▪ Cognitive Dysfunction
▪ Liver Disease	▪ Septic Embolic

Underlying medical conditions, such as depression or other mental disorders may influence initiation or continuation of substance use ("self medicating" depression). The prolonged use of drugs in this setting can exacerbate, rather than improve these problems. Female drug users, as a group are more likely to suffer from depression and anxiety disorder than the general population, or other medical groups. The strong association between drug use and mental health disorders is evident in environmental and genetic predisposition to addictive, impulsive and compulsive behaviors and personality disorders. A conservative estimate is that 53% of drug abusers have one or more mental health diagnoses. Successful treatment of the drug addiction is unlikely until their mental illness is treated.

The cognitive effects of drug use may result in unrecognized disease exposure. These cognitive effects include impaired decision-making or a reduced ability to understand or evaluate one's actions. Drug effects, such as disinhibition, are known to decrease compliance with safer sex precautions or drug paraphernalia hygiene. Crack use is associated with high-risk sexual behavior, other drug use, and the exchange of sex for money and/or drugs. Although IDU-related HIV transmissions is most closely associated with the sharing of injection equipment, a significant portion is related to sexual risk. Sex and drug related HIV risk behaviors are strongly associated in women. Women acquire HIV, Hepatitis B and STDs through sexual partnerships with injection drug users. Prevention intervention strategies for women at risk must include both contextual relevance (e.g. dealing with an IDU sexual partner) and real world appropriate planning like condom use strategies in the setting of drug/alcohol intoxication. Also important are treatment and prevention of co-morbid conditions like STDs and Hepatitis C, which facilitate sexual and perinatal HIV transmission.

Signs and symptoms of drug addiction, HIV and other infectious or medical diseases often overlap, complicating surveillance and early identification efforts, as well as care. Cognitive dysfunction, neuropathy, liver disease, and various infections may be caused by drug use or co-morbid conditions, complicating appropriate and timely diagnosis and management. Among IDUs, important presenting symptoms include thrombophlebitis, endocarditis, pericarditis, septic emboli, cellulitis and pneumonia.

Although women have lower rates of drug use than men, they are more likely to become infected with HIV and other infections by their own drug use habits and sexual contact with their partners. About sixty percent of AIDS cases in women are drug-related. Although minority groups constitute about 26% of the U.S. population, about half of drug-related female AIDS cases are among black women, for whom AIDS has been the leading cause of death since 1993. (Krieger, 1997) Co-morbid diseases among HIV infected drug-using women are likely to occur more often and progress more rapidly, complicating treatment. Drug use and related co-morbid conditions influence a number of other health outcomes in HIV+ women, including mortality and maternal fetal HIV transmission.

In both substance abuse treatment programs and primary care clinics, strategies are needed to identify and manage HIV and other co-morbid problems like tuberculosis, sexually transmitted diseases (STD), Hepatitis B and C, as well as mental health and social/economic problems.

Primary care providers are uniquely positioned to identify early indications of drug-use related HIV risks and signs of other comorbidities and to engage drug users in treatment at earlier stages of drug dependence. New and younger initiates to injection drug use engage in particularly high-risk behaviors for acquisition and transmission of infectious diseases and HIV. (Carneiro, 1999) In primary care settings, interventions can be put in place to prevent further transmission (Anderson, 1996) of HIV or other infections. Misconceptions about the legal, social and health implications of testing positive for HIV reduce early detection efforts, are particularly among patients at high risk. (Harvey)

IV. SUBSTANCE ABUSE IN WOMEN

Women have different risk factors for initiating drug use, require different diagnostic approaches to detect drug use and should have treatment plans and care sites which address their personal, social and familial needs. Historically however, most treatment and diagnostic paradigms for addiction treatment were based on experience in treating male users. Stigma, family circumstances, community environment and social status affect the treatment of substance abuse, especially for women. Very few facilities accommodate women who are pregnant or have small children. It is now clear that care sites should be able to address medical, drug use and living circumstance problems simultaneously.

The relationship of drug use to the spread of infectious diseases such as HIV, can be challenging to assess, particularly when, as in many cases, no specific risk factor for exposure is reported. (Warner, 1995) It is possible that pressures of stigma and fear associated with drug abuse may cause some individuals, particularly women, to be reluctant in identifying injection drug use as a risk factor. For this reason, many women are not identified as having health or drug use problems until very late in the natural history of these diseases.

V. IMPACT OF SOCIETAL PERCEPTIONS AND BELIEFS

There are numerous social, moral, personal and situational beliefs adversely affecting a drug using woman's health. Historically, the U.S. society's response to drug addiction is punitive, stigmatizing and prejudiced against drug users and their families. The negative public sentiment surrounding illicit and injection drug use is especially evident in criminal justice sentencing practices. Health providers often share these views of drug users as unreliable and noncompliant. Value-laden judgments may impact provider willingness to treat this population and influence the care provided and therapeutic regimens prescribed. Providers may be also being reluctant to raise the subject of substance abuse or treatment with patients because of misconceptions about the effectiveness of treatment.

Women with substance abuse are more likely to experience poor health and are less likely to access services, receive treatment or seek health care, partially because of the stigma of drug use. Suspicion, fear and distrust of the health care system result in reluctance among drug users to disclose medically necessary information. Negative sanctions, such as mandatory HIV testing during pregnancy and incarceration of drug using pregnant women for child abuse, have intensified fears about contact with the health system. For economically disadvantaged women with HIV and drug abuse problems, the fear of discrimination, retribution, loss of housing or loss of children may become more important than seeking or engaging in health services (Sly, 1997) and may keep them from receiving personally tailored prevention messages.

Individuals who are drug dependent, even though they may exhibit dysfunctional behavior, retain the right to be evaluated as individuals and to be treated with respect and equality, regardless of conflicts in values or beliefs between patient and physician.

VI. IDENTIFICATION OF SUBSTANCE USE

A. DIAGNOSIS BY HISTORY

Identification of substance use can be a challenge, given the myriad of illnesses it can mimic. However, the biggest barrier to identification is denial. Given the stigma associated with substance use, as well as the stereotypes associated with substance use, health care providers must entertain the diagnosis in *all* patients. Substance use must be a diagnosis to be excluded in the differential diagnoses of many medical conditions. Table 10-5 lists clues to a possible substance use diagnosis. These clues include erratic behavior, agitation, disorientation, doctor 'hopping', child custody loss and frequent unexplained accidents.

TABLE 10-5: CLUES TO SUBSTANCE USE		
MEDICAL HISTORY	*BEHAVIORAL CLUES*	*SOCIAL HISTORY CLUES*
■ HIV infection infection ■ Endocarditis ■ Hepatitis B or C infection ■ Septic Embolic ■ Septic thrombophlebitis	■ Agitation ■ Somnolence ■ Disorientation ■ Erratic behavior ■ Doctor "hopping" ■ Frequent unexplained accidents	■ Inability to retain employment ■ Child custody loss ■ Seemingly unexplainable financial difficulties

The diagnosis of drug addiction is made by taking a careful history of drug use, as well as a directed medical and psychosocial history; performing a complete physical evaluation; and laboratory testing for the presence of drugs or the complications of drug use. Providers must also be aware of the variable duration of time drug metabolites are present in blood and/or urine. Hence, if the index of suspicion is high, a single negative lab result should not exclude the diagnosis.

The most commonly used instruments to detect and assess drug and alcohol use are the CAGE survey, the *Diagnostic and Statistical Manual of Mental disorders, Fourth Edition* (DSM IV) substance abuse diagnostic criteria, and the Addiction Severity Index (ASI).

If the provider cannot get a sense of the patients drug use from unstructured questions, the CAGE survey offers a non-threatening alternative approach. The CAGE survey is a four-question format intended to be used in primary care and other non-substance abuse-related health care facilities.

1. Have you felt that you ought to **C**ut down on your drinking or drug use?

2. Have people **A**nnoyed you by criticizing your drinking or drug use?

3. Have you ever felt bad or **G**uilty about your drinking or drug use?

4. Have you ever had a drink or used drugs first thing in the morning (**E**ye opener) to steady your nerves, get rid of a hangover, or to get the day started?

This type of screening test though simplistic is very useful for getting substance addicted patients into a trajectory for drug use care. Otherwise, they may be seen in different parts of the health care system for other problems, while the substance abuse is not addressed.

Finally, some patients will come to medical attention due to substance intoxication or withdrawal. As with substance abuse, entertaining the diagnosis, as well as recognition of the constellation of signs and symptoms is critical to recognition of intoxication and withdrawal syndromes. Alcohol intoxication maybe characterized by inebriation, sedation, ataxia and slurred speech. However, this extreme of behavior is witnessed in a subset of patients of the 113 million Americans age 12 and older who reported alcohol use, 33 million reported binge drinking (meaning they drank 5 or more drinks on one occasion 5 or more days during the past 30 days). (SAMHSA, 1999) Alcohol withdrawal can vary from agitation, to the more florid syndromes associated with the delirium tremens. This includes labile blood pressure, autonomic instability, visual hallucinations and death. It should be noted that delirium tremens is associated with a 10–15% fatality risk.

Opiate intoxication is associated with sedation, including somnolence or 'nodding.' There has been a resurgence in heroin popularity, with and estimated 81,000 new heroin users in 1997. (SAMHSA, 1999) Opiate withdrawal is characterized by the loss of CNS depression. These signs include piloerection, vomiting, diarrhea, agitation, irritability and sweating. Cocaine, and its alkaline cheaper form, crack, are highly addictive. Intoxication with cocaine is associated with euphoria, as well as profound hypertension (secondary to the vasoconstrictive effects). Increased pulse rate and dilated pupils are also associated with cocaine intoxication. Cocaine/crack withdrawal is associated with irritability, agitation, and mood liability.

The DSM IV criteria for drug addiction are developed for the 11 classes of
abused drugs and include 7 major criteria (Table 10-6). DSM IV criteria determine addiction by finding evidence of physical or psychological dependence on
a drug or tolerance to it, disruption of social life patterns, and disregard of the
negative medical consequences of using drugs. A person is considered to be
drug addicted if they fulfill 3 of the 7 criteria within the previous 12 months.

TABLE 10-6: DSM IV DRUG ADDICTION CRITERIA
▪ Presence of drug use withdrawal
▪ Escalation of drug doses
▪ Persistent inability to reduce or control drug use
▪ Increased time obtaining the drug
▪ Personal and business activities are reduced by drug use
▪ Development of drug tolerance
▪ Knowledge of drug use's negative health and personal effects, yet continuing to use drugs
Source: Adapted from DSM IV, 4th edition, 1994.

The Addiction Severity Index (ASI) (Assessing Client Needs Using the ASI,
1995) is most commonly used to help health caregivers assess the severity of
the drug addiction in persons who are already determined to have a drug use
problem and for whom a treatment plan must be developed. The ASI is a
detailed one hour assessment of environmental, historical, physiologic and drug
related factors contributing to that individual's drug use. The specific areas of
evaluation include: drug and alcohol use, psychiatric problems, legal problems,
family/social issues, and employment/support concerns. Physical and psychological signs of drug use, and changes in medical and mental health status are
also assessed. The data accumulated by ASI information is useful for developing treatment plans that include lifestyle change goals. The ASI is also a useful
instrument for assessing progress at different follow-up points because it is
time-based and yields quantitative composite scores for each problem area.

B. DIAGNOSIS BY LABORATORY AND CLINICAL EXAMINATION.

Substance abuse disorders are erratically diagnosed on physical examination
because of caregivers' lack of interest or awareness of drug use symptoms or
because the symptoms may be subtle. The majority of drug addicted persons
have jobs and lead a "normal" life, without the stereotypic dysfunction of
severe injection- and non- injection users. Cocaine snorting can be suspected
by seeing a damaged nasal mucosa; hypodermic marks or "tracks" suggest
injection drug abuse, although the absence of visible marks does not rule this
out. The single most useful examination is of the eyes. Nystagmus is often
seen in abusers of sedatives/hypnotics or cannabis. Mydriasis is often seen in
persons under the influence of stimulants or hallucinogens or in withdrawal

from opiates. Miosis is a classic hallmark of opioid effect. Evidence of multiple minor (or past major) injuries can also be a clue to possible substance abuse.

Drugs may be detected in almost any fluid or tissue in the body. The most commonly samples for drug tests are urine, blood, saliva, hair, sweat and breath samples. (Wolff, 1999) Urine testing is the most available and useful testing format. There are test kits which may be used in offices and at home and require simple collection of a urine sample. Urine test limitations however are numerous. These limitations include the ability to detect only recent drug use as seen in Table 10-7. Furthermore, the samples can be adulterated, drug detection changed by the acidity of the urine and it is unable to quantitatively analyze drug use. Blood testing is available to many caregivers but is more expensive and more cumbersome than urine analysis. Blood testing is more accurate at quantitative detection of drugs in the user. Saliva may also be useful and correlates well with drug levels in the blood. However, to use the saliva assay, complex test standardization assays and calculations are needed to verify that saliva and blood drug levels are comparable. Hair analysis is a more recent technology which may be a future tool for drug detection. It has the advantage of detecting drug use over a 1 to 3 month period of time depending on a person's hair growth rate. The reasons that the test is not used widely are that cosmetic hair treatments, i.e. hair bleaching, may change drug level results as well as other factors such as hair pigmentation and hair growth rate. Sweat testing is another non- invasive test which is more useful for monitoring drug relapse during drug treatment. It is designed to continuously monitor a person's drug use over a period of time by placing a special absorbant pad on the skin. The pad continuously collects microscopic amounts of sweat produced by the body over time and is analyzed later for presence of drugs. Breath testing is commonly used to estimate the concentration of blood in a alcohol user and is a reliable reflection of blood alcohol. In research settings, marijuana may also be detected using breath testing. (Manolis, 1983)

TABLE 10-7: DURATION OF DRUG DETECTION

DRUG	DURATION OF DETECTION
Alcohol	48 hours
Amphetamines	12 hours
Barbiturates	10–30 days
Valium	4–5 days
Cocaine	24–72 hours
Heroin	24 hours
Marijuana	3–30 days
Methaqualone	4–24 days
Phencyclidine (PCP)	3–10 days
Methadone	3 days
Sex, Food, Gambling	N/A

Overall, The urine tests are the most reliable tests for clinicians to use. However, test results may be difficult to interpret for the inexperienced care giver because the results may be confounded by secondary drug exposures, chemical characteristics of the drugs to be detected, drug level variations in different body tissues and fluids and test method variations. Drug testing properly used, is a useful adjunct to clinical and behavioral drug use assessment and a useful but limited drug use screening tool. Drug tests should not be used as the sole criteria for detecting substance abuse but properly used is helpful during drug use, therapy and follow up.

VII. TREATMENT READINESS/HARM REDUCTION

Readiness for treatment involves a desire for drug abstinence. The motivating factors for treatment readiness in women are most commonly associated with difficulty in raising their children or in response to interventions by social services departments. (Brady, 1999) Unlike men, women are more likely to express their treatment readiness in non-substance use settings, especially in mental health care sites. (Lex, 1991) For that reason, drug use readiness should be evaluated in all health care settings for any drug.

For persons who are not ready for addiction treatment, caregivers can provide harm reduction interventions, aimed at reducing the damaging effects or harm resulting from risk behaviors and practices such as the sharing of syringes and other drug injection equipment and/or unsafe sex practices resulting from the use of drugs. (Des Jarlais. 1995) Comprehensive strategies that can effectively target high risk populations consist of a hierarchy of risk reduction approaches that, depending on the composition and needs of the populations being served, may include needle exchange programs or community outlets providing condoms. (Sumartojo, 1996) Sexually transmitted disease prevention programs, education programs, social and work skills building programs, health and drug use treatment health access programs should be provided through community resources. Programs targeting drug use populations and sub populations are all useful in preventing diseases such as HIV, STDs, Hepatitis and Tuberculosis and should eventually lead to encouraging the drug user to seek help in stopping drug use. (Needle, 1997)

A patient's history and behavior may be more predictive of treatment readiness and potential for engaging in care and adhering to therapeutic regimens than provider judgments based on gender, racial or ethnic background. There is a direct relationship between patient adherence with substance abuse treatment and the quality of the patient-physician relationship; however, the lack of physician training in the care of injection- and other drug abusers and the negative attitudes about drug use pose significant barriers. (Laine, 1998)

VIII. TREATMENT OF SUBSTANCE ABUSE

A. TREATMENT PROGRAMS

The most effective treatment programs are comprehensive and multi-dimensional and can be effectively delivered in outpatient, inpatient, and residential

TABLE 10-8: COMPONENTS OF DRUG USE TREATMENT

PERSONAL NEEDS	TREATMENT NEEDS
■ Family services	■ Behavioral therapy
■ Housing and transport	■ Clinical and case management
■ Financial services	■ Intake and processing
■ Legal services	■ Treatment plans
■ AIDS/HIV services	■ Pharmacotherapy
■ Educational services	■ Continuing care
■ Medical services	■ Substance use monitoring
■ Vocational services	■ Self-help/peer support groups
■ Child care services	

settings. In addition to behavioral (counseling, cognitive therapy or psychotherapy) and/or pharmacological therapies, the patient may need other medical services, family therapy, family planning, violence prevention, parenting instruction, vocational rehabilitation, and social and legal services (Table 10-8).

Treatment programs should also provide repeated assessments for HIV, AIDS, hepatitis B and C, tuberculosis, and other infectious diseases, as well as non-infectious diseases like diabetes and hypertension, and counseling and referral for relevant mental health treatment.

The most successful treatment occurs when the environmental, social, behavioral, medical and addiction problems are found early and treated over a long period of time (more than a year). Though it would be desirable to detect and treat drug use early after onset, when patterns of drug use are more easily treated or modified (Coates, 1998), most drug treatment modalities target more advanced stages of dependence, when medical or legal interventions are needed. Women's drug use problems tend to occur at an older age of onset and develop more rapidly than men. Women also learn of their HIV infection and other co-morbid conditions much later than men. The late diagnosis of drug use and other diseases often results in shorter survival. The confluence of factors which complicate health care for female drug users underscores the importance of early engagement and retention of women in care.

Effective treatment of drug dependence produces reductions in drug use by 40–60%, and significant decreases in criminal activity during and after treatment, and increases full-time employment. Establishment of accessible care in primary care settings offer countless opportunities to initiate prevention and treatment interventions targeted to adults, adolescents and other population groups at risk for drug abuse and associated problems. Easy health access for women is particularly important since their motivation for drug use is most often to cope with negative mood or anxiety. (McCaul, 1999) Providers should be accessible and should monitor individual triggers for stress and levels of stress sufficient to produce drug use complications or relapse.

B. PHARMACOLOGICAL INTERVENTIONS

Today even the most severe physical withdrawal symptoms can be managed with appropriate pharmacological treatments, reducing the emphasis on physiologic dependency as the focus of treatment of drug addiction. Drugs for alcoholics and sedative-hypnotic addicts are important for controlling and preventing serious medical consequences of drug withdrawal while other medications like methadone can help stabilize a patient and facilitate a return to productive functioning. Other important pharmacological interventions include the treatment of comorbid conditions common in drug using populations. Use of anti depressants in mentally ill drug users are as important as therapies directed to the effects of the drugs of abuse.

The pharmacological treatments for drug use are well known but not well understood by many health care givers. There are several classes of medications which maybe used to treat, modulate or prevent drug use.

OPIATE ADDICTION

Opiate agonist drugs like methadone, 1-alpha-acetyl-methadol (LAAM) and buprenorphine are used as opiate substitutes for opiate-dependent addicts. These 3 drugs, used to treat addiction, block the ability of the illicit drugs to attach to opiate receptors therefore decreasing a person's craving for the drug without causing euphoria. This is the most misunderstood medical approach to addiction treatment. Although methadone, LAAM and buprenorphine are addictive, they are successful helping the addict stop their negative and harmful drug use associated behaviors and begin to concentrate on developing the skills to discontinue drug use entirely. It is the drug craving which is associated with drug use relapse and criminal behavior and it is its prevention that makes substitution medications work successfully as part of a drug use treatment program. Methadone suppresses withdrawal for 24 hours (four to six times the duration of the effects of heroin) and decreases or eliminates drug craving; it is not sedating and can be dosed once a day. Furthermore, it is medically safe even when used continuously for 10 years or more.

LAAM is a newer synthetic opiate resembling methadone. LAAM can block the effects of heroin for up to 72 hours with minimal side effects when taken orally. Its long duration of action permits dosing just three times per week, thereby eliminating the need for daily dosing and take-home doses for weekends.

These substitution medications are not a cure for addiction but important adjunct to care. It has been shown that while an opiate user is on methadone, she is much less likely to commit a crime and more likely to succeed in completing a drug use program.. However, when combined with behavioral therapies or counseling and other supportive services, these pharmacologic approaches are highly effective for treating heroin addiction, particularly in those with long-term addiction.

Antagonist medications like Naloxone and naltrexone block the effects of morphine, heroin and other opiates. As antagonists, they are especially useful as antidotes. Naltrexone, with a duration of action ranging from 1 to 3 days depending on the dose, blocks the pleasurable effects of heroin and is useful in treating some highly motivated individuals, such as professionals who do not want to lose their jobs. It is also successful in preventing relapse by former opiate addicts released from prison on probation.

ALCOHOL ADDICTION

Antabuse (disulfiram) is used in alcohol abusers by causing negative side effects when the patient tries to consume alcohol. The drug interferes with alcohol metabolism, causing the production of acetaldehyde, a noxious chemical which causes severe flushing, nausea, and vomiting. The effectiveness of therapy is dependent on patient adherence to a daily medication dose. Acamprosate (Putzke, 1996) is a newer drug currently used in Europe which also decreases the desire to drink alcohol by affecting gamma aminobutyric acid and glutamate brain receptors causing decreased alcohol craving.

COCAINE ADDICTION

There are no effective medications for treating cocaine addiction but in some cases treating comorbid mental health problems may improve a cocaine or crack addict's chances of stopping cocaine use. Pharmacologic therapies have been specifically targeted at decreasing the dysphoric effects of cocaine withdrawal. Unfortunately, studies examining anti depressant medications targeting numerous neuron targets and multiple generations of antidepressant medications such as fluoxetine, sertraline, maprotilene, phenelizine, trazodone and lithium have not been proven successful in assisting a person in permanently stopping cocaine or crack use. (McCance, 1997) Dopaminergic agents such as bromocriptine, amantadine, haloperidol, bupropion and others have also not been proven to be effective. However, in a studies using desipramine, carbamazine and bupropion , the drugs' effects on the mental health of the affected patient were clinically helpful for a patient's successful drug cessation in drug use treatment program. (Kranzler, 1999)

DETOXIFICATION

Addiction detoxification is used to either prevent serious medical or psychologic complications of drug withdrawal from alcohol or sedative hypnotics or is used to ease the symptoms of withdrawal from the other drugs which do not have withdrawal syndromes with any significant morbidity or mortality (all other drugs of abuse). (Prater, 1999) In either case, detoxification protocols are not treatments for drug use but are part of a drug use treatment strategy.

Detoxification of alcoholics and sedative hypnotic users will prevent severe and sometimes fatal complications of drug withdrawal. For alcoholics, chlordiazepoxide (Librium) sedation is an important part of patient therapy. In most cases, the treatment should be done in hospital settings and if a woman is pregnant, Librium should not be used. Alternative medications especially for persons with severe liver disease are lorazepam (Ativan), oxazepam (Serax) and phenobarbital. In conjunction with the sedatives, thiamine to prevent Wernicke-Korsakoff syndrome and clonidine or beta blockers may be helpful to control noradrenergic symptoms in individuals. Withdrawal from sedative hypnotics is characterized by severe, chronic anxiety which may need one year of controlled, tapering doses of sedatives. Carbamazine (Tegretol) and valproic acid have also be used to control anxiety in sedative-hypnotic patients. (Eickelberg, 1998)

Detoxification for other types of drug abuse are useful for diminishing the symptoms of drug withdrawal but do not have any long lasting beneficial effect on the drug user. For example, clonidine (Gold, 1979) and Lofexidine (Bearn, 1996) are used in this way because they decrease the adrenergic symptoms of opiate withdrawals. These measures are short term and do not address the true underlying problems of drug use. Even though the effects of detoxification are only short term, it is one of the few drug use interventions which is reimbursable in most health systems. (O'Brien, 1997)

NEW PHARMACOLOGIC APPROACHES

The combined use of antagonist-agonist medications has been evaluated for drug treatment, with the biological objective of preventing activation of opiate receptors with two medications blocking the activation of opiate and other drug use- related cell receptors. Recent research has found that treating nicotine addicted persons with mecamylamine prevents smoking relapse. (Rose, 1994) This may be a useful adjunct therapy for persons in tobacco cessation programs.

Anticraving medications are used to prevent a person from wanting to take the drug. The biology and psychology of craving and its prevention is not well understood but it has been proven to be effective in treating addiction to nicotine. Buproprion (Wellbutrin), a anti depressant medication, has been successfully used to treat cigarette craving. (Ferry, 1999)

Vaccines against addictive drugs are intended to block the binding of illicit drugs to their cellular receptors. Though no vaccines are currently available for human use, there is evidence that a vaccine against cocaine may be possible to develop. Much future research is planned in this area.

C. COGNITIVE/BEHAVIORAL INTERVENTIONS

Behavioral and cognitive interventions are not as well known as the pharmacologic approaches, but are a vital part of drug addiction treatment and prevention. Cognitive-behavioral therapies are based on the assumption that learning processes play an important role in the development of drug use and dependence and therefore is important for efforts to reduce use and dependence. Behavioral methods are employed to identify high-risk relapse situations, create an aversion to drug use, develop self-monitoring of use behavior, and establish competing coping responses. By learning to recognize situations conducive to drug use, patients can develop individual coping strategies to avoid circumstances that place them at risk for relapse. Perhaps the single most important factor for short- and long-term relapse prevention is the learning and application of individual coping skills. Avoidance of other drug users and drug use environments are key tools for maintaining abstinence.

There are at least 11 research-validated therapies (Table 10-9) using a variety of behavioral, social, and incentive based systems to treat drug use. (Principles of Drug Addiction Treatment, 1999) The objectives of the different programs include removing patients from stressful environments to get care (short and long term residential homes); providing alternatives to pharmacologic treatment (outpatient drug free programs); and providing community specific interventions (community based programs for drug users and recently released criminals). There are several psychotherapy programs, based on the patient's willingness to recognize drug use as a problem and to stay off drugs, with or without incentives.

TABLE 10-9: NON-PHARMOLOGIC DRUG ADDICTION TREATMENTS
■ Supportive — Expressive Psychotherapy
■ Individualized Drug Counseling
■ Motivational Enhancement
■ Behavioral therapy for adolescents
■ Multi-systemic Therapy
■ Combined Behaviroal and Nicotine Replacement Therapy
■ Community Reinforcement Approach
■ Voucher-based Reinforcement Therapy (Methadone Maintenance)
■ Day Treatment with Abstinence Contingencies and Vouchers
■ Matrix Model
Source: Adapted from Principles of Drug Addiction, NIH publication No. 990-4180, 1999.

The 12 step self help drug use problems are important non medical, behavioral drug use intervention and prevention programs which are used by 10 to 15 million Americans in 500,000 or more groups. (Goldsmith, 1989) These programs emphasize fellowship and provide support for maintaining drug abstinence from alcohol, other drugs or addictive behaviors like overeating. These programs are not intended to replace medical and behavioral drug use treatments but are meant to add to their effectiveness. The largest 12 step groups are Alcoholics Anonymous, Narcotics Anonymous, for all drug users including alcoholics, Al Anon, to support family and friends of alcoholics and drug users and Overeaters Anonymous. (Chappel, 1999) In 1976, Women for Sobriety was established as a 12 step program to help women when it was recognized that Alcoholics Anonymous did not address adequately the specific needs of alcoholic women. (Katkulas, 1996)

IX. PREDICTORS OF DRUG TREATMENT RETENTION AND THE DURABILITY OF TREATMENT GAINS

Predictors of treatment retention include high motivation, legal pressure, receiving psychological counseling while in treatment, no prior violations of the law, and an absence of other psychological problems. (NIDA, 1998) Specific characteristics such as: IV drug use, age, race, socioeconomic status, level of education and occupation are actually poor predictors of adherence to drug treatment programs. The most accurate predictors of drug program retention and medication adherence are health care beliefs, health care access, familiarity of the treatment setting, availability of social support, perceived support from the clinical staff, and simplicity of the treatment.

Provider and patient recognition of the chronic nature of drug addiction and the need for treatment is essential to successful and durable addiction care. It has also been recently shown that lasting reductions in drug use are greater for patients who remain in treatment for 3 months or longer (Drug Abuse Treatment Outcome Study, 1997) and are treated with a combination of medical, behavioral and cognitive treatments.

Available treatment options continue to expand, providing therapeutic combinations that, when appropriately matched to patients' specific treatment problems, can increase the patient's chances of staying drug free. (McClellan, 1997) Treatments taking care of a patient's specific social and personal needs, increases an individual's chances of successfully completing the treatment program, and have improved post-treatment outcomes. Treatment for women that is woman-focused and targets the unique needs of women, including their children, interpersonal, cultural and contextual issues, and employment and housing considerations are also known to increase effectiveness. (Metsch, 1995) Participation in these programs provides women with children to develop stronger life and social skills to insure stable independent living practices. (Hughes, 1995)

X. RELAPSE

Drug addiction is a chronic disease characterized by periodic drug use relapses. Although many treated addicts relapse, it is wrong to conclude that treatment has failed or that the addict is hopeless. Like diabetes or hypertension, the individual with a substance abuse problem will need frequent and long-term follow-up to maintain a drug free state. Not surprisingly, simultaneous treatment for co-occurring medical, mental health and drug use problems offers significantly higher rates of success. The interventions that successfully address co-morbidity maximize linkages between school, community, clinic and other health service delivery systems. Woman- focused HIV prevention interventions include overcoming gender, cultural and power barriers that increase risks, such as learning negotiation strategies for gaining partner acceptance for condom use, dealing with parenting responsibilities and interpersonal conflicts. The relative success and durability of approaches that have multiple and mutually reinforcing outcomes depends on coordination among professional and material resources in a rational, systematic, and cost-effective manner.

Treatment should be judged by the same criteria used for other chronic disease interventions: Will it help lengthen the time between relapses, ensure the individual can function in society, and minimize long-term physical damage?

XI. SUBSTANCE ABUSE IN PREGNANCY

It is difficult to determine the true prevalence of substance abuse by pregnant women. Stigma, criminal laws regarding child endangerment and denial all contribute to the epidemiological conundrum. Cross sectional studies at large urban center, given the high risk populations served, may overestimate community drug use health problems. In 1990, a Centers for Disease Control and Prevention study in Rhode Island revealed a statewide prevalence of 6.5%. A cross-sectional study the same year in Pinelen County in Florida revealed that 15% of unselected women had evidence of recent drug use. (Chasnoff, 1990) Despite 1975 data demonstrating the improvement in women's health and pregnancy outcomes, punitive approaches to the problem of substance abuse during pregnancy risk threatening privacy rights. This treat further serves as a deterrent to health seeking behavior, and may further threaten the health of women and children.

The sequelae of substance use in pregnancy is beyond the scope of this chapter, however, a few specific drugs will be highlighted.

Alcohol use in pregnancy is associated with fetal alcohol syndrome (FAS). This congenital syndrome is characterized by 3 findings: growth retardation, facial abnormalities, and central nervous system dysfunctions. Skeletal abnormalities structural cardiac defects are also seen in the FAS, but it is the performance deficits that are most obvious. Decreased IQ, fine motor dysfunction and hyperactivity are all common findings. (ACOG, 1994)

Cocaine use in pregnancy poses maternal as well as fetal hazards. Some of these stem from the intense vasoconstriction associated with cocaine (malignant hypertension, cardiac arrthymias and cerebral infarction). Cocaine has been associated with premature rupture of membranes, pre-term labor and delivery, growth retardation, cognitive development delays and placental abruption. There are also documented cases of in-utero fetal cerebral infarction. (MacGregor, 1987)

Opiate addiction during pregnancy also poses serious risk to the mother, as well as the fetus. Newborn infants of narcotic addicted mothers are at risk for several complications, including the potentially fatal narcotic withdrawal syndrome. Withdrawal syndromes may appear 24 hours after birth, but may be delayed as long as 10 days after birth. (Levy, 1993)

X

XII. ANTIRETROVIRAL THERAPY IN SUBSTANCE ABUSERS

There is often a lack of compassion toward people who have contracted HIV through stigmatized behavior, such as drug use. (Hajela, 1998) Such sentiments are compounded by perceptions about adherence among drug users and the threat to public health associated with non-adherence leading to multi-drug resistant strains of HIV or other infectious diseases. (Gourevitch, 1996) These assumptions may lead to blanket denial of appropriate antiretroviral therapy to individuals with a past or current history of substance abuse.

Although active substance abuse (including alcohol, cocaine, or heroin) are associated with non-adherence, patient readiness for antiretroviral therapy must be carefully assessed on an individual basis, and those who have been treated for drug dependence may even be more adherent than the general population or other medical groups. However, drug users are less likely to receive care, with IDUs being among the least likely to receive antiretroviral therapies even when these treatments are available and free. (Shapiro, 1999) In fact, active IDUs may be up to 3 times less likely to receive HAART. (Carrieri, 1999)

XIII. CRIMINAL JUSTICE SETTINGS

Women are the fastest growing segment of the prison population, and their drug-related crimes are increasingly more serious. (FBI, 1997) Criminal justice reports show that substance use is implicated in the incarceration of 80% of men and women in state, federal and local prisons. Persons either violated drug laws, stole property to buy drugs, or have a history of substance abuse or addiction, or engaged in some combination of the above. (Maruschak, 1997) The more prior convictions an individual has, the more likely s(he) is to be drug dependent.

The most serious offense for 40% of women in state and federal prisons is the violation of drug laws. The enactment of mandatory sentencing policies has been associated with a ten-fold increase in the number of women incarcerated for drug crimes between 1986 and 1996.

Statistics show alcohol present in 31% of crimes, a combination of alcohol and other drugs in 16%, and other drugs alone 8.8%. A recent study confirms what many criminologists have long known: alcohol is associated with more violent crime than any illegal drug, including crack, cocaine, and heroin. Twenty-one percent of violent felons in state prisons committed their crimes while on alcohol alone. Only 3% were high on crack or cocaine alone, and only 1% were using heroin alone.

State officials have estimated that 70% to 85% of inmates need some level of substance abuse treatment; however only about 13% actually receive treatment. (Harlow, 1997) Those individuals with substance abuse histories also have an increased likelihood of a history of physical and sexual abuse. (National Minority AIDS Council, 1997) Criminal Justice reports attribute the overwhelming majority of AIDS cases among inmates to injection drug use, with an incidence of new AIDS cases among inmates 17 times higher than that in the general population.

Inmates who have received appropriate treatment in prison are 50 to 60 percent less likely to be arrested again during the first 18 months after release. For each offender who successfully completes treatment and returns to the community as a sober citizen with a job, it is estimated that reduced crime, arrest prosecution and incarceration costs, health care savings and potential earnings accrue in the first year after release. (Califano, 1998) One study found that total savings can exceed costs by a ratio of 12 to 1, another that for every $1 invested in drug treatment, there is a return of up to $7. Levels of criminal activity have also been shown to decline by two-thirds from the period before treatment to a comparable period after treatment.

REFERENCES

ACOG Technical Bulletin 1994 195: 825–831

Anderson MD, Hockman EM, and Smereck G. Effect of a nursing outreach intervention to drug users in Detroit, Michigan. *Journal of Drug Issues* 26(3):619–634, 1996.

Assessing Client Needs Using the ASI: Resource Manual, National Institutes of Health Publication No. 95-3620, 1995

Bearn J, Gossop M, Strang J. Randomised double-blind comparison of lofexidine and methadone in the in-patient treatment of opiate withdrawal. *Drug Alcohol Depend.* 1996 43(1–2):87–91.

Brady KT, Randall CL. Gender Differences in Substance Use Disorders. 1999 *Psychiatr Clin North Am* Jun;22(2):401–23.

Califano, J, Behind Bars: *Substance Abuse and America's Prison Population,* The National Center on Addiction and Substance Abuse (CASA) Columbia University, 1998.

Carneiro M, Fuller C, Doherty MC, Vlahov D. HIV Prevalence and Risk Behaviors among new initiates into injection drug use over the age of 40. *Drug Alcohol Dependence,* March 1999. 1:54(1):83–6.

Carrieri MP, Miotti JP, Vlahov D, Obadia Y, Reynaud-Maurupt C, Chesney M. Access to antiretroviral treatment among French HIV infected injection drug users: the influence of continued drug use. MANIF 2000 Study Group. *Journal of Epidemiology and Community Health,* January 1999 53(1):4–8.

Chappel JN, DuPont RL. Twelve-Step and Mutual Help Programs for Addictive Disorders. *Psychiatr Clinc North Am.* 1999 22(2): 425–446.

Chasnoff IJ, Handress HJ, Barrett ME. The prevalence of illicit-drug or alcohol use during pregnancy and discrepancies in mandatory reporting in Pinellas County, Florida. *N Engl J Med.* 1990 Apr 26;322(17):1202–6.

Coates TJ and Collins, C. Preventing HIV Infection: Altering behavior is a primary way to control the epidemic. *Scientific American* July 1998.

Des Jarlais, D. Harm reduction a framework for incorporating science into drug policy. *American Journal of Public Health.* January 1995, Vol. 85, No. 1.

Drug Abuse Treatment Outcome Study (DATOS), Special Issue of *Psychology of Addictive Behavior,* vol. 11, 1997.

Eickelberg SJ, Mayo-Smith MF. Management of Sedative Hypnotic intoxication and withdrawal. Graham AW, Schultz TK, eds. *Principles of Addiction Medicine,* 2d ed., Chevy Chase, Md.: American Society of Addiction Medicine. 1998:452–453.

Federal Bureau of Investigation *Uniform Crime Reports,* 1997.

Ferry, LH, Non-nicotine pharmacotherapy for smoking cessation. *Prim Care.* 1999 26(3):653–69.

Gold MS, Redmond DE, Kleber HD. Noradrenergic hyperactivity in opiate withdrawal supported by clonidine reversal of opiate withdrawal. *Am. J. Psychiatry* 1979 136(2): 100–102

Goldsmith MF. Proliferating "Self Help" Groups Offer Wide Range of Supports Seek Physician Rapport. *JAMA* 1989 261:2474–2475.

Gourevitch MN, Wasserman W, Panero MS, Selwyn PA. Successful adherence to observed prophylaxis and treatment of tuberculosis among drug users in a methadone maintenance program. *Journal of Addictive Diseases.* 1996 15:93–104.

Hajela R. The stigma facing drug abusers impedes treatment. *CMAJ.* 1998 May 19;158(10):1265–6.

Harlow CW. HIV in U.S. prisons and jails, special report (NCJ-143292). Washington, DC. Bureau of Justice Statistics, 1997.

Harvey D and Wyatt G. Study Tracks HIV-Positive Women's Psychosocial Issues: Women and Family Project.UCLA and Drew University medical centers.

Hughes, PH, Coletti, SD, Neri, RL et al. Retaining cocaine-abusing women in a therapeutic community: The effect of a child live-in program. *American Journal of Public Health* 1995 85(8):1149–1152.

Katkulas LA. Pathways to Self Help among Women for Sobriety. *Am J Drug Alcohol Abuse* 1996 22:259–280.

Kranzler HR, Amin H, Modesto-Lowe V Oncken C. Pharmoacologic Treatments for Drug and Alcohol Dependence *Psychiatr Clin North Am* 1999 22(2):401–23.

Krieger N, Zierler S. Reframing Women's Risk: Social Inequalities and HIV Infection. *Annu. Rev. Public Health* 1997 18:401–436.

Laine C., Markson LE, McKee LJ, Hauck WW, Fanning TR and Turner BJ. The relationship of clinic experience with advanced HIV and survival of women with AIDS. Clinic-focused features and prevention of pneumocystis carnii pneumonia. *Journal of General Internal Medicine,* January 1998 13(1):16–23.

Levy M, Spino M. Neonatal withdrawal syndrome: associated drugs and pharmacologic management. *Pharmacotherapy.* 1993 May–Jun;13(3):202–11. Review.

Lex BW. Gender differences and Substance Abuse. 1991 *Adv Sub Abuse* 4:225–96

MacGregor SN, Keith LG, Chasnoff IJ, Rosner MA, Chisum GM, Shaw P, Minogue JP. Cocaine use during pregnancy: adverse perinatal outcome. *Am J Obstet Gynecol.* 1987 Sep;157(3):686–90.

Manolis A, McBurney LJ, Bobbie BA. The Detection of delta 9- tetrahydro cannibinol in the Breath of Human Subjects. *Clinical Biochemistry* 1983 16:229–232.

Maruschak L. HIV in prisons and jails in 1995. Bureau of Justice Statistics Bulletin, 1997.

McCance EF. Overview of Potential Treatment Medications for Cocaine Dependence. 1997 National Institute on Drug Abuse Research Monogram. No. 175:36–72

McCaul, ME, Svikis, DS, and Feng T. Pregnancy and Addiction: Outcomes and Interventions. *Maryland Medical Journal* 1999 40:995–1001.

McClellan, AT, Grissom, GR, Zanis, et al. Problem-service "matching" in addiction treatment: A prospective study in four programs. *Arch Gen Psychiatry.* 1997 54(8):730–5.

Metsch LR, Rivers JE, Miller M, Bohs R, McCoy CB, Morrow CJ, Bandstra ES, Jackson V, Gissen M. Implementation of a family-centered treatment program for substance-abusing women and their children: barriers and resolutions. *J Psychoactive Drugs.* 1995 Jan–Mar;27(1):73–83.

National Household Survey on Drug Abuse (NHSDA) 1998, Summary of Findings, Department of Health and Human Services, Substance Abuse and Mental Health Administration, Office of Applied Studies.

National Minority AIDS Council, Special Report. *Women of Color and HIV/AIDS Policy, Trends in HIV AIDS Among Women of Color.* March 1997.

Needle RH, Coyle SL, Normand J, Lambert E. Cesari H. HIV Prevention with Drug-Using Populations Current Status and Future Prospects: Introduction and Overview. *Public Health Reports* 1997;113 (Supplement 1):4–18

NIDA Administrative Report. *Drug Abuse and Addiction Research.* November, 1998.

O'Brien, CP. A Range of Research Based Pharmacotherapies for Addiction. *Science* 1997 278:66–70

Prater CD, Miller KE, Zylstra RG. Outpatient Detoxification of the Addicted or Alcoholic Patient. 1999 *Am Fam Physician* ;60:1175–83.

Principles of Drug Addiction Treatment, A Research-Based Guide, 1999 NIH Publication No., 99–4180

Putzke, R, Spanagel, TR., Tolle W, Zieglansberger. The anti-craving drug acamprosate reduces c-fos expression in rats undergoing ethanol withdrawal. *Eur. J.Pharmacol* 1996 317(1) :39–48.

Rose, JE, Behm FM, Westman EC, Levin ED, Stein RM, Ripka GV. Mecamylamine combined with nicotine skin patch facilitates smoking cessation beyond nicotine patch treatment alone. *Clin Pharmacol Ther.* 1994 56(1):86–99.

SAMHSA FACT SHEET — August 1999. The 1998 National Household Survey on Drug Abuse, pages 1–5

Shapiro MF. *Disparities in AIDS Treatments among IDUs,* HCSUS HIV Cost and Services Utilization Study, RAND Corporation 1999.

Sly DF, Quadagno D, Harrison DF, Eberstein I, Rischman K. The association between substance use, condom use and sexual risk among low-income women. *Family Planning Perspectives* 1997;29:132–6.

Sumartojo E, Carey J, Doll L, Gayle H. Targeted and general population interventions for HIV prevention: Towards a comprehensive approach. *AIDS* 1996;11:1201–9.

Wolff K, Farrel M, Marsden J, Monteiro MG, Ali R, Welch S, Strang J. A Review of Biological Indicators of illicit Drug Use, Practical Considerations and Clinical Usefulness. *Addiction* 1999 Sept;94(9):1279–98.

Warner L, Kessler R, Hughes M, Anthony J, Nelson C. Prevalence and correlates of drug use and dependence in the U.S.: Results of the National Co Morbidity Study. *Archives of General Psychiatry.* 1995:52:219–29.

This *Guide* is a PRELIMINARY EDITION.

We need YOUR HELP to make the NEXT EDITION as useful as possible!

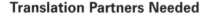

Please send your
comments
criticisms
corrections
suggested changes, and
other guidance
to one of the addresses below. Be sure to include in your letter/note an address (fax, e-mail, or postal) where you can be reached for follow-up.

Translation Partners Needed

Write to us if you can help us find partners to help us have this *Guide* translated into your native language. For instance, provide us with a contact who works with translation in your country's Ministry of Health, or tell us about a group at a medical school that translates medical texts.

Send Us Your Comments

E-mail: womencare@hrsa.gov

Fax to the attention of "Womencare": 301-443-0791 (USA)

Postal address: Womencare
Parklawn Building, Room 11A-33
5600 Fishers Lane
Rockville, Maryland 20857
USA

Note that this and subsequent editions of
A Guide to the Clinical Care of Women with HIV
will be available online.

Go to the HIV/AIDS Bureau Web site
and click on the publication *Women's Guide*:
http://www.hrsa.gov/hab

XI: ADOLESCENTS[1]
Donna Futterman, MD

Adolescence is a time of significant cognitive, emotional and physical development and is often characterized by exploration and experimentation. As adolescents explore intimacy, sexuality and develop autonomy, it is also a time of
heightened vulnerability, including risk for HIV infection. This chapter focuses
on young women as it reviews the epidemiology of HIV/AIDS in adolescents
and provides guidelines for HIV counseling and testing, medical and psychosocial care and strategies for linking HIV-infected and at-risk youth to care.

I. EPIDEMIOLOGY

Adolescents are at high risk for HIV infection. Worldwide, one out of every
two new cases of HIV — half of 5.8 million new infections during the past
year — occurred in youth ages 15–24. In developing countries, women are
becoming infected at significantly younger ages than men, with more young
women in their teens and early twenties becoming infected than women in
any other age groups. In the U.S., (CDC, 1999) more than half (53%) of
adolescents newly infected with HIV are female, and 25% of all new infections, or some 10,000 new cases per year, are estimated to occur in youth
ages 13 to 21. In addition, 19% of U.S. AIDS cases are reported in young
adults in their 20s. Given a ten-year period, on average, from initial infection
to clinical manifestations of AIDS, most of these young people were likely
infected during their teens.

Compared with adults, female adolescents represent a much higher proportion of HIV/AIDS cases. In 1998, adolescent girls ages 13–19 years
accounted for 51% of incident adolescent AIDS cases while female adults
comprised 23% of incident adult AIDS cases. Between 1988 and 1993, estimated HIV prevalence increased 36% among young women aged 18 to 22,
while dropping 27% among young men in the same age group. At highest risk
are African-American youth, who comprised 58% of incident teen cases in
1997, while representing only 15% of the U.S. adolescent population.

[1] This article was adapted with permission from a 2 part series that appeared in the *AIDS Clinical
Care* February and March 1999 issues: Chabon, B and Futterman, D. Adolescents and HIV. *AIDS
Clinical Care* 11(2):9–16; Hoffman ND, Futterman D, Myerson A. Treatment Issues for HIV+
Adolescents. *AIDS Clinical Care* 11(3):17–24.

XI

A. SEXUAL RISK

The majority of adolescent females (52%) with AIDS were infected through heterosexual intercourse. Moreover, an additional 15–20%, who are classified as having "no identified risk" because they were unable to identify their partners' risk, are also assumed to have been infected through heterosexual encounters. This is consistent with widespread lack of awareness of their potential risk for HIV infection among sexually active adolescents and adult women. For example, of adolescents known to be HIV positive, 75% of young women are unable to identify their partners' risk factors. (Futterman, 1993) A much smaller proportion of female youth (13% of 13–19 year olds and 27% of 20–24 year olds) were infected through injection drug use, compared with 44% of adult women with AIDS. Adolescents who were infected perinatally account for a small but growing number of adolescents with HIV/AIDS, and some are not diagnosed until adolescence.

Clinicians working with adolescents have noted additional risk factors for youth. A significant proportion of adolescents with HIV have experienced childhood sexual abuse; of adolescents screened at the Adolescent AIDS Program (AAP) at Montefiore Medical Center, 25–40% report having been sexually abused. (Futterman, 1993) Childhood sexual abuse has been associated with subsequent feelings of powerlessness in sexual situations and increased risk for unsafe sexual activity.

Moreover, 20% of sexually infected HIV+ youth seen in an Adolescent Program reported having a parent who is also HIV-infected. (Chabon, 1997) Further research is needed to assess parental influence on their children's HIV status. Nevertheless, children of parents with HIV generally live in the same high prevalence neighborhoods as their parents and may also face increased risk as a sequela of parental illness, or substance abuse. Clinicians should ascertain a history of sexual abuse or forced sex as well as parental HIV history when taking a history with adolescents.

B. SEXUALLY TRANSMITTED DISEASES AND PREGNANCY

Sexually active teens are also at risk for pregnancy and other STDs. According to the 1997 Youth Risk Behavior Survey, nearly half of all U.S. female high school students are sexually active (including 62% of 12 graders), and 9% report having been pregnant. (CDC, 1998) Approximately one million teens become pregnant each year, 74–85% of them unintentionally. Both STDs and pregnancy are markers for unsafe sexual activity and, in addition, STDs (both ulcerative and inflammatory) increase susceptibility for HIV infection. Two-thirds of the 12 million cases of STDs reported in the U.S. each year occur in youth under age 25, and 1 out of 4 are reported in adolescents. Younger teens, particularly females, are least likely to be considered at risk or to be screened, particularly if they are asymptomatic, which is the case with the majority of STDs in women. For example, chlamydia is asymptomatic in three-fourths of infected women, while approximately half of gonorrhea infections in women have no symptoms. This is especially salient since adolescent women have the highest age-specific incidence rates for both gonorrhea and chlamydia; 79% of reported cases of chlamydia occur in young women (46% in 15–19 year olds and 33% in 20–24 year olds).

C. HEIGHTENED VULNERABILITY FOR INFECTION

Adolescents are at risk for HIV and STDs as a result of the interplay between behavioral, biological and socioeconomic factors. (IOM, 1997)

BEHAVIORAL RISK

During adolescence, sexual activity is often initiated, risk taking and experimentation are normative, and many sexually active adolescents fail to take appropriate prevention precautions, despite basic knowledge of HIV transmission and prevention. During their last sexual encounter, nearly half of 9–12 grade girls did not use condoms, while one 1 in 7 (14%) reported having more than 3 sexual partners. Many teens follow a pattern of sexual "serial monogamy" and may not consider themselves as having multiple partners. Nearly 1 in 5 (19%) reported using alcohol and drugs which can impair judgment and increase potential for high risk behaviors. Most high school seniors have used alcohol, and 1 out of 3 students report having five or more drinks at least once during the past 30 days. More than 25% smoke marijuana, 16% report using inhalants and nearly 1 in 50 have injected illegal drugs. (CDC, 1998)

Specific populations of teens are at especially high risk, including adolescents who are lesbian, bisexual and transgender, homeless or runaway, injection drug users, mentally ill and youth who have been sexually or physically abused, incarcerated or in foster care. These youth experience increased vulnerability and multiple health and social problems as a result of abuse and neglect and lack of services and care. Lesbian and bisexual youth may view themselves at lower risk but those who are sexually active with gay male peers are at risk for infection due to higher HIV prevalence among gay males.

BIOLOGICAL RISK

Several biological factors also contribute to heightened risk in adolescent females. During puberty, the cervix undergoes physical maturation that makes the cellular lining less susceptible to infection as the single-layer columnar epithelium of the cervix is replaced with thicker multilayered squamous cells. Until this occurs, the cervix is much more vulnerable to STDs, particularly chlamydia and gonococcus, which have an affinity for columnar cells and have also been shown to facilitate STD transmission. At the same time, male to female transmission of STDs is much more efficient than female-to-male transmission given the larger surface area of the lower female genital tract and mechanics of sexual intercourse, which can result in mucosal trauma to women. In addition, STDs in women are more likely to remain asymptomatic and thus, unrecognized and untreated, for a longer period of time.

XI

Socioeconomic Risk

Adolescents are the most uninsured and underinsured group in the United States and are the least likely to receive office-based medical care or to use primary care services. Twenty-five percent of youth ages 15–29 have no health insurance and approximately 1 in 5 suffers from at least one serious health problem. Poverty, poor access to care and lack of education and prevention skills further increase vulnerability to HIV. Additional barriers include mistrust of the health care system, fear of inappropriate disclosure and providers' lack of understanding of adolescent rights to confidentiality and care without parental consent for sensitive health issues.

Moreover, many adolescents use emergency and walk-in facilities for acute care needs. As a result, they lack a primary care provider who can ensure ongoing care and address prevention and health promotion needs. Because adolescence is a time when help-seeking behaviors and attitudes about health and self-care are formed, the experiences adolescents have with health care providers are especially important. They form the basis for future provider-client interaction, communication patterns and relationships.

II. HIV CARE FOR ADOLESCENTS

Cornerstones of adolescent care include consent policies, confidentiality, accessibility, outreach and linkage to care and prevention. Even though youth prefer health care settings that are geared to their needs, most teens will not receive care in adolescent programs. Although most facilities are unable to offer the ideal "one stop shopping" for teens, quality care can be provided by identifying a staff member and/or provider team who wants to work with adolescents and by adapting adult and family programs to meet an adolescent's needs. This can be done by accommodating walk-ins since youth do not often plan ahead, addressing payment barriers and providing flexible appointments that will not conflict with school or work.

A. CONFIDENTIALITY AND LEGAL ISSUES

All states have laws that allow minors to consent to treatment without parental consent for specific health services including emergency care, STDs or reproductive health and substance abuse treatment services. In many, but not all states, this includes the right to consent for HIV counseling and testing. However, not all providers are aware of these rights or understand their significance for adolescents and these rights vary by state and the medical service provided. Most importantly, lack of confidentiality may cause adolescents to avoid or delay needed care. Even though parental consent may not be needed to provide an HIV test or HIV-related care, providers should carefully assess an adolescent's cognitive capacity to understand the implications of having HIV disease and should encourage them to involve a supportive adult in their care.

B. COUNSELING AND TESTING

Although most youth do not think they are at risk for HIV infection, they pre-fer providers to initiate discussion concerning HIV prevention and risk assess-ment. All adolescents should receive HIV prevention education, and sexually active adolescents should routinely receive HIV counseling and be offered HIV testing with informed consent. This enables providers to identify positive youth and provide ongoing medical care and support services, while relieving anxiety and reinforcing preventive behaviors for youth who are HIV negative. For adolescents who are not sexually active, counseling provides an opportu-nity to talk about sexual readiness, delaying intercourse and low risk ways to explore intimacy.

New testing options such as those that test for antibodies in oral fluids or urine are helpful with youth who are afraid of needles and allow providers to offer testing in a variety of settings including mobile vans, school-based clinics and drug treatment programs. Same-day testing may also be useful by eliminat-ing the need for a return visit for results, but will require careful planning for the delivery of HIV-positive results. Meeting adolescent needs for flexibility, accessibility and low or no fee HIV testing is important in overcoming primary barriers to accessing care and can serve as an entry point to care. Like other underserved populations, adolescents are generally diagnosed with HIV/AIDS late in the course of illness, relatively few receive care for HIV disease and most do not know they are infected. Thus, ensuring access to HIV counseling and testing is essential in enabling adolescents to receive ongoing treatment and care.

Although counseling and testing for adults has generally been based on one initial pre-test counseling session with providers, a "one-shot" approach to counseling is not effective with all at-risk youth. Two short counseling sessions prior to testing, using personalized risk reduction plans, can increase condom use and prevent new HIV and other STD infections. Pre- and post-test coun-seling provide an opportunity to promote preventive health behaviors and to assess substance use and family planning needs, while providing basic informa-tion on HIV, obtaining consent and conducting a comprehensive risk assess-ment. (Table 11-1, on the following page) More extensive guidelines are also available for adolescent HIV counseling and testing in all health settings. (Chabon, 1998) Because adolescents may have misconceptions about aspects of HIV transmission and prevention, providers should assess their capacity to understand basic concepts of HIV disease and viral transmission. Effective HIV counseling for adolescents should be culturally sensitive and tailored to an adolescent's developmental needs. In addition, providers should take special precautions to ensure confidentiality in institutional settings such as foster care, residential treatment or detention.

Knowledge of appropriate condom use and widespread availability of condoms are especially important in promoting risk reduction behaviors among youth. All facilities that provide health care for adolescents should make condoms available and providers should demonstrate condom use with

XI

TABLE 11-1: TEEN AIDER (ASSESS, INQUIRE, DISCUSS, EDUCATE, READINESS) INTERVIEW FOR HIV COUNSELING, TESTING AND RISK REDUCTION

ASSESS AND INQUIRE

Create a confidential atmosphere

- Assure youth about confidentiality of visit and ability to consent for testing per local laws
- Assure youth that testing is their choice
- Acknowledge that it can be embarrassing to discuss sexual behaviors
- Help youth to identify supportive adult who is aware that youth is being tested

HIV/AIDS Knowledge

- Allow adolescent to verbalize understanding of HIV, clarify misconceptions and fill in gaps in knowledge
- Assess feelings about testing and previous HIV testing experiences
- Inquire if youth knows anyone with HIV/AIDS (e.g., sexual partner, family member)

Sexual Risk Assessment

- Assess sexual behaviors without making assumptions about sexual orientation, not all youth are heterosexual and not all youth who have engaged in same sex behavior self-identify as lesbian or gay
- Assess number of partners, age differential and partner's known risks
- Assess frequency of substance use in the context of sexual behavior
- Assess consistency of condom use and obstacles to use such as unassertiveness, desire to become pregnant, fear of violence and religiosity
- Assess for history of sexual abuse or rape

Substance Use and Other Risk Assessment

- Assess level of drug and alcohol use and reasons and context in which use occurs
- Review risk of impaired judgement that may result leading to unsafe sex
- Assess potential need for drug treatment
- Assess violence and substance use in home and community

Table continues . . .

anatomical models. Adolescents have difficulty using condoms during intercourse for several reasons, including: 1) lack of knowledge about effective use; 2) lack of communication and social skills; 3) lack of availability of condoms at the time of sexual activity; and 4) impulsive behavior exacerbated by drug or alcohol use. Gender and power imbalances in relationships make condom use especially difficult for adolescent women whose partners are older and who are just beginning to develop communication and negotiation skills. Helping youth identify their personal values may increase self-esteem and help them resist pressures to engage in sexual risk behaviors. (Table 11-2)

C. PREVENTION

Promoting risk reduction among adolescents is especially challenging since developmental characteristics encourage concrete, short term thinking and experimentation and increased reliance on peers. Thus, successful primary and secondary programs for adolescents are those that provide interventions to

---

TABLE 11-1: TEEN AIDER (ASSESS, INQUIRE, DISCUSS, EDUCATE, READINESS) INTERVIEW FOR HIV COUNSELING, TESTING AND RISK REDUCTION (continued)

DISCUSS AND EDUCATE

- Discuss sexual activities that don't involve exchange of body fluids (outercourse)
- Demonstrate proper male condom, female condom and dental dam use on anatomical model and provide opportunity for practice
- Rehearse effective ways to communicate risk reduction with sexual partner (s)
- Discuss harm reduction strategies for youth using drugs
- Develop a personalized risk reduction plan
- Discuss postponing sex for youth who are not sexually active
- Determine referral needs (e.g., Medical, Psychosocial, School /Vocational, Substance Abuse, Reproductive Health, Legal, Housing, Psychiatric)

READINESS FOR HIV TESTING AND REFERRAL

- Adolescent should be informed about both anonymous and confidential testing
- Provide education about Partner Notification programs and other options for disclosure to partners
- Assess understanding of meaning of a positive and negative test result
- Assess understanding of benefits of early intervention
- Determine with youth if testing should occur at this time and obtain informed consent
- Strategies for coping (how to relieve stress and anxiety during the testing process)
- Arrange follow-up appointment and method for confidentially contacting youth, if needed

Source: Reprinted with permission from: Chabon, B and Futterman, D. Adolescents and HIV. *AIDS Clinical Care.* Vol. 11:2, pp. 9–16, February 1999.

TABLE 11-2: FACTORS ASSOCIATED WITH CONDOM USE

ENCOURAGES USE	DISCOURAGES USE
■ Knowledge about condoms	■ Drug/alcohol use
■ Belief in effectiveness	■ Relationship power imbalances
■ Discussion with health care provider	■ Peer pressure may discourage use
■ Self-esteem/self-efficacy	■ Lack of effective sex education
■ Communication/negotiation skills	■ Lack of media/cultural support of
■ Availability/accessibility	condom use

IX

increase self-esteem and self efficacy, build social skills and provide basic information geared to the adolescent's developmental level, using a peer support model. For high risk youth, the AIDS Risk Reduction Model (Catania, 1990) has been widely used to foster primary and secondary prevention, based on the premise that behavior must first be acknowledged as risky before youth will initiate change.

School-based programs that provide comprehensive health education in conjunction with school health clinics offer optimal opportunities to reinforce positive health behaviors and ensure routine screening for a range of health and mental health concerns. But they are especially important in reducing risk and identifying sexually active youth who are at risk for STDs and pregnancy. A comprehensive review of school-based programs designed to reduce risky behavior in teens found that adolescents who received AIDS education were less likely to engage in sexual activity and more likely to practice safer sex than peers who lacked AIDS education in school. (Kirby, 1998) In particular, successful programs include skills building, reinforcement of values and norms to prevent unprotected sex that are based on age and experience levels, and discussion of social influence and pressure. School clinics also offer an important venue for access to condoms and appropriate instruction on condom use. Although not widely available, school clinics provide an important site for HIV counseling and testing for in-school youth, given new rapid testing options. Ultimately, successful prevention must also involve society and the media – until youth see condom use and safer sex discussions incorporated into sex scenes in music videos and movies, they will not believe that this is a social norm.

D. LINKING YOUTH TO CARE

Linking at risk youth to care is essential in meeting their needs for risk reduction education and appropriate ongoing HIV medical and psychosocial care. Most HIV-infected youth do not know they are infected, and many providers are not aware of available community service agencies that can help address their multiple mental health and social service needs. Community outreach is a primary component in ensuring access to care for youth with HIV disease. Peer-based outreach services are frequently employed, as adolescents are more likely to listen to their peers. Unlike adult women who have more opportunities to obtain HIV testing and to access care related to their reproductive health needs, adolescents who are not pregnant require proactive outreach efforts to promote HIV testing and engage them in care. This includes citywide campaigns to encourage testing and to make it more widely available, with direct linkages to adolescent health care facilities. One such initiative — a social marketing campaign spanning the continuum from HIV prevention through testing to care — was developed by the Adolescent AIDS Program at Montefiore Medical Center in New York City in1996. "HIV. Live with it. Get Tested" was designed with marketing experts, health providers and most importantly youth themselves, to combine media advertisements such as posters, radio and TV ads with community outreach in settings where at-risk youth access information and are likely to congregate. Using teen language for sexual activity (e.g., "Knockin' Boots" or "Hittin' the Skins") to promote testing and care services through a coalition of adolescent HIV programs and community based youth agencies, the initiative is intended to help adolescents link having sex with HIV risk and the importance of HIV testing. Now in its third year, the initiative focuses annual activity around a "Get Tested! Week" launched with a youth-led Town Hall meeting and peer outreach. The campaign's success has also resulted in a national initiative that during 1999 took place in 5 additional cities — Baltimore, Los Angeles, Miami, Philadelphia and Washington, D.C. — within the NIH- and HRSA sponsored Adolescent Medicine HIV/AIDS Research Network (AMHARN) Network. In each city, new coalitions were successfully built, increased numbers of youth were tested, and HIV-positive youth were identified and linked to care. (Futterman, 2000)

E. HIV CLINICAL AND PSYCHOSOCIAL CARE

Although the natural history of HIV infection in adolescence is still being defined, the course of disease appears to follow that of adults. A national prospective study with sites in 13 cities — AMHARN — has been funded by the National Institutes of Health and the Health Resources and Services Administration to identify the course of disease in adolescents, including its spectrum, manifestations, effects of puberty, and developmental and psychosocial interactions. (Rogers, 1998) Initial findings suggest that adolescents may have greater potential for immune reconstitution than adults as a result of residual thymic function, which underscores the need for aggressive outreach efforts and access to early effective treatment and has also identified a high prevalence of sexually transmitted disease in this population.

Physical Exam, Laboratory Tests and Immunizations

Physical examinations for adolescents should follow guidelines for adults, however, providers should use Tanner staging of puberty (characterizing breasts, genitalia and pubic hair) to interpret blood values and prescribe medications. (Schneider, 1998) Because sexually active adolescents are at very high risk for STDs, providers should routinely screen with cervical cytology, and for chlamydia, gonorrhea, syphilis, and hepatitis B and C, as well as follow Tuberculosis screening guidelines for adults with HIV infection. Pregnancy testing should be performed when indicated by history or exam findings, but should always be considered with missed menses, abnormal bleeding or development of pelvic pain. Adolescents require more immunizations than adults. (Table 11-3) Since immunizations may briefly boost viral load, they should be

XI

TABLE 11-3: Immunizations for Adolescents
▪ Measles, Mumps and Rubella (MMR) booster
▪ Diphtheria-Tetanus toxoid (dT) booster
▪ Hepatitis B Vaccine (3 in series)
▪ Hepatitis A Vaccine (2 in series) (not routine; recommended for males who have sex with males)
▪ Influenza (yearly)
▪ Pneumococcal vaccine
▪ HIB (optional)
▪ Varicella zoster vaccine for contacts (not currently approved for HIV+ persons)
Source: Reprinted with permission from: Hoffman ND, Futterman D, Myerson A. Treatment Issues for HIV+ Adolescents. *AIDS Clinical Care.* Massachusetts Medical Society. Vol. 11:3, 17–24, March 1999.

scheduled on the same day or after viral load measurements. At present, CD4 counts and viral load measurements are interpreted as for adults and used to guide treatment.

HIV TREATMENT

Information from clinical trials is limited since few adolescents have participated in existing clinical trials. Although adolescent trials are under development, HIV and opportunistic infection treatment and prophylaxis recommendations for post-pubertal adolescents currently follow clinical guidelines for adults. Because pubertal changes may affect pharmacokinetics, dosage is based on Tanner staging, rather than age. For example, pediatric dosing should be used for adolescents who have entered/are in early puberty (Tanner stage I/II), while dosing for adolescents in mid-puberty (Tanner III/IV) should be based on whether or not they have completed the growth spurt. Adolescents who have completed puberty, (Tanner V) should receive adult dosages.

Treatment adherence, which is challenging for adults, can be especially challenging for adolescents who struggle with a range of developmental tasks that require them to balance dependence with increasing autonomy. As with any successful work with adolescents, the first step in promoting adherence is establishing a solid therapeutic alliance. Providers must develop a systematic approach that facilitates adherence by addressing four areas of interaction, including building trust, assessing and facilitating readiness, helping teens initiate and practice the new treatment regimen and providing ongoing support for adherence. (Table 11-4) This approach addresses barriers to maintaining a complex medication schedule for adolescents, such as lack of privacy in school, home or residential settings, the need to develop a reminder system, and the incongruity of having a serious illness while exhibiting few visible indicators of disease. For example, the most common reasons for missing medication by youth in a Los Angeles adolescent HIV/AIDS program include: forgetfulness, side effects, the inconvenience of having to take so many pills, and the fact that taking the medication is a continual reminder of being HIV infected. (Belzer, 1998)

AMHARN has designed a multi-level adherence initiative: Project TREAT (Treatment Regimens Enhancing Adherence in Teens) to address medication adherence in adolescents. A monograph describing the model has been developed for providers and is available from HRSA. (Schietinger, 1999) Based on Prochaska and DiClemente's Transtheoretical Model of Change, Project TREAT acknowledges the uniqueness of each adolescent's readiness for treatment. The model has developed specific interventions and materials (video and audio tapes and booklets) for each stage of readiness to facilitate successful adherence. (The Stages of Change are: Precontemplation, Contemplation, Preparation, Action, Maintenance and Relapse.) Practice regimens with vitamins help youth rehearse their medication regimen, while enabling them to problem-solve potential barriers without risking under-dosing. Medications

Table 11-4: Adherence: Using your EARS

Engage

- Establish therapeutic alliance and build trust; goal is active participation by adolescent in all aspects of treatment
- Address immediate needs (health, housing, insurance, family, and partners)
- Educate about HIV infection: transmission, disease course and benefits of medications

Assess

- Stage HIV infection
- Assess mental health and cognitive abilities
- Assess physical ability to take medicines
- Assess support systems and disclosure issues: family and friends
- Assess readiness to begin medications

Readiness

- Decide with adolescent on regimen that integrates clinical needs with lifestyle — show different pills/combinationss
- Solidify support systems: family and/or treatment buddy
- Pratice chosen regimen with surrogate vitamins; distribute medications into a weekly medication planner, program one-day pill timer with the adolescent
- Address adherence barriers discovered in practice run

Support

- Provide ongoing support with frequent clinic visits and phone contact
- Acknowledge and address side effects
- Develop strategies to ensure tolerability and regularity
- Facilitate interactions with other youth taking medications

Source: Reprinted with permission from: Hoffman ND, Futterman D, Myerson A. Treatment Issues for HIV+ Adolescents. *AIDS Clinical Care.* Vol. 11:3, 17–24, March 1999.

must be integrated into the adolescent's daily routine. Ideally, adolescents should be prescribed a daily or twice-daily medication regimen. Many providers also initiate treatment without using protease inhibitors (PI); these are incorporated into later regimens after the adolescent has demonstrated effective adherence, to avoid risking potential cross-resistance to PIs.

Psychosocial Issues

The Adolescent AIDS Program has identified five key issues that adolescents with HIV/AIDS must address in coping with their changing health status. These include: 1) receiving an HIV diagnosis; 2) disclosing an HIV status to parents, partners and others; 2) coping with HIV disease; 4) becoming symptomatic; and 5) preparing for death. (Kunins, 1993)

1. **Receiving an HIV Diagnosis:** Providers should instill a sense of hope and encouragement when giving adolescents an HIV diagnosis. Asymptomatic youth must learn to balance healthy denial and preoccupation with HIV infection. Concrete thinking makes it difficult for some youth to integrate the concept of disease latency and

asymptomatic infection. Support is essential in helping youth integrate
this life changing information. Individual and peer group interventions
with psychologists and social workers can help facilitate adjustment.
Psychotropic medication may be needed to manage pre-existing psychiatric problems and for anxiety and depression that may accompany
the diagnosis.

2. **Disclosure of HIV Status:** After learning their diagnosis, adolescents
must decide who to inform and when to disclose their HIV status.
Telling their parents is difficult for many adolescents who fear losing
their love and support. Fear of rejection and loss of confidentiality is
also a concern in disclosing to sexual partners. Providers should offer
to help with disclosure and offer guidance in determining when it is
safe and appropriate for the youth to disclose her HIV status. Role
playing and working through scenarios ahead of time can help the
adolescent manage potential fears and concerns.

3. **Coping with HIV:** Adolescents also need guidance in learning how
to interpret changes in their viral load and CD4 counts. Since fluctua-
tion in results may cause some youth to panic, providers can help by
explaining that variation is common and significant changes will not
prevent them from leading satisfying and productive lives.

4. **Becoming Symptomatic:** The appearance of HIV-related symptoms
can be especially disturbing for adolescents who may have only super-
ficially acknowledged their HIV status. For some youth, becoming
symptomatic may encourage them to fight HIV and may enhance
treatment adherence and self-care. Others, however, may feel overwhelmed and may lose their motivation to live. When symptoms
occur, providers should explore their meaning, correct misconceptions
about their significance and ensure that adequate services and support
are available.

5. **Preparing for Death:** Many adolescents have limited experience with
death and have naive perceptions about what to expect. Introducing
the topic by talking about living wills and health care proxies before
HIV becomes too advanced is a practical way to help youth begin to
deal with issues related to death. When clinically appropriate,
providers can help adolescents explore their feelings about dying by
discussing options for dying in the hospital or at home, talking about
funeral or memorial services, and exploring child custody or permanency planning with adolescent parents.

Mental Illness and Substance Use

Mental illness and substance abuse are important co-morbidities for HIV-positive adolescents. Accurate screening and diagnosis are essential in helping adolescents cope with their disease and successfully maintain their treatment
regimen. Case studies of adolescents and young adults with HIV indicate a

high prevalence of depression, bipolar disorder and anxiety, often pre-dating their HIV diagnosis. Similarly, many adolescents with HIV report alcohol and drug abuse. Of adolescents in the REACH study, 14% percent of females and more than 25% of males report weekly use of alcohol during the past three months. During the same period, 7% of females and 20% of males reported using hard drugs. (Rogers, 1998) In addition, as already noted, a high proportion of HIV+ male and female youth report childhood sexual abuse. (See Chapter I on Epidemiology and Natural History) which has many psychological and behavioral sequelae, including depression, post traumatic stress disorder, substance abuse, suicidality and risk for HIV infection.

III. SUMMARY

The high risk of adolescent females for HIV infection makes the development of realistic prevention programs a vital necessity. This includes wider availability of prevention skills building and the routine offering of HIV counseling and testing to sexually active teens in all programs that provide adolescent care. While most youth will not receive services in adolescent programs, services can be readily adapted to provide a "youth-centered" approach, by such basic accommodations as offering flexible hours and low or no payment for services and care as well as providers who are knowledgeable about adolescents. Relevant clinical trials should be made available to adolescents, and there should be wide dissemination of information to health care providers about providing adolescent-related HIV care, such as use of Tanner staging for assessing test results and determining appropriate dosage. Youth at high risk for HIV should be identified and engaged in primary care as soon as possible and outreach programs are an important component for programs that seek to link HIV-positive youth to care. Adolescents with HIV need intensive individual and group support to maintain health and reduce transmission to others. Health care providers in all settings that serve adolescents need to assist in making services visible, flexible, affordable, confidential, culturally appropriate and available for all adolescents.

XI

REFERENCES

Belzer M, Slonimsky G, Tucker D. Antiretroviral adherence issues among HIV+ youth. Presented at the Annual Meeting of the Society for Adolescent Medicine 1998, *J Adol Health* 22:160, 1998.

Catania JA, Kegeles SM, Coates TJ. Toward an understanding of risk behavior: An AIDS risk reduction model. *Health Education Quarterly* 17: 53–72, 1990.

Centers for Disease Control and Prevention. *HIV/AIDS Surveillance Report* 11 (No. 1): 1–42, 1999.

Centers for Disease Control and Prevention. Youth risk behavior surveillance — United States 1997. *MMWR* 47(SS-3), 1998.

Chabon B, Futterman D, Jones C. Adolescent HIV counseling and testing protocol. In Ryan, C. and Futterman, D. *Lesbian and Gay Youth: Care and Counseling.* New York: Columbia University Press, 1998, pp. 152–161.

Chabon B, Hoffman N, Hershey B, Futterman D. High prevalence of HIV among parents of HIV+ youth. Presented at the Annual Research Meeting of the Society for Adolescent Medicine, San Francisco, CA, March 1997.

Futterman D, Rudy B, Peralta L, et al. Social Marketing to Promote HIV Counseling and Testing to Youth: A Six City Initiative. Presented at the Annual Meeting of the Society for Adolescent Medicine, 2000, Washington, DC.

Futterman D, Hein K, Reuben N, et al. Human immunodeficiency virus-infected adolescents: The first 50 patients in a New York City program. *Pediatrics* 91:730–35, 1993.

Institute of Medicine. *The Hidden Epidemic: Confronting Sexually Transmitted Diseases.* Washington, DC: National Academy Press, 1997.

Kirby D, Short L, Collins et al: School based programs to reduce sexual risk behaviors: a review of effectiveness. *Public Health Reports* 109:339–360, 1994.

Kunins H, Hein K, Futterman D. et al. A Guide to Adolescent HIV/AIDS Program Development. *J Adolesc Health*, Special Suppl., 1–168, July 1993.

Rogers AS, Futterman DC, Moscicki AB, et al. The REACH project of the Adolescent Medicine HIV/AIDS Research Network: Design, methods, and selected characteristics of participants. *J Adol Health* 22:300–311, 1998.

Ryan C and Futterman D. *Lesbian and Gay Youth: Care and Counseling.* Columbia University Press, New York, 1998.

Schietinger H, Sawyer M, Futterman D, et al. *Helping Adolescents with HIV adhere to HAART.* TREAT Monograph: Rockville, MD: HRSA/HAB, 1999.

Schneider M. Physical Examination. In Friedman S. et al. *Comprehensive Adolescent Health Care.* St. Louis: Mosby-Year Book, 1998.

XII: PALLIATIVE AND END-OF-LIFE CARE
Carla Alexander, MD

I. INTRODUCTION

This chapter is meant to provide ideas for coping with symptoms which impact quality of life throughout HIV disease and to prepare for issues faced near the end of life. Aggressive palliative care anticipates, prevents, and relieves suffering on emotional and spiritual levels as well as the physical. Because of gaps in traditional medical education related to end-of-life issues (Weissman, 1998; Field, 1997), information in this chapter focuses on care near the end of life. (Hanson, 1997) The newer definitions of palliative care used in women with chronic illness does not only refer to "end-of-life" care. As a comparatively new field, palliative medicine, which has been largely an oral tradition continues to be in need of research and literature. The challenge to readers is to share successes and failures in order to expand the literature especially for those living in countries with fewer resources.

Hospice, an early form of palliative care, developed in London during the late 1960's when Dame Cicely Saunders proposed using an *inter*disciplinary team to focus on the "relief of suffering" rather than simply on long-term survival for persons living with advanced cancer. This care was ideally delivered *in the home* and focused on *relieving physical symptoms* which might impede successful psychosocial and spiritual life closure prior to death. (Saunders, 1989) In 1980, the World Health Organization defined palliative care as:

> "The active total care of patients whose disease is not responsive to curative treatment. [It] . . .affirms life and regards dying as a normal process, . . . neither hastens nor postpones death, . . . integrates the psychological and the spiritual aspects of care, . . . offers a support system to help patients live as actively as possible until death, . . . and offers a support system to help the family cope during the patient's illness and in their own bereavement." (Doyle, 1998)

There are many differences between patients with cancer, who eventually learn that their disease is no longer being contained by treatment and persons with HIV/AIDS who suffer from a more episodic illness with very difficult to predict end-points. In HIV disease palliative care is best woven into the general fabric of care from the time of diagnosis. A small group of HIV providers, invited by the Health Resources and Services Administration

XII

(HRSA) of the Department of Health and Human Services which oversees the Ryan White CARE Act, have attempted to define what this care should be in HIV disease:

"... that care which is patient and family-centered and optimizes quality of life by active anticipation, prevention, and treatment of suffering through respectful and trusting relationships formed with an interdisciplinary team throughout the continuum of illness: addressing physical, intellectual, emotional, social, and spiritual needs and facilitating patient autonomy, access to information, and choice." (HRSA staff, 1999)

As HIV disease becomes a chronic rather than terminal illness, management must be accomplished in the overall context of life. (Breitbart, 1996) Good supportive care means "to be safe and not to be hurt, to be given refuge or sanctuary, to be comforted and accepted, to belong, and to give and receive love." (Standards Comm, N.H.O., 1997) Adjusting goals may be challenging for health care workers who use only a "cheerleading" approach to support. Involving the patient and her support system in decision-making affords her a sense of control over her disease which ultimately extends to the end-of-life. (Fogel, 1993; Newsham, 1998; Sanei, 1998) All staff must learn to value the impact of symptoms on the woman's daily life as much as they do viral load and the CD4 cell count.

HIV disease has been associated with shame and a negative stigma (Abercrombie, 1996; Chung, 1992; Sowell, 1999) resulting in the isolation of many who are infected but especially of women. Those who suffer from the disease are frequently without social support or the financial means, including health insurance, necessary for coping with their disease.(Cohen, 1998; Chung, 1992; Nannis, 1997; Pergami, 1993; Sowell, 1997.) As the traditional care-giver, a woman may not have anyone else to provide her own care. She may have also suffered many personal losses leaving her emotionally drained and unable to provide care for someone else. (Sarna, 1999) She must cope with knowing that she will one day be dying herself and that she must make provisions for her children and other dependents who will be left behind.

II. QUALITY OF LIFE

The overarching goal of palliative care is to relieve or reduce suffering and promote quality of life. With HIV disease, the unpredictable and episodic course of illness makes it difficult to estimate an individual's prognosis. Use of combination therapy has decreased mortality rates by 23–90% depending on the population examined. (Pezzotti, 1999 ; Sendi, 1999) Quality of life (QoL) alone has become an important outcome measure and providers now need to pay more attention to pain, fatigue, anorexia and other symptoms which can be present even when the disease markers are improving. (Barrosa,1999; Van

Servellan, 1998) Each provider must become adept at anticipating symptoms related to therapies and offering the woman a mechanism for preventing or controlling these side effects.

In spite of prolonged survival, physical and spiritual distress; psychological pain; and grief remain a part of the illness. (O'Neill, 1997) There does come a point in illness when quality of life becomes more important than *quantity* of life. (Harris, 1985) The transition away from aggressive, curative care can be as difficult for members of the health care team as it is for patients and families. (Finucane, 1999)

Several studies have specifically considered QoL in women with HIV disease. (Sewell, 1997; Farsides, 1995; Rosenfeld, 1996) Sewell found that social, and particularly psychological, symptoms have a major impact. Quality of life has been affected by "HIV treatment, physical symptoms, psychological well-being and [change in] role functioning." (Hays, 1992) Sarna found that problems arise in four domains: physical, psychological, social, and sexual. Schag, however, noted that financial concerns were the number one disrupter.. This is followed by "worry about family," "distress at losing others," and "worry about progression of disease."

Routinely measuring QoL throughout the disease (1) alerts health care providers to changes and stresses which may not always be obvious during a busy clinic visit. Completing questionnaires every 3–4 months or at the time of a clinical change may help the woman communicate with her providers. These answers can assist providers by monitoring problems and targeting interventions more specifically. (Sarna, 1999) Quality of life scales have traditionally reflected functional status, for example, the Karnofsky Performance Status assigns a global ranking which reflects activity during any given day. The Medical Outcomes Study (Wu, 1997) is frequently used in the HIV population and has been shortened for easier use in the clinical setting. However, many of these scales, because they are function based, may not be as useful as the woman becomes more debilitated and approaches end of life. (Pratheep-awanit, 1999)

In advanced disease one's focus is often directed to psychosocial and spiritual concerns which can be addressed even while bed-ridden. When we are healthy, not being able to leave the bed might seem unbearable. Approaching death, priorities shift; relationships and momentary pleasures become more important. In fact, it is not unusual for people to feel that their quality of life is better during this period because they are able to avoid mundane tasks and to focus on personal goals. The Missoula-Vitas Quality of Life Instrument (available through Vitas Healthcare Corporation, phone 305-350-6033) has recently been developed specifically for those with deteriorating functionality. With this form the patient notes the importance of each domain and scoring reflects how the change in each characteristic, such as symptom control and sense of well-being, affects the woman.. It is always useful simply to ask the woman how she would rank her own quality of life and what things are most important to her at the present time.

III. SYMPTOMS THROUGHOUT DISEASE

Three symptom surveys of outpatients with HIV/AIDS (Ferris, 1995; Sims, 1992; Carr, 1994) are summarized in Table 12-1. As disease advances it may not be possible to eliminate the cause of a symptom but the woman and her family should be educated about symptom management, and thus be empowered to master these symptoms.

TABLE 12-1: COMMON SYMPTOMS IN HIV DISEASE

SYMPTOM	# 1	# 2	#3
Anorexia/Weight Loss	91%	31%	61%
Fatigue/Weakness	77%	50%	
Pain	63%	52%	total 84%
Shortness of Breath	48%	22% (respiratory problem)	11% (dyspnoea)
Nausea/GI upset	35%	28%	21%
Cough	34%	27%	19%
Anxiety /Depression	32%	24% (Depression) 40% (Anxiety)	20% (Depression)
Skin Breakdown	24%	24% (Skin Problem)	42% (Skin Problem)
Diarrhea		24%	18%
Confusion/Dementia	43%		29%
Constipation	24%		18%
Fever	13%	27%	

#1 Ferris F and Flannery J eds. *A Comprehensive Guide for the Care of Persons with HIV Disease: Module 4: Palliative Care.* Mount Sinai Hospital/Casey Hospice Toronto, 1995.

#2 Carr, DB, ed. *Pain in HIV/AIDS,* (La Douleur du SID/HIV), Robert G. Addison, publisher, 1994

#3 Sims R. and Moss VA. *Palliative Care for People with AIDS,* 2nd ed. Edward Arnold, London, 1995.

Fatigue, pain, and difficulty with sleep are three symptoms which occur throughout the course of HIV disease (van Servellan, 1998; Whalen, 1994) and are often over-looked by providers. Patients believe they "must put up with" these problems and may avoid acknowledging them to providers. Women do not want to appear less courageous in coping with their disease or to distract the provider. Women who have a history of past or current substance abuse may fear being labeled as "drug-seeking" or may fear relapse if given pain medication. On the other hand, providers often do not inquire about these symptoms because they may not know how to manage them or feel inadequate to address them.

Dame Cicely Saunders, the founder of modern-day hospice at St. Christopher's in London, introduced the term "total pain" (Saunders,1966) which is a model for how to approach all symptoms. She recognized that each complaint has a physical, emotional, and even spiritual component. If pain, or another symptom, is difficult to relieve with usual measures it may be that the woman has assigned special meaning to the symptom. She may be afraid her disease is getting worse or that "it is God's punishment." Both of these beliefs can exacerbate any symptom. (Hankes, 1998) Particularly when a symptom seems difficult to control, it is useful to ask the patient: "What does the pain (or nausea or shortness of breath) mean to you?" or "Why do you think you have this symptom?"

A. IDENTIFYING AND DEFINING THE PROBLEM

Instead of a "review of systems," it may be useful to think of a "review of symptoms" moving from the head down to the feet. All symptoms can be approached similarly (MacDonald, 1999) by asking about the character (what does it feel like); the location (including radiation to other parts of the body); what makes it worse, what makes it better; and are there any other symptoms associated. It is also useful to ask how symptoms limit or affect daily activity. Asking these questions lets the woman know that you are interested in the particulars of how this effects her life, that her perception of her daily comfort is as important to you as is her viral load.

In cancer patients with symptoms such as fatigue, it has been shown that just the act of asking and being aware of the importance of this symptom to the patient provides some relief from it. A problem often worsens when the patient tries to deal with it alone and her fear of what is causing it grows. Routinely using a checklist of symptoms such as the Memorial Symptom Assessment Scale (Bookbinder, 1995) will alert the practitioner to issues facing the patient. A review of symptoms will also alert the provider to the appearance of new symptoms which might herald progression of disease.

B. QUANTITATING SYMPTOMS

Two simple methods can be used to quantify symptom severity: 1) on a scale of zero to ten, where zero means the absence of any symptom and ten is the very worst it can be, how would the patient score her pain or fatigue" 2) the visual analog scale (VAS) is a straight, ten-centimeter line upon which the patient can make a mark representing how severe the symptom feels with the left end of the line representing "not at all" and the right being "the worst." Distance along the line can be measured in centimeters resulting in a numeric figure to record in the medical record for comparison purposes. Actual numbers are unique to the individual reflecting her perception and should not be

XII

used to compare her with other patients. Quantification is a mechanism for judging effectiveness of therapy and may alert the provider to a change in disease status.

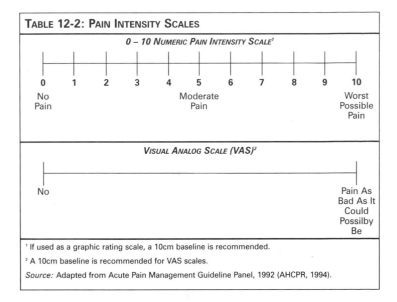

TABLE 12-2: PAIN INTENSITY SCALES

0 – 10 NUMERIC PAIN INTENSITY SCALE[1]

| 0 | 1 | 2 | 3 | 4 | 5 | 6 | 7 | 8 | 9 | 10 |

No Pain — Moderate Pain — Worst Possible Pain

VISUAL ANALOG SCALE (VAS)[2]

No — Pain As Bad As It Could Possilby Be

[1] If used as a graphic rating scale, a 10cm baseline is recommended.

[2] A 10cm baseline is recommended for VAS scales.

Source: Adapted from Acute Pain Management Guideline Panel, 1992 (AHCPR, 1994).

C. MANAGEMENT OF INDIVIDUAL SYMPTOMS

Effective symptom management is based on a thorough understanding of the symptom and education of the patient and family, allowing them to anticipate crisis episodes with appropriate planning. It requires a multidisciplinary approach. The goal is to help the patient "move from a feeling of helplessness to a feeling of supremacy over the symptom" and to develop and retain as much control over her life and illness as possible through the use of practical advice and emotional support. (W.H.O., 1998) Symptoms can be managed with medications and/or non-pharmacologic interventions. In general, the oral route for medications is preferred to the parenteral; treatment regimens are tailored to the individual.

FATIGUE

Scope of the Problem

This is the most frequent complaint of persons with HIV disease in a number of different series.(Laschinger, 1999; von Servellan, 1998) Seventeen to sixty per cent of persons, even before they are diagnosed with AIDS, have this complaint. (Breitbart, 1998; Groupman, 1998; Piper, 1993) "Chronic fatigue" is present when symptoms of disproportionate tiredness, unrelated to activity or exertion last for one month or more. Patients complain of "lack of energy, stamina, or endurance." (Piper, 1993) Women with fatigue have complained of decreased stamina at work, lowered quality of work, and frequent absenteeism possibly putting their jobs at risk. (Semple, 1993)

Once the problem and its meaning to the woman are well-delineated it is important to rule out and treat correctable etiologies. Anemia, depression, fear of the unknown, hypothyroidism, adrenal testosterone insufficiency (even in women), occult infection (particularly abscess or MAC), end-stage renal, pulmonary, or cardiac disease, malnutrition, lack of exercise, and disease progression itself all cause asthenia and fatigue. (O'Dell, 199 ; Groupman, 1998; Piper, 1998) In HIV disease, it is often a combination of these factors.

TABLE 12-3: TREATABLE CAUSES OF FATIGUE

■ Adrenal/hormonal insufficiency	■ Insomnia
■ Anemia	■ Lack of exercise
■ Depression	■ Malignancy
■ Disease progression	■ Malnutrition
■ End-stage organ disease	■ Medications
■ Fear of the unknown	■ Metabolic (low K/Mg)
■ Hypothyroidism	■ Occult infection (abscess/MAC)

In a study of 438 ambulatory patients in New York (52% of these had intravenous drug use as an exposure factor), Breitbart showed a significant correlation between fatigue and the presence of pain ($p < 0.0001$); higher psychological distress and poorer QoL ($p < 0.0001$); more depressive symptoms on the Beck depression Inventory (BDI) ($p < 0.0001$ and greater hopelessness on the Beck Hopelessness Scale ($P < 0.0001$). (Breitbart, 1998)

Approach to Management

It is important to work with the woman on ways to manage her fatigue even while the work-up is being pursued:

1. Showing interest in alleviating this symptom offers her emotional support which helps relieve the fatigue itself.

2. Referring her for a physical therapy assessment and prescription of simple strengthening exercises not only physically attacks the problem but allows her to begin to rebuild her own self-esteem.

3. Keeping a diary of what helps minimize her fatigue and what she can accomplish in a day as well as a daily numeric score (see quantitating symptoms) involve her in her own improvement and provide a better picture of how this symptom affects her daily life.

4. As each possible etiology is addressed, remind the woman to have realistic expectations in order to avoid becoming discouraged by false hopes.

XII

5. Using a positive, encouraging tone and setting small goals are helpful.

6. Nurses are adept at helping women find ways to eliminate or modify activities which are energy-consuming.

7. For many people, addressing spiritual issues or supportive counseling at this time may also provide comfort and encouragement.

8. Making use of other health care practitioners not only helps the woman to cope with this exhaustion but also releases the provider to concentrate more on those physical aspects of management which need to be addressed.

Pharmacologic treatments include methylphenidate 2.5–5.0 mg in the morning and repeated in early afternoon or high dose prednisone followed by a rapid taper. These therapies are usually needed in very advanced disease when the concern for further long-term immunosuppression is not the most important aspect of management.

PAIN

Scope of the Problem

Breitbart (1996) recently reported that pain in women with HIV disease is "prevalent, often severe, and highly distressing." Laschinger, (1999) in reporting a phenomenological study, states that the "pain experience embodies more than physical pain" (not unlike the "total pain" of Saunders). For this reason, understanding and controlling pain in women with HIV disease can be quite difficult as the practitioner must tease out the myriad components in order to optimally manage this symptom.

Surveys of ambulatory populations with HIV disease have documented that the prevalence of pain is 40–60%. (Lebovits, 1989; Breitbart, 1996; O'Neill, 1993; Singer,1993) For those who have more advanced disease and may be bedridden, these figures increase to as much as 83%. However, of those who do have pain, only about 40% are actually treated (Holzemer) and of those treated only about 40% (Holzemer) ever have adequate pain relief and can still rate their pain as a "seven out of ten" in severity. (Anand, 1994) These findings are universal and not limited to those with a history of substance abuse.

In HIV disease, pain can be caused by the disease itself, by therapies used to treat the disease, or by unrelated problems. The most frequent types of pain are abdominal pain and peripheral neuropathy (Anand, 1994; Newsham, 1998) or those caused by infections such as oral, esophageal, or genital/perineal herpes or fungus. Medications for treatment are based on location and type of pain.

As in cancer patients, up to 80% of persons with HIV disease having pain will experience more than one pain simultaneously. (Singer,1993) It is not unusual for a patient who has obtained relief from one pain to notice another type of pain which has been masked by the now-relieved pain. It is important to listen to and believe the patient. Carefully document all pain components and their characteristics to avoid a picture of "pseudoaddiction" or a label of "drug-seeking" in which an individual who is only partially treated continues to ask for pain medication. (Weissman, 1989)

One approach to pain management often neglected in the literature is the "phenomenological" which means understanding the human experience of pain from the perspective of the patient. Prior to the use of protease inhibitors, Laschinger (1999) conducted a qualitative study of 22 Canadian patients predominately gay men but with the one woman who had parallel experiences. They identified four substantive themes as components of pain: physical pain, painful losses, pain of not knowing, and social pain. The one additional factor found in the woman was that she also had concerns related to her children.

"Physical pain" included joint pain, headache, neuropathic and abdominal pain, as well as skin and mouth lesions. "Losses" referred to loss of energy, time, independence, and relationships. "Not knowing" meant the added anxiety of fearing that the pain might be life threatening. And "social pain" reflected inability to continue to participate in usual activities. The woman's fears had to do with how the knowledge of her disease might impact her children's schooling and how her death would impact their futures. This is a small but important study because it records the actual feelings of patients as opposed to asking for a provider's perception of what pain means to the patient. Although only one woman was represented, the findings are in keeping with our clinical experience.

Barriers to Pain Relief

There are many reasons offered by providers throughout the world for not prescribing adequate pain relief. (Am Pain Soc, 1999) Many societies fear "addiction" or diversion of medications. Health care workers often approach pain management with inadequate training in pain management skills. (Fields, 1998; Portenoy, 1994) Without appropriate knowledge of the pathophysiology either of pain or of its relief, providers may have the same fears as the public, believing that treating pain can "cause" addiction or that they must "save" powerful pain killers for a time when they might be "more needed." Also there may be the conviction that one should "bear the pain" to show strength or religious faith. All of these notions, while widely believed, have no basis in fact.

Principles of Pain Management

Pain, as with any symptom, should be described, quantitated, treated, and promptly re-evaluated with appropriate dose modification of therapy. The

---

TABLE 12-4: BARRIERS TO PAIN MANAGEMENT

PROBLEMS RELATED TO HEALTH CARE PROFESSIONALS

- Inadequate knowledge of pain management.
- Poor assessment of pain.
- Concern about regulation of controlled substances.
- Fear of patient addiction.
- Concern about side effects of analgesics.
- Concern about patients becoming tolerant to analgesics.

PROBLEMS RELATED TO PATIENTS

- Reluctance to report pain
  - Concern about distracting physicians from treatment of underlying disease.
  - Fear that pain means disease is worse.
  - Concern about not being a "good" patient.
- Reluctance to take pain medications.
  - Fear of addiction or of being thought of as an addict.
  - Worries about unmanageable side effects.
  - Concern about becoming tolerant to pain medications.

PROBLEMS RELATED TO THE HEALTH CARE SYSTEM

- Low priority given to cancer and AIDS pain treatment.
- Inadequate reimbursement.
  - The most appropriate treatment may not be reimbursed or may be too costly for patients and families.
- Restrictive regulation of controlled substances.
- Problems of availability of treatment or access to it.

Source: Adapted from AHCPR Clinical Practice Guideline, Number 9, *Management of Cancer Pain*, p.17, 1994.

AHCPR *Guidelines for the Treatment of Cancer Pain* recognize that pain experienced by those with HIV disease is comparable to the chronic pain experienced by persons with cancer which often requires management with opioids. Unlike blood pressure which might be regulated over weeks, pain should be controlled within the shortest time possible to prevent the development of long-term symptoms such as depression and anhedonia.

It is useful to start with the W.H.O. ladder approach which uses non-opioids initially and progresses through combinations of therapies and next to stronger opioids depending on the patient's response. (See Table 12-5) However, in HIV pain, opioids are frequently needed because of the severity of the pain and there is growing literature that *the use of the "second step, or weak opioids" might best be eliminated in HIV-related pain.* This second step includes "combination" pain medications, those containing an opioid plus aspirin or acetaminophen, which may increase the risk of hepatotoxicity or bleeding in women on HAART therapy. Becoming familiar with one or two agents for pain relief makes pain management easier.

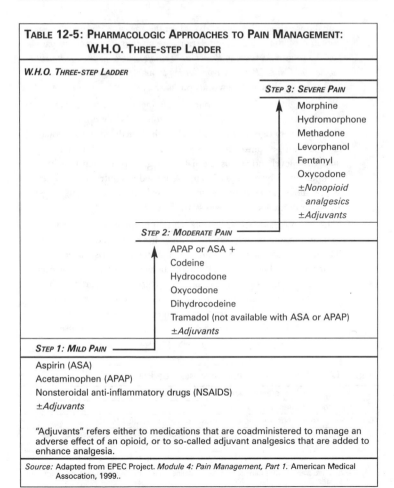

TABLE 12-5: PHARMACOLOGIC APPROACHES TO PAIN MANAGEMENT: W.H.O. THREE-STEP LADDER

W.H.O. THREE-STEP LADDER

STEP 3: SEVERE PAIN

Morphine
Hydromorphone
Methadone
Levorphanol
Fentanyl
Oxycodone
±Nonopioid
   analgesics
±Adjuvants

STEP 2: MODERATE PAIN

APAP or ASA +
Codeine
Hydrocodone
Oxycodone
Dihydrocodeine
Tramadol (not available with ASA or APAP)
±Adjuvants

STEP 1: MILD PAIN

Aspirin (ASA)
Acetaminophen (APAP)
Nonsteroidal anti-inflammatory drugs (NSAIDS)
±Adjuvants

"Adjuvants" refers either to medications that are coadministered to manage an adverse effect of an opioid, or to so-called adjuvant analgesics that are added to enhance analgesia.

Source: Adapted from EPEC Project. *Module 4: Pain Management, Part 1.* American Medical Assocation, 1999..

The following guidelines are helpful in prescribing pain medication: (American Pain Society, 1999)

1. Use a grading system (such as the scale of 0–10) to document pain severity and relief from pain for monitoring the effectiveness of therapy.

2. Start with a dose that will acutely relieve the pain. This may be given intravenously or sub-cutaneously to achieve a rapid response. Care should be taken to observe for any signs of respiratory depression in opiate-naive patients.

3. Next, begin a low dose every three to four hours (based on the half-life of the drug) "around-the-clock" and not on a PRN basis. The

XII

initial dose should be chosen based on the age, size, and renal/hepatic function of the patient. (Suggestions are given in any standard pain-management text such as *Principles of Analgesic Use in the Treatment of Acute and Cancer Pain, Fourth Edition* available from the American Pain Society at **http://www.ampainsoc.org**)

4. This dose given every four hours should include a supplemental, or "breakthrough," dose of about 1/6 of the total daily opioid dose to be given every one–two hours between the scheduled doses should the pain not be controlled. This allows for development of a steady state drug level and avoids alternation of great pain intensity with somnolence. This is the same approach used to control hyperglycemia with a sliding scale of regular insulin based on glucometer readings; these doses are based on pain scores.

5. When pain is fairly well-controlled, it is appropriate to change the patient to a long-acting pain medication for ease of administration. The dose is calculated by adding together the total dose taken in 24 hours and dividing by the half-life of the new preparation. For example, for a medication meant to be given every 12 hours: divide the total dose by two and this number will be your dose every twelve hours. Don't forget the breakthrough dose. This is a short-acting opioid, preferably of the same type as the long-acting one for use at times that the pain is not adequately controlled.

TABLE 12-6: MNEMONIC FOR ASSESSMENT OF PAIN
A — Ask about pain regularly; Access systematically
B — Believe the patient and family
C — Choose treatment options appropriate to patient and setting
D — Deliver medications on an "around-the-clock" basis with adequate "breakthrough" doses
E — Evaluate results frequently; Empower patients and families to control
Source: Adapted from AHCPR Clinical Practice Guideline, Number 9, *Management of Cancer Pain*, 1994.

6. Liquid formulations are useful for those with difficulty swallowing as well as rectal suppositories, "sprinkles" which can be mixed with soft food, or patches which can be absorbed through the skin.

Side Effects

Opioids usually cause drowsiness in the first 24–36 hours and patients should be advised that this will resolve. Use a low dose to initiate therapy but be prepared to increase the dose over the next 48 hours based on the patient's pain scores. Nausea is another common side effect in those first few days and can be treated with an anti-emetic such as prochlorperazine or lorazepam. All opioids slow bowel motility and patients should be given a stool softener when pain medication is prescribed.

Many prescribers will use an anti-emetic or methylphenidate to counteract these symptoms over a few days. Prolonged sleeping after the initial dosing may simply reflect the woman's need for rest which has not been possible because of the pain. If side effects are pronounced over a longer period, it is best to talk with the woman about what else is going on and it may be useful to discuss with a pain specialist and involve other team members.

Although many providers fear respiratory depression, this is unusual unless an opiate-naive patient is given a large, parenteral dose initially. Most pain (85-90%) can be controlled with oral medications. If the patient is having severe pain in a controlled situation such as a hospital or hospice, an initial subcutaneous injection of morphine or hydromorphone may control the pain more rapidly. Once a patient is on an appropriate dose, side effects (except for the slowed bowel motility) generally resolve and patient's return to their usual level of functioning, or even improved activity, because the pain is relieved.

TABLE 12-7: COMMON SIDE EFFECTS OF OPIOID ANALGESICS

CONSTIPATION	Requires prescription of stool softener at the time of prescribing opioid; *tolerance* does NOT develop
DROWSINESS	Resolves after 24-36 hours; extended sleeping can be from exhaustion; may need psycho-stimulant e.g. methylphenadate
NAUSEA	Prescribe anti-emetic with first prescription; resolves in several days – may need around-the-clock dosing
URINARY RETENTION	Uncommon side effect; change opioids or adjuvants
ITCHING/TWITCHING	May indicate toxic levels due to decreased elimination; lengthen interval; rotate opioids.

With very high doses, twitching or myoclonus may occur and in this case, it is possible to alternate two different opioids (referred to as "rotating") or to change to another drug entirely. (Galer, 1992) If twitching develops, the patient may have decreased renal or hepatic clearance. In this case the dosing interval should be lengthened or different opioids can be used in an alternating fashion.

Opioid Conversions

There are many opioid preparations available. These drugs are not equivalent on a milligram-to-milligram basis and it is possible to see what appears to be "drug-seeking behavior" if the conversion dose chosen is too low. When changing from one medication to another, use a conversion chart to find the total dose in morphine-equivalent units and convert according to the table. There is "no ceiling effect" with opioids as there is with other medications such as acetaminophen, aspirin or tricyclics; i.e., there is no toxic dose and the patient should be given whatever dose relieves her pain. Just as pain scores are individual, so are ultimate doses. It may be useful to seek the guidance of someone knowledgeable in pain management if you as the provider are not experienced with these medications.

XII

TABLE 12-8: DOSE EQUIVALENTS FOR OPIOID ANALGESICS IN OPIOID-NAÏVE ADULTS AND CHILDREN ≥ 50KG BODY WEIGHT

DRUG	APPROXIMATE EQUIANALGESIC DOSE		USUAL STARTING DOSE FOR MODERATE TO SEVERE PAIN	
ORAL	PARENTERAL	ORAL	PARENTERAL	
OPIOID AGONIST				
Morphine	30 mg q 3-4 h (repeat around-the-clock dosing) 60 mg q 3-4 h (single dose or intermittent dosing)	10 mg q 3-4 h	30 mg q 3-4 h	10 mg q 3-4 h
Morphine, controlled-release (MS Contin, Oramorph)	90-120 mg q 12 h	N/A	90-120 mg q 12 h	N/A
Hydromorphone (Dilaudid)	7.5 mg q 3-4 h	1.5 mg q 3-4 h	6 mg q 3-4 h	1.5 mg q 3-4 h
Levorphanol (Levo-Dromoran)	4 mg q 6-8 h	2 mg q 6-8 h	4 mg q 6-8 h	2 mg q 6-8 h
Meperidine (Demerol)	300 mg q 2-3 h	100 mg q 3 h	N/R	100 mg q 3 h
Methadone (Dolophine, other)	20 mg q 6-8 h	10 mg q 6-8 h	20 mg q 6-8 h	10 mg q 6-8 h
Oxymorphone (Numorphan)	N/A	1 mg q 3-4 h	N/A	1 mg q 3-4 h
COMBINATION OPIOID/NSAID PREPARATIONS				
Codeine (with aspirin or acetaminophen)	180-200 mg q 3-4 h	130 mg q 3-4 h	60 mg q 3-4 h	60 mg q 2 h (IM/SC)
Hydrocodone (in Lorcet, Lortab, Vicodin, others)	30 mg q 3-4 h	N/A	10 mg q 3-4 h	N/A
Oxycodone (Roxicodone, also in Percocet, Percodan, Tylox, others)	30 mg q 3-4 h	N/A	10 mg q 3-4 h	N/A

Source: Adapted from AHCPR Clinical Practice Guideline, Number 9, *Management of Cancer Pain,* p.52, 1994.

Pain Management with a History of Substance Abuse

Those who have used opioids in the past may have a higher tolerance and thus require higher than usual doses. "Addiction" is a psychological craving and the use of drugs "to get high" or despite personal harm and should not be confused with tolerance. When treating someone who has previously (or is currently) abused drugs, it its useful to discuss the full plan ahead of time. The patient should understand that this is a two-way interaction, that she must be truthful about her pain and its severity/relief as the provider will endeavor to control the pain. Most people with an addiction history who have legitimate pain are thankful to have it dealt with in an adult manner and understand that this is not a time to engage in manipulative behavior. In fact, many are afraid to take narcotics for fear of relapse.

Seeking a higher dose of drug does not necessarily mean that the patient is "drug-seeking." "Losing" or forging prescriptions, stealing from or having them "stolen" by others, visiting multiple providers for duplicate prescriptions and injecting oral formulations (Portenoy, 1994) are signs that the patient may not be using the medication appropriately. She must understand that she will be given adequate drug to last for a clearly described interval; she cannot obtain refills on weekends; and that there is only one provider who can write her prescriptions. Situations involving tampering with prescriptions or selling medication should be turned over to legal authorities and will sever the patient-provider supply of medication. Written contracts are used in some clinics but a well-documented discussion in the medical record is adequate.

Women with a history of substance abuse are often poorly emotionally defended and may have inadequate coping skills for even minor frustrations. Low self-esteem and little self-confidence can impact pain and make it worse. Breitbart noted that pain in women is more intense and that those with a history of opportunistic infections or intravenous drug use are "more likely to experience pain.?" (Breitbart 1995a)

Management of pain is not easy and requires a great degree of trust on both sides. Being consistent, open, and fair are important attributes for the provider to model. Providing positive feedback, reducing harm through education, and attempting to understand individual circumstances are most helpful to the patient. Clearly, as a patient approaches the end of life, old habits and fears often resurface and, at this time, the patient may need more support than usual.

Gender Differences

There is a growing literature suggesting that pain in women is under-treated. Breitbart recently reported that women with HIV disease appear to have "higher levels of pain intensity . . . [and are] more likely than men with AIDS to have their pain under-medicated." (Breitbart 1995b)

SLEEP DISTURBANCE/INSOMNIA

Scope of the Problem

Insomnia and excessive daytime sleepiness are primary complaints in persons with HIV disease regardless of stage. (Lashley, 1998) Cohen et al (1996) reported that fully two thirds of patients with AIDS have difficulty falling asleep without correlation with CD4 count. Insomnia includes difficulty falling asleep, difficulty staying asleep, and early morning awakening.

For women fatigue is not necessarily related to sleep patterns although it is important to document what the sleeping pattern is. Using questions similar to those in the table, try to determine the pattern of sleep problems, the frequency, associated events, as well as other factors listed below. Treatment should be tailored to the etiology. If you see patients in a busy setting, it is useful to have then fill out a card recalling specific characteristics of the symptom. A nurse can help the patient complete this card, leaving the provider to focus on therapy and documentation.

Assessment

Having the patient keep a sleep diary; bringing a family member to appointments to comment on sleep patterns; and clearly documenting bedtime, how long it takes her to go to sleep, and how long she can stay asleep provide the best picture of this problem. Include a full history of caffeine and alcohol intake and describe the environment and other factors which might affect sleep. (Lashley, 1998) Review current medications to eliminate these as a possible etiology which may cause insomnia particularly NNRTIs and selective serotonin reuptake inhibitors (SSRIs) taken at bedtime. Remember that injections drug users may have night sweats and abdominal pains as signs of withdrawal. Simple sleep-wake reversal may herald liver damage. Sleep disorder, classically early-morning wakening, may be a symptom of depression. (Nokes, 1999)

TABLE 12-9: SLEEP PROBLEMS (SAMPLE QUESTIONNAIRE FOR OFFICE USE)	
Do you have trouble ❑ falling asleep? Or ❑ staying asleep?	
Do you take naps during the day? ❑ Yes ❑ No How many hours _____ ?	
Do any of the following wake you up?	
❑ headache	❑ fever/night sweats
❑ bad or vivid dreams	❑ leg cramps
❑ problems breathing	❑ fear
❑ chest pain/heartburn	❑ another person in the house
❑ abdominal pains	❑ other _____
❑ need to pass urine	_____
❑ need to move bowels	_____
What have you tried for sleep?	
❑ Drug store product	❑ Counting sheep
❑ Sleeping pill from friend	❑ Warm bath
❑ Hot milk	❑ other _____
❑ Reading	_____
❑ Music	_____

Management of Insomnia

Treat the underlying problem whenever possible starting with simple environmental modifications e.g. fresh air; quiet (may need white noise emitter); avoiding exercise, heavy meals, large amounts of alcohol or arguing just before bed. Plain acetaminophen or aspirin in low doses if not contraindicated may be helpful, as well as short-acting hypnotics or sedating antidepressants e.g. trazedone 50 mg qhs. When underlying depression is identified, appropriate treatment with an SSRI or a tricyclic antidepressant is indicated. (See Chapter IX on Psychiatric Issues) Short-acting benzodiazepines are useful acutely but should be avoided long-term or in patients with dementia since they may increase confusion. (Phillips, 1999) Physical interventions such as massage, relaxation exercises, and deep breathing are also beneficial.

PRURITUS/ITCHING

Generalized pruritus without a rash may be secondary to dry skin, hepatic dysfunction, or an allergic reaction. The rash with scabies in an immunocompromised host may be diffuse and might require biopsy if symptoms do not respond to empiric therapy.

Along with specific therapy for scabies, the patient should be given an antihistamine to break the cycle of itching. Low doses of an opioid are not uncommmonly required to conquer this symptom. If the symptoms have been present for weeks, it may be necessary to follow the night-time scabies treatment with 1% hydrocortisone lotion each morning..

If the itching is thought to be secondary to hepatic dysfunction, holding hepatotoxic agents and using an H2 blocker such as around-the-clock cimetidine for several days is helpful. As the hepatic enzymes return to normal, medications can be resumed at lower doses and/ or with longer dosing intervals. This is true if the underlying pathology is not related to the lactic acidosis associated with some anti-retroviral therapies. In this case consult a liver specialist before re-introducing medications. These patients are partially relieved with a 1% hydrocortisone lotion containing menthol.

HICCUPS/HICCOUGHS/SINGULTUS

When intractable this symptom can lead to poor oral intake and weight loss as well as to depression because of an interruption of all normal activity. Simple mechanical measures such as drinking out of the "wrong" side of the glass and swallowing up-hill against gravity may transiently interrupt these symptoms. The usual medical treatment is low-dose (12.5–25 mg) chlorpromazine orally. Metachlopramide, baclofen, amantadine, benzodiazepines and haloperidol (Kaye, 1989; Woodruff, 1999) have also been described as useful although there is little evidence base for these recommendations. One treatable cause for this symptom is persistent and severe esophageal candidiasis which

XII

requires aggressive therapy of this infection for relief. Malignancy impinging on the phrenic nerve can also cause hiccough and a chest x-ray is recommended to rule out a mass.

XEROSTOMIA/DRY MOUTH

This condition can be secondary to medications such as antidepressants, anticholinergics, or HIV medications such as ddI or ddC. It is generally reversible if noticed soon enough and drug is stopped. However, if this condition persists without detection and treatment, it may become permanent. Direct invasion of the salivary gland with HIV can also cause dry mouth. Treatment should be directed at the etiology.

Artificial saliva, drinking extra fluids with meals, and fluoride treatments administered by a dentist may be necessary to reverse this symptom. If it is not noticed in a timely manner can lead to tooth decay and gingival disease may occur, resulting in caries and "sore" teeth. Left untreated, the patient may withdraw from society and become quite depressed because of the inability to be comfortable during a meal with others. Pilocarpine drops taken orally four times per day have been useful in this syndrome. (LeVeque, 1993) However, the onus is on the provider to ask about the presence of this symptom on a regular basis in order to detect, treat, and reverse the problem.

DYSPNEA/SHORTNESS OF BREATH

In the original hospice studies in this country, dyspnea was one of the five symptoms correlated with a shortened life expectance even when patients had no demonstrable disease in the cardiovascular or pulmonary systems. Dyspnea is an uncomfortable feeling of not being able to breathe although the oxygen saturation may be normal. Treatment should be directed at the presumed etiology using bronchodilators, diuretics, and steroids as necessary. In the hospice literature morphine has been used anectdotally as an aerosol with significant relief although this has not been formally proven to be useful; subcutaneous morphine or oral can also be used (start with 5mg every 3–4 hours). Clinical trials are needed to compare aerosolized morphine with saline nebulizers, which some authors have found equally useful.

Benzodiazepines are desirable to interrupt the cycle of dyspnea and panic which set in when an individual is having difficulty breathing. A long-acting drug such as lorazepam 0.05mg can be given around-the-clock every 6–8 hours to minimize the anxiety in this setting.

IV. PROGNOSIS

The use of combination, or highly active antiretroviral therapy (HAART), and the ability to measure the existing human immunodeficiency viral burden have significantly impacted the course of HIV disease. With improved antiretroviral therapy, use of prophylaxis for opportunistic infections, and treatment by providers who are knowledgeable about HIV disease, patients can look forward to living longer and healthier lives. However, particularly in resource-poor nations, most will die of this disease. In order to set realistic goals, the provider must have some sense of the individual's expected survival time.

Being able to give the patient and family a realistic appraisal of life expectancy, particularly near the end of life, is an important adjunct to disease management. For example, if the woman has several months to live, this may be the best time to review and clarify who will help with decision making should she become acutely or seriously ill. It is also a time to investigate and make decisions about guardianship as well as to make a will and determine general advance directives. Deciding which medications to discontinue and when depend upon the providers projection of how long the patient has to live.

While overall prognosis may be difficult to estimate, there are general signs which reflect advanced disease or failure of the immune system. (N.H.O., 1996) For example, repeated episodes of opportunistic infections, uncontrollable weight loss, or frequent hospitalizations all suggest that the woman is no longer "doing well." Once this decline begins and all antiretrovirals have been exhausted or the woman opts for no further aggressive therapy, it is reasonable to focus on issues related to life closure. As the woman becomes weaker, certain therapies may be withdrawn and attention should be directed toward psycho-social and spiritual tasks.

In 1996, prior to widespread use of combination therapies, the National Hospice Organization published *Medical Guidelines for Prognosis in Non-Cancer Diseases, 2nd Edition* (Standards Comm, N.H.O., 1996) which described indicators for a shortened life expectancy in several chronic diseases including HIV/AIDS. When several of these indicators are present, one should consider the prognosis to be limited unless the use of new or unapproved therapies is possible.

Wasting syndrome based on loss of lean body mass (Kotler, 1989) and anemia are both independent risk factors for decreased survival. (Moore, 1999) Median time to death can be related to the severity of each. Persistent oral thrush is also an independent predictor of progression of AIDS. Concurrent unresponsive malignancy or end-stage organ failure shortens the prognosis. Worldwide, hepatitis C is rapidly becoming a leading cause of death.

Although it is not well-documented, the woman's personal goals may significantly affect life expectancy. The experience in hospice care is that people must have completed psychosocial and spiritual goals before being able to peacefully "let go." For women with children this may mean making reasonable guardianship arrangements. For others it may mean resolving a relationship or coming to terms with her life events or accomplishments. Saying goodbye to loved ones and to care providers is a last necessary step before death.

XII

TABLE 12-10: FACTORS ASSOCIATED WITH SHORTENED LIFE EXPECTANCY

■ CD4 persistently low	■ Advanced disease: < 50 cells/cc
■ Viral burden remains 100,000 copies/ml	■ Despite combination therapy
■ Functional Status < 50 (Karnofsky Performance Status)	■ Spending > 50% of day in bed
■ Failure of optimized therapy	■ Multi-drug resistence or failure
■ Desire to forego more therapy	■ Often occurs after multiple hospitalizations
■ Anemia (Hemoglobin < 12)	■ Persistent oral thrush
■ Significant wasting	■ Loss of > 30% lean body mass
■ Progressive hepatitis C	■ Hepatic failure; drug intolerance
■ Progressive multi-focal leukoencephalopathy (PML)	■ Progressive dependencies; dementia
■ Unresponsive Kaposi's sarcoma involving an organ	■ Progression despite therapy
■ End-stage organ disease	■ Renal, hepatic, or cardiac failure
■ Persistent diarrhea > 1 mo.	■ No response to treatment
■ Unresponsive lymphoma/ other malignancy	■ Progression despite therapy
■ Desire of patient for death	■ Acknowledgment by patient and family of poor prognosis

Source: Adapted from *Medical Guidelines for Prognosis in Non-cancer Diagnoses,* 2nd Ed., 1997 Moore, AIDS, 1999.

V. TRUTH-TELLING AND BREAKING BAD NEWS

Communication skills are particularly important as the woman's health begins to decline. Being a good listener is paramount and there are concrete skills which can be learned. When discussing emotionally-laden issues or breaking bad news, it is best to ask what the perceptions are of those present whether you are addressing the woman alone or her friends and family. "Before I talk, tell me how you think you are [she is] doing" "What are your concerns at this time" Not only does this help the provider to know where to begin but it provides a vocabulary to use in this discussion.

Baile and Buckman discuss how to talk about difficult topics described in Table 12-11. (Baile, 1998) They note the importance of paying attention to the physical environment when having serious discussions with patients and fami-

TABLE 12-11: MNEMONIC FOR BREAKING BAD NEWS

S — Setting and listening Skills
P — Patient & family Perception of condition
I — Invitation to patient to determine how much Information he/she wants to know
K — Knowledge; reviewing the facts
E — Explore Emotions & Empathize
S — Summary & Strategy

Source: Adapted from *Pocket Guide to Communications Skills in Clinical Practice,* 1998, (1-800-757-4868).

lies. It is important to have privacy, quiet and lack of interruptions as much as possible. The provider should sit down to talk with whatever "family" the patient wishes to include. The use of touch may be comforting although it is important to gain permission first. Body language and eye contact are a part of the setting.

Initially, it is useful to find out what the patient or family perceives to be the current condition. "Before I talk, tell me how you think you are [or she is] doing" Their answers will help the provider know where to begin. Words used by them will suggest vocabulary as well as degree of comprehension. Avoiding jargon or strictly medical terms is helpful. In the case of bad news, it is useful to provide a *warning statement* such as "I have some bad news for you" or "This is a very difficult time and I want you to be prepared." Once the facts have been communicated, it is important to determine what the reaction is to this news. Providing a period of silence may help those involved to gather their thoughts before speaking. (Weissman, 1999)

Listening skills include asking open-ended questions and repeating the last comment made by patient or family member to clarify what has been said. *Acknowledge emotions* by using empathic responses even if the feelings themselves are unimaginable to you. After a period of discussion, develop a *strategic plan* with the patient or family by discussing expectations and goals. Use this time to reassure that there will be future conversations. *Summarize* what has been discussed and ask for any remaining questions.

TABLE 12-12: Making Plans Ahead of Time

1. Appointment of Power of Attorney for health matters and for financial matters	These are two different issues; the healthcare POA does not last beyond the death; therefore, all plans must be made and executed ahead of time.
2. Appointment of guardian for children	Be certain that children & guardian are both aware of these plans.
3. If there are children left behind	Many people make a scrap book, write a letter, or even make a video to remind younger children who their mother was.
4. Make a will if there is anything you own that you would like to leave to a particular person	This includes money, a home, dishes from your grandmother, or jewelry that has a special meaning to you.
5. Discuss with family or friends how and where you would like to die	You can be involved in planning a funeral or memorial service; can pick out your clothes and pallbearers.
6. Discuss desires regarding care before death: ■ For nutrition and hydration ■ For cardiopulmonary resuscitation ■ For being kept alive on machines	It may be helpful to think about what you might want in different situations. For example, if you would be bed-bound; if you were no longer able to care for yourself; if you would not be able to recognize people or carry on normal conversations.

XII

IV. REALISTIC GOAL SETTING AND ADVANCE CARE PLANNING

We must all learn to think ahead to a time when we may not be healthy and able to care for ourselves. Women, in particular, need to make provisions for others they care for such as children or an elderly parent. Thinking ahead prevents confusion and also assures that no one person will be burdened with matters near the time of death. Each woman needs to select someone who will be able to accomplish her legal affairs and also someone to make medical decisions for her should she not be able to do so. This may be two different people but it is important for the woman to discuss her own wishes with that person early in her illness. By doing it at a time when she feels well, she can remain in control and make her own choices.

A. IMPORTANCE OF MAINTAINING HOPE

To provide the most supportive and sensitive care throughout illness, the provider must understand the overall goals of the patient. As the woman moves through her disease it is necessary to intermittently discuss these preferably while the patient is feeling well and able to feel more in control of her disease. Just as quality of life evolves, so do desired outcomes. Many medical providers seem to fear that having these discussions might "take away hope."

Hope is not false expectation. It can be re-defined in an acceptable way for the individual. Whereas hope for a long life may no longer be possible, hope for being able to leave good memories behind for children may be fulfilled by making a scrapbook, audio tape, or even a video. One can simply hope for days that are meaningful. (Bennett, 1995) Multiple studies document that having a sense of spiritual (not necessarily religious) well-being has a positive effect on health. (Colman, 1999)

Hope "... is the emotion upon which all the other emotions of elation are grounded... shaped by a glimpse of something not yet clearly within sight... always looks toward creative changes... an expression of the will to live... of an individual's trust in life... even terminally ill persons express the feeling that things will somehow get better... that as long as we live, we live for a better future." (Kast, 1996) It is not a commodity that one person gives to another but is within the individual and can be modified accordingly. Ernst Bloch (19) in *The Principle of Hope* wrote

> "What matters is learning to hope. Hope does not abandon its post. It is in love with success rather than failure. Hope, superior to fear... reaches out; it broadens rather than narrows."

He apparently "saw hope in daydreaming, fantasy, and imagination." Albert Schweitzer also believed that imagination was what allows the human to tolerate the present.

B. PERSONAL GOALS

In discussing goals, it is useful to ask the woman, "What aspects of your life are most important to you? What have you accomplished in your life that makes you feel proud?" This is also a time to determine which other persons she cares about and who provides her support. Frequently, it is a family anniversary or event, such as the birth of a grandchild, that comprise the woman's true goals.

Each of us has dreams. It is up to the provider or other members of the team to discover those and help the woman to see how they might be achieved. With HIV disease the young woman may not have had time to realize her dreams. In this case, the team must help her value the life she has had and to discover and acknowledge what it is that she wishes remembered about her life. She can also be assisted in grieving the loss of future. Sharing a funny story or memory of a special event helps the young woman know that she has left her mark.

C. ADVANCE CARE PLANNING

Once the provider understands what is important to the woman, it is much easier to talk about the kind of care she would like to receive near the end of life. Being able to hold her grand-daughter may be more important than living another year. Once broad goals cans be identified, the team needs to shift from a tactical approach to care to a more strategic one. (NEJM, 1996) Bennett (1995) refers to this as changing from a "cure-based approach to a psychosocial model." It means to target an overall goal rather than to get bogged down in correcting the electrolytes. Being at home may be more pertinent than having the last potassium adjusted or receiving the final days of a course of intravenous antibiotics. Being free of pain and in a dry bed with loved ones present may be the ultimate goal.

While the term "advance directive" makes sense to those in the health care environment, these words may be essentially meaningless to the woman and those who make up her support system. In trying to determine what the patient wants it is necessary to use concrete and explicit terms when discussing this topic. Clark (1989) stresses the importance of developing a "psychosocial success" register where psychosocial desires and resolutions can be formally recognized; this might be done during a case conference with staff.

VII. END OF LIFE ISSUES

A. PHYSICAL COMFORT NEAR THE END OF LIFE

When the patient is bed-ridden, it is comforting to be surrounded by photos or objects that remind her of events and people she would like to remember or that make her happy. Being in a home-like environment is the desired

XII

resting place for many. (American Health Decisions, 1997) Attention to reducing noise, providing a fan or some means of air movement, serving small portions of food several times throughout the day rather than three large meals, and playing music or reading stories may all provide comfort. If the patient has a favorite pet or small children she might enjoy short visits with them.

Complementary therapies such as massage, guided imagery, or acupuncture are widely used and can provide comfort to those for whom they are familiar. Others may not appreciate being touched by strangers and it is always important to discuss these methods before introducing them. Likewise, incense or

---

TABLE 12-13: PHYSICIAN'S CARD

Side One

COMFORT MEASURES AT LIFE'S END

L — **LIPS,** mouth & eyes moistened; ice chips; artificial saliva /tears

I — **INCONTINENCE** of bowel & bladder expected - use Foley/Texas; bed pad

F — **FEVERS** expected: around the clock antipyretics (po or supp)

E — **ELIMINATE** all but essential meds

S — **SYMPTOM** management - be aggressive

E — **EATING** less is expected; diet as desired

N — **NURSING** call orders--revise

D — **DECUBITUS**/skin care/turning q 2 hrs.

Side Two

Making the decision to write **"Do Not Resuscitate"** orders is often difficult but it does not mean that there is "nothing else to be done." Once the order **"No CPR"** is written *reverse your thinking* and write **orders for RPC:**

R — **REASSURANCE**
- you will continue to care for the patient and family
- symptoms which interfere with good quality of life will be controlled
- there are effective ways for coping with stresses and for grieving
- patient and family concerns will direct how and where care is provided

P — **PRESENCE**
- be there to hold conversations
- visit on a regular basis
- sit down and hold a hand
- listen respectfully

C — **CARING**
- provide comfort measures
- honor the individual
- share laughter and touch

Facilitate "life review" & these important conversations:
- **Thank you**
- **Please forgive me**
- **I forgive you**
- **I love you**
- **Goodbye**

Source: © University of Maryland, Baltimore, 1999 Palliative Care Program, Permission to reproduce for educational purposes granted.

---

peppermint oil may be used to mask unpleasant odors; activated charcoal on a gauze pad or chlorophyll tablets can accomplish the same result.

Cultural beliefs and rituals become very important at this time. Use the rest of your team to discover what practices must be respected as ignorance of these might inhibit a peaceful transition as well as leave bad memories for families and friends. For example, some cultures or religions require that the patient receive fluids or that the healthcare workers give the appearance of performing resuscitation attempts or efforts to prevent the actual death. Knowing these beliefs ahead of time will allow the staff to prepare and conversations to be held which might preclude misunderstanding.

Once the patient and family have made the final decision for "No cardiopulmonary resuscitation (CPR)," many health care workers are at a loss for exactly what to do. Although fluids and antibiotics may be withheld, there are still many techniques which staff can employ to support the patient and family as a unit. Dr. Linda Emmanual of the Ethics Institute of the American Medical Association has suggested that "Orders to Intervene" should be offered.

Alexander, Perrone, and Reiss have developed a mnemonic for remembering simple medical orders which might be implemented as an example of these interventions. (See Table 12-13) The care provider should recognize that despite the end of curative interventions, there is always something which can be done to comfort both patient and family. By reversing "No CPR" and writing orders for "RPC" the team can continue to offer support. *Reassurance* of continued involvement by the health care team, *presence* at the bedside on a predictable basis, and an attitude of *caring* which respects individual goals and comfort are the least that can be done. *The Oxford Textbook of Palliative Medicine, 2nd Edition* contains a wealth of knowledge for those who desire to give good supportive care.

B. CLINICAL TREATMENT

Treatments which have been used throughout active disease may need to be modified as the woman comes closer to dying. Using complex diagnostic procedures and prolonged courses of therapy may not be necessary at the end of life and may be a significant burden to the patient. Short bursts of antibiotics may be all that is needed to arrest a symptom. Such judgements must be based on realistic prognosis as discussed earlier in this chapter. For example, a woman resistant to oral antifungal agents may need a brief course of intravenous therapy if this offers the quickest relief of her symptoms.

If there are high fevers and sweats presumed secondary to MAC she may no longer tolerate the usual combination of drugs and single agent or short burst doses may be adequate to control symptoms at a time when a reduced pill count is the over-riding goal. One of the difficult aspects of managing the end stages of illness is knowing when it is appropriate to discontinue certain therapies. Much of this decision making is based on the provider ability to

XII

provide realistic prognostic information to the patient and family. For example, prophylactic therapies might be discontinued in the last 3–4 weeks of life as they can easily be resumed should the woman become symptomatic.

C. CONVERSATIONS FOR THE END-OF-LIFE

Families often fear that discussing death might "scare" the dying person. However, most people know when they are dying and are relieved at being able to discuss their fears or beliefs. Women in particular, often feel a need to "protect" those around them and may be more comfortable talking about their impending death with someone who is not a family member. Although most people feel awkward around someone who is very ill or dying because they "don't know what to say" there are a number of things to talk about.

Most people near the end of life want to know that their time on earth has been worthwhile. They want to know that they have been loved, that they will be remembered, and that they are forgiven for things they may have done wrong. One simple method for achieving these goals is to "do life review" which means to ask to hear stories of the person's life: what she is most proud of, what is the funniest thing that ever happened to her, what she is ashamed of or wishes she hadn't done. By asking these questions, the listener can reassure the person that those memories will stay alive. By talking about negative events, they can be minimized or forgiven.

An anonymous hospice nurse once said that there are five important conversations for the dying person to have to assure a peaceful death. These are "Thank you," "Forgive me," "I forgive you," "I love you," and "Goodbye." The last of these is the most difficult both for the dying woman and for those who will be left behind. But, this is the most important conversation because the dying need to feel reassured that those left behind will be able to take care of themselves. This is especially true of women regarding spouses and children; it

is accentuated when the woman is young and there are young children involved. Those being left behind must also say goodbye by giving the dying woman "permission to go" which represents their acceptance of the finality of the death. This permission must also be verbally granted by health care providers who may have become like family members near the end of a long illness.

TABLE 12-14: FIVE IMPORTANT CONVERSATIONS TO COMPLETE FOR A "PEACEFUL" DEATH
▪ Thank you.
▪ I forgive you.
▪ Please forgive me.
▪ I love you.
▪ Goodbye.

Forgiveness and reconciliation are spiritual as well as personal issues. (Hall, 1998) Depending on the belief-system of the woman, it may be important to have a priest, a pastor, a rabbi, or other spiritual representative present throughout the last month of life. In societies where large numbers of women are dying, there may be insufficient care givers since this is a role often assumed by women. It is important to find someone to sit with the dying woman to provide comfort and security in her last hours. Simple presence without conversation represents real support and caring.

Christina Puchalski defines spirituality as " whomever or whatever gives one a transcendent meaning in life." She suggests doing a spiritual assessment of the woman at the same time that other historical information is gathered. The mnemonic FICA is useful for remembering what questions to ask.

TABLE 12-15: SPIRITUAL ASSESSMENT – FICA	
F — Faith or beliefs	Do you consider yourself spiritual or religious? What things do you believe in that give meaning to your life?
I — Importance and Influence	What influence does it have on how you take care of yourself? What role do your beliefs play in re-gaining your health?
C — Community	Is there a person or group who are really important to you? Are you part of a religious community?
A — Address	How would you like your health care providers to address these issues?

D. TIME OF DEATH

At the time of death it is important to be familiar with the woman's customs. Friends and family present may want to hold hands or stand in a circle around the bed. A prayer or song may be said or sung together. In many cultures, the women, or men, depending upon the belief system will want to wash the body, perhaps apply oils, and to wrap the body in appropriate garments. Staff should be aware of these practices and allow the family as much time as is needed to complete these rituals. It may be necessary to wait for other friends or family members to arrive to say their own goodbyes. Children should not be kept from participating and will understand the death within their own age-related construct.

E. GRIEF AND BEREAVEMENT

Grief is the process and work of adjusting to the irrevocable loss of persons, objects, relationships, and dreams. The grieving period often begins before death (anticipatory grieving) but may appropriately extend for two years or more after death depending upon the nature of the relationship. Grief is a normal response to loss and includes such symptoms as sadness, crying, withdrawal from other friends and family, loss of drive or ability to concentrate, and fears of "losing ones mind" or experiencing physical symptoms similar those of the person who died. The grieving person requires significant support such as brief visits, phone calls, or invitations to simple social events. Many community hospice programs can provide this type of support.

One role of the palliative care team is to assure that care is given to those left behind, the bereaved. Because of the concentration of activity near the

XII

time of death, the bereaved may not feel the full impact of the death for at least two weeks after the actual event. Contact at this time is helpful as is remembering the person on important anniversaries such as one month after the death, holidays, and days particular to the individual who died such as a birthday or wedding anniversary. The first and tenth year anniversaries of the death are a often a difficult time for families and friends. Many cultures have rituals related to the date of death which continue to comfort those surviving. Coping strategies that have been useful throughout the disease can also be applied after the death of a loved one.

MULTIPLE LOSS

Having to mourn a second or third person soon after the death of the first is generally more than any individual is able to cope with alone. Dean (1995) found a direct relationship between the number of bereavement episodes suffered by one person and the development of "stress response" symptoms or as Rando says "psychic numbing." (Rando, 1993) Although the phenomenon of "multiple loss" has been acknowledged in association with natural disasters and concentrations camp survivors, there has been little published about how to cope with and resolve the issues raised by multiple loss.

Many survivors of multiple loss are afraid to openly grieve for fear of losing control of their emotions. Holding onto this grief produces a syndrome similar to that seen with "burn-out." (Bennett, 1998; Price, 1984) Emotional numbing, withdrawal from others, mis-directed anger, a lack of pleasure in anything, and resorting to use of drugs or alcohol are all common elements of this syndrome. Kastenbaum (1969) called this series of consecutive losses "bereavement overload." More recently Nord has delineated four stages of response to multiple AIDS-related loss. These are not mutually exclusive stages and may occur at random rather than in a linear fashion. These stages include: a) shock and denial; b) overload and confusion; c) facing reality; and d) re-investment and recovery.

The traditional bereavement model is inadequate for grieving the multiple losses experienced by survivors of AIDS-related loss. Care of persons with AIDS is complicated by the fact that the care-giver may himself or herself be infected and facing death. It is important to be able to refer the care-giver for appropriate medical care and counseling. Depression is not unusual and, particularly in those who are also infected, should be treated appropriately and aggressively, even at the time of death of the loved one.

Not only members of the gay and hemophiliac communities (which have been decimated by the epidemic), but mothers of inner city minority youth who may have experienced the death of more than one child and are often alone in trying to resolve their grief, are at risk for complicated mourning. "When multiple deaths occur, the people to whom the mourner would ordinarily go for support are gone." (Rando, 1993) Therefore, new models for dealing with these losses need to be developed. Survivors of multiple loss might be helped by a referral for professional counseling.

A time-honored hospice technique has been to attempt to make the sufferer aware of the many manifestations of grief by verbalizing that thoughts of "going crazy" are not unusual and by reassuring those grieving that they, as survivors, are and will be OK. According to Nord, "social support, community involvement, and fostering a sense of purpose are useful" toward achieving the goal of empowerment which helps reduce the role of victim. Achieving a sense of balance in life and pursuing a "life outside of AIDS" give survivors a necessary source of detachment. Physical exercise, meditation, and trips away from the usual environment are acceptable methods used to care for the care provider. An active sense of humor is also helpful.

"Bearing witness" means keeping the memory alive; the AIDS quilt is a good example. The quilt is also an example of the power and importance of ritual. Making a quilt panel is a shared experience which provides support for the makers as for the viewers. Memorial services on a regular basis can be comforting and assist the survivor in bringing closure for an individual death.

TABLE 12-16: METHODS FOR COPING WITH MULTIPLE LOSS
■ Acknowledge the loss
■ Normalize feeling of "going crazy"
■ Physical exercise; adequate sleep
■ Community service; foster "sense of purpose"
■ Keep the memory alive
■ Perform rituals e.g. quilt panel; memorial service

GUIDELINES FOR AFTER THE DEATH

Mallinson has outlined guidelines for addressing grief which might be useful in working with those who are surviving loss from HIV disease. Simply rehearsing words or phrases ahead of time make it easier for the health care team to interact with survivors during a time which many find awkward.

■ Acknowledge the death: "I understand that your [partner; spouse] died last week. How is this going for you?"

■ Validate the importance to the survivor: "You knew her for a long time, and the two of you were very close. What was she like?"

■ Speak of the deceased when appropriate: "I remember when Tommy was first born. This would have been his second birthday this week. How are you feeling?"

■ Note the existence of multiple losses: "Since you have been coming to clinic, you have lost your partner, your best friend, and now, your daughter. I can't imagine what it is like. How do you handle the grief?"

■ Learn about grief and loss: Take courses, attend workshops, read research and acquire therapeutic communication skills.

VIII. CARE OF THE CARE PROVIDER

Palliative care is difficult work because it requires that team members suspend personal needs or beliefs in deference to the desires of the patient and family. It requires a degree of emotional maturity and insight regarding personal feelings/beliefs which might interfere with the work. One must develop coping skills for both external and internal stressors. (Bennett, 1998) "Debriefing" is important and must be a recognized part of this care.

Although "support groups" often seem like a useful mechanism, they can be burdensome themselves and are not helpful for everyone. Staff must have a recognized way to "take a time-out" and be flexible enough to "cover" for a colleague who needs a bit of time to "re-group." (Puckett, 1996) Many who do hospice work have learned to take breaks, or mini vacations; to develop outside interests or to do community service of another type. Without conscious support of all members of the team the burn-out rate would undoubtedly be high. (Price, 1984)

TABLE 12-17: FACILITATING THE GRIEVING PROCESS

1. Share your thoughts
2. Make time for enjoyable activities
3. Exercise regularly
4. Treat yourself to little extras
5. Work through your grief gradually

Source: Leash, M. *Death notification: a practical guide to the process.* Upper Access, Hinesberg, Vt. 1994.

TABLE 12-18: MNEMONIC FOR LIFE'S END

L — **LIPS,** mouth & eyes moistened; ice chips; artificial saliva /tears

I — **INCONTINENCE** of bowel & bladder expected - use Foley/Texas; bed pad

F — **FEVERS** expected: around the clock antipyretics (po or supp)

E — **ELIMINATE** all but essential meds

S — **SYMPTOM** management - be aggressive

E — **EATING** less is expected; diet as desired

N — **NURSING** call orders — revise

D — **DECUBITUS**/skin care/turning q 2 hrs.

Source: © University of Maryland, Baltimore, 1999 Palliative Care Program, Permission to reproduce for educational purposes granted.

REFERENCES

Abercrombie, PD. Women living with HIV infection. *Nursing Clinics of North America* 1996; 31(1):97–105.

AHCPR *Clinical Practice Guideline # 9: Management of cancer pain.* Dept of Health and Human Services, Washington, DC, 1994. (Publication # 94-0592).

American Health Decisions. The quest to die with dignity: an analysis of American values, opinions, and attitudes concerning end-of-life care. American Health Decisions, Atlanta, Ga. 1997.

American Pain Society. Principles of Analgesic use in the treatment of acute and cancer pain, 4th ed. Glenview, Ill., 1999. http://www.ampainsoc.org.

Anand A. et al. Evaluation of recalcitrant pain in HIV-infected hospitalized patients. *J AIDS* 1994; 7:52–56.

Barroso, J. A Review of fatigue in people with HIV infection. *Journal of the Association of Nurses in AIDS Care.* 1999; 10(5):42–49.

Bartlett JG. *1999 Medical Management of HIV Infection.* Baltimore, MD: Johns Hopkins University, 1999.

Bennett, L AIDS Health Care: Staff stress, loss and bereavement. *Grief and AIDS.* 1995; 6:87–102.

Bloch, Ernst. *The Principle of Hope.*

Bloomer, SC. Palliative Care. *Journal of the Association of Nurses in AIDS Care.* 1998; 9(2):45–47.

Breitbart, W. et al. Pain in ambulatory AIDS patients. I: Pain characteristics and medical correlates. *PAIN*, 1996; 68:315–321.

Breitbart W, McDonald MV, Rosenfeld B, Monkman ND, and Passik S. Fatigue in ambulatory AIDS patients. *J Pain and Sympt Man* 1998; 5(3):159–167.

Brown, GR. The Use of methylphenidate for cognitive decline associated with HIV Disease. *Int'l. J. Psychiary in Medicine.* 1995; 25(1):21–37.

Bruera E, MacDonald S. Audit methods: The Edmundton Symptom Assessment System" in Higginson I, ed. *Clinical Audit in Palliative Care.* Oxford: Radcliffe Medical Press, 1993.

Byock, IR. Dying Well: *Peace and Possibilities at the End of Life.* New York: Riverhead Books, 1997.

Carr, DB, ed. *Pain in HIV/AIDS* (La Douleur du SID/HIV). Washington, DC: Robert G. Addison, 1994.

Cassell, Eric J. Diagnosing suffering: a perspective. *Ann Intern Med.* 1999;131(7) 531–4.

Cassel, EJ. *The Nature of Suffering and the Goals of Medicine.* Oxford University Press, New York, 1991.

Chlebowski, RT, et al. Nutritional status, gastrointestinal dysfunction, and survival in patients with AIDS. *American Journal of Gastroenterology.* 1989; 84(10):1288–1293.

Chung, JY. A Group approach to psychosocial issues faced by HIV-positive women. *Hospital and Community Psychiatry.* 1992; 43(9):891–894.

Cohen, FL. et al. Sleep in men and women infected with human immunodeficiency virus. *Holist Nurs Pract* 1996; 10(4):33–43.

Cohen, MAA. Psychiatric care and pain management of persons with HIV infection. *AIDS and Other Manifestations of HIV Infection*, Third Edition. 1998; 19:475–503.

Colman, CL. Spirituality, psychological well-being, and HIV symptoms for African Americans living with HIV disease. *Journal of the Association of Nurses in AIDS Care.* 1999; 10(1):42–50.

Dean, L The epidemiology and impact of aids-related death and dying in New York's gay community. *Grief and AIDS* 1995 Ch. 2:29–42.

Doyle D, Hanks GWC, and MacDonald N, eds. *Oxford Textbook of Palliative Medicine.*, 2nd ed. Oxford: Oxford Univ Press, 1998.

Dudgeon DJ, Raubertas RF, Doerner K, O'Connor T, Tobin M, Rosenthal SN. When does palliative care begin? *J Pall Care.* 1995; 11(1):5–9.

XII

Farsides, CCS. Allowing someone to die. *Grief and AIDS* 1995 Ch. 7:103–12.

Ferris F and Flannery J eds. *A Comprehensive Guide for the Care of Persons with HIV Disease: Module 4: Palliative Care.* Toronto: Mount Sinai Hospital/Casey Hospice, 1995.

Field, MJ and Cassel, CK Eds. *Approaching Death: Improving Care at the End of Life.* Washington, DC: National Academy Press, 1997.

Fowler, MG et al. Women and HIV — Epidemiology and global overview. *Obstetrics and Gynecology Clinics of North America* 1997; 24(4):705–728.

Friedman M. Treatment of aphthous ulcers in AIDS patients. *Laryngoscope* 1994; 104:566–570.

Galer BS, Coyle N, Pasternak GW, et al. Individual variability in the response to different opioids: report of five cases. *PAIN* 1992; 49:87–91.

Greenspan D. HIV-related oral disease. *Lancet* 1996; 348:729–733.

Hall, B. Patterns of spirituality in persons with advanced HIV disease. *Research in Nursing & Health*, 1998; 21:143–153.

Hanson, LC, et al. Can clinical interventions change care at the end of life? *Ann Intern Med.* 1997; 126(5):381–388.

Holzemer

Kast V. *Joy, Inspiration, and Hope.* 199

Kasterbaum R.. Death and bereavement in later life. In AH Kutscher, ed. *Death and Bereavement.* Springfield IL: Charles S. Thomas, 1969.

Kaye P. Notes on symptom control in hospice and palliative care. Hospice Education Institute, Essex, Conn, 1989.

Keithley, J. Nutrition-related changes. *HIV Nursing and Symptom Management — Unit 2,* Chapter 10:291–309.

Laschinger, SJ The experience of pain in persons with HIV/AIDS. *Journal of the Association of Nurses in AIDS Care* 1999 Sept/Oct; 10(5):59–67.

Lebovits A. The prevalence and management of pain in patients with AIDS: a review of 134 cases. *Clin J Pain* 1989; 5:245–248.

LeVeque F. A multicenter, randomized, double-blind, placebo-controlled, dose-titration study of oral pilocarpine for treatment of radiation-induced xerostomia in head and neck cancer patients. *J of Clin Onc* 1993; 11(6):1124–1131.

Libbus, MK. Women's beliefs regarding persistent fatigue. *Issues in Mental Health Nursing*, 1996; 17:589–600.

McDaniel, JS et al. An assessment of rates of psychiatric morbidity and functioning in HIV disease. *General Hospital Psychiatry* 1995; 17:346–352.

MacDonald, N. *Palliative Medicine: A Case-based Mmanual.* Oxford: Oxford University Press, 1998.

McCormack J. Inadequate treatment of pain in ambulatory HIV patients. *Clin J of Pain* 1993; 9: 279–283.

Mead, SCW. Crisis of the psyche: psychotherapeutic considerations on aids, loss and hope. *Grief and AIDS* 1995; 8:115–126.

Moneyham, L. Depressive symptoms and HIV disease. *Journal of the Association of Nurses in AIDS Care* July/August 1999; 10(4):93–94.

Moore, J et al. Severe adverse life events and depressive symptoms among women with, or at risk for, HIV infection in four cities in the United States of America. *AIDS* 1999, 13:2459–68

Nannis, ED. Coping with HIV disease among seropositive women: psychosocial correlates. *Women & Health* 1997; 25(1):1–22.

Newshan, G. Is Anybody Listening? A phenomenological study of pain in hospitalized persons with AIDS. *Journal of the Association of Nurses in AIDS Care* March/April 1998; 9(2):57–67.

Nokes, KM et al. Exploring the complexity of sleep disturbances in persons with HIV/AIDS. *Journal of the Association of Nurses in AIDS Care* May/June 1999; 10(3):22–29.

Nord D. Issues and implications in the counseling of survivors of multiple AIDS-related loss. Death *Studies* 1996;20:389–413.

O'Neill, JF and Alexander, CS. Palliative Medicine and HIV/AIDS in Primary Care 1997; 24(3):September, 607–615.

O'Neill W. Pain in human immunodeficiency virus disease: a review. *PAIN* 1993; 54:3–14.

Pergami, A et al. The Psychosocial Impact of HIV infection in women. *Journal of Psychosomatic Research* 1993; 37(7):687–96.

Pezzotti P et al. Increasing survival time after AIDS in Italy: the role of new combination antiretroviral therapies. *AIDS* 1999;13:249–255.

Phillips, KD. Physiological and pharmacological factors of insomnia in HIV disease. *Journal of the Association of Nurses in AIDS Care* September/October 1999;10(5):93–97

Portenoy RK: Opioid therapy for non-malignant pain. In Fields HL and Liebeskind JC, eds. *Pharamcological approaches to the treatment of chronic pain: new concepts and critical issues. Progress in pain research and management,* Vol. I. Seattle: IASP Press, 1994.

Portenoy RK, Thaler HT, Kornblith AB, LePore JM, et al. The Memorial symptom assessment scale: an instrument for the evaluation of symptom prevalence, characteristics and distress. *European J of Cancer* 1994;30A:1326–36.

Price, DM et al. Staff burnout in the perspective of grief theory. *Death Education* 1984; 8:47–58.

Puckett, PJ et al. Who supports you when your patient dies? *RN* October 1996: 48–52.

Puchalski CM. Et al FICA: a spiritual assessment, *J of Palliative Care*, 1999. (in press).

Rando, TA. *Treatment of Complicated Mourning.* Champaign, Illinois: Research Press, 1993.

Reidy, M. AIDS and the Death of a Child. *Grief and AIDS* 1995; Ch.12:181–210.

Rosenfeld, B et al. Pain in Ambulatory AIDS Patients. II. Impact of Pain on Psychological Functioning and Quality of Life. *PAIN* 1996; 68:323–28.

Rabkin JG, Wagner GJ, Rabkin R Testosterone therapy for human immunodeficiency virus-positive men with and without hypogonadism. *J Clin Psychopharmacol.* 1999; 19(1): 19–27.

Russell, GC. The Role of Denial in Clinical Practice. *Journal of Advanced Nursing* 1993; 18:938–40.

Sarna L, van Servellen G, Padilla G, and Brecht ML. Quality of life in women with symptomatic HIV/AIDS. *J Advanced Nursing,* 1999; 30(3):597–605.

Saunders C. Terminal patient care. *Geriatrics.* 1996; 21(12):70–4.

Sendi PP et al. Estimating AIDS-free survival in a severely immunosuppressed asymptomatic HIV-infected population in the era of antiretroviral triple combination therapy. *JAIDS* 1999; 20:376–381.

XII

Sherr, L. The Experience of Grief — Psychological Aspects of Grief in AIDS and HIV Infection. *Grief and AIDS* 1995; CH 1:1–26 2.

Sims R. and Moss VA. *Palliative Care for People with AIDS*, 2nd ed. Edward Arnold, London, 1995.

Singer E. Painful symptoms reported by ambulatory HIV-infected men in a longitudinal study. *PAIN* 1993;54:15–19.

Sowell, RL et al. Quality of life in HIV-infected women in the south-eastern United States. *AIDS Care* 1997; 9(5):501-1.

Sowell, RL. Stories of Violence and Shame. *Journal of the Association of Nurses in AIDS Care* July/August 1999; 10(4)15–16.

Standards and Accreditation Committee, 1995–1996. *A Pathway for patients and families facing terminal illness.* Arlington, VA: National Hospice Organization, 1997.

Standards and Accreditation Committee: Medical Guidelines Task Force. *Medical Guidelines for Determining Prognosis in Selected Non–Cancer Diseases.* Arlington VA: National Hospice Organization, 1996.

Teguis, A. Dying with AIDS. *Living and Dying With AIDS* 1992 Ch 9:153–177.

Torres RA and Barr M. Impact of combination therapy for HIV infection on inpatient census. *NEJM* 1997; 336:1531–1532.

van Servellen, G. Women with HIV: Living with symptoms. *Western Journal of Nursing Research* 1998; 20(4):448–64.

Weissman, DF & Haddox, JD. Opioid Pseudoaddiction: An Iatrogenic Syndrome. *Pain* 1989; 36:363–66.

Weissman, DE. A Survey of Competencies and Concerns in End-of-Life Care for Physician Trainees. *Journal of Pain and Symptom Management* February 1998; 15(2)82-90.

Whalen, CC et al. An Index of Symptoms for Infection with Human Immunodeficiency Virus: Reliability and Validity. *J Clin Epidemiol* 1994; 47(5):537–46.

Woodruff, R. *Palliative Medicine: symptomatic and supportive care for patients with advanced cancer and AIDS.* Victoria, Australia: Asperula Pty. Ltd, 1999.

World Health Organization. Symptom Management. Geneva: W.H.O., 1998.

Wu AW, Hays RD, Kelly S, Malitz F, and Bozette SA. Applications of the Medical Outcomes Study health-related quality of life measures in HIV/AIDS. *Quality of Life Res* 1997; 6:531–554.

Zakrzewska, JM. Women as dental patients: Are there any gender differences? *International Dental Journal* 1996; 46(6)548–57.

XIII: OCCUPATIONAL EXPOSURE

Rani Lewis, MD

I. INTRODUCTION

The risk of HIV transmission to medical personnel has been recognized since 1984, with the first reported case of HIV transmitted to a health care worker (HCW) following needle stick injury. (Anon, 1984) Since that time, information regarding occupational exposure and outcomes has been collected. As of October, 1998 , there have been 187 reported cases in the medical literature of HIV transmission in the United States (CDC, 1998a) and 264 cases worldwide (Ippolito, 1999), presumably related to occupational exposure. A HCW is defined as any person whose activities involve contact with patients or with blood and/or body fluid from patients in a health care setting or laboratory setting. An exposure is defined as a percutaneous injury (needlestick or other cut with a sharp object), mucous membrane or nonintact skin (e.g., chapped or abraded skin, dermatitis), or prolonged contact and/or contact involving an extensive area with blood, tissue, or certain other body fluids. Table 13-1 list types of exposure that yield a significant health care risk for HIV transmission. Table 13-2 lists body fluids with their relative relationship to risk to exposure. Table 13-3 lists the occupations of people who have been suspected of infection from occupational exposure. When possible, biomolecular assays, including nucleic acid sequencing, have been used to determine the similarity in viral strain between the infected HCW and the possible source. (Diaz, 1999)

TABLE 13-1: TYPES OF EXPOSURE ASSOCIATED WITH TRANSMISSION[1]	

Percutaneous	■ Needle stick
	   ● Diameter of needle
	   ● Visible contamination of device
	   ● Placement of needle[2]
	   ● Emergency situation
	■ Sharp object

Skin	■ Non-intact skin
	   ● Abraded
	   ● Chapped
	■ Mucous membrane
	■ Intact skin[3]
	■ Other[3]

[1] Not all these modes of exposure are associated with a significant transmission risk requiring PEP	
[2] Involving needles that had been placed in an artery or vein of the index patient	
[3] There is a theoretical but undocumented risk to HCW from saliva, tears and amniotic fluid, and with intact skin	

XIII

TABLE 13-2: Body Fluids and Risk of Exposure Requiring PEP

High Risk of Transmission	Poorly Defined Risk of Transmission	Low Risk*
■ Blood, serum ■ Semen ■ Sputum, phlegm ■ Vaginal Secretions	■ Amniotic Fluid ■ Cerebrospinal Fluid ■ Pleural Fluid ■ Peritoneal Fluid ■ Pericardial Fluid ■ Synovial Fluid	■ Cervical Mucous ■ Emesis ■ Feces ■ Saliva ■ Sweat ■ Tears ■ Urine

* Unless visibly contaminated with blood.

Source: CDC. Public Health Service Guidelines for the Management of Health-Care Worker Exposures to HIV and Recommendations for Postexposure Prophylaxis. MMWR 47(RR-7):2-3, 1998.

TABLE 13-3: U. S. Health Care Workers with Documented and Possible Occupationally Acquired HIV Infection and AIDS, Reported Through June 1998

Occupation	Documented	Possible
Dental Workers		6
Embalmer/Morgue Technician	1	2
Emergency Medical Technician/Paramedic		12
Health aide/attendant	1	14
Housekeeper/maintenance worker	1	12
Laboratory technician (clinical)	16	16
Laboratory technician (nonclinical)	3	
Nurse	22	33
Physician (nonsurgical)	6	11
Physician (surgical)		6
Respiratory therapist	1	2
Technician (dialysis)	1	3
Technician (surgical)	2	2
Technician/therapist other than above		10
Other health care occupations		4
Total	**54**	**133**

Source: CDC-NCHSTP- Division of HIV/AIDS Prevention, Fact Sheet-Preventing Occupational HIV Transmission to Health Care Workers

In 1995, the Centers for Disease Control and Prevention (CDC) published a report of known cases of occupational exposure in France, the United Kingdom, and the United States. (CDC, 1995) This retrospective case-control study gave improved information regarding risk factors for transmission. An important finding in this document was that post-exposure prophylaxis (PEP) with zidovudine (ZDV) was associated with an overall 79% reduction in transmission with the use of ZDV (OR=0.21, 95% CI of 0.06–0.57) decrease in the risk of seroconversion. This prompted the formation of a United States Public Health Service interagency working group, comprised of members from the CDC, the Food and Drug Administration, the Health Resources and Services Administration, the National Institutes of Health and other expert consultants, who developed guidelines for the use of PEP for HCWs after occupational HIV exposure; these recommendations were updated in 1997. (CDC, 1996; CDC, 1998b) (Table 13-4)

This chapter will review risk factors for transmission and the magnitude of risk for HIV transmission from an occupational exposure, prevention of exposures, and post-exposure management, including PEP with antiretroviral medications.

TABLE 13-4: BASIC AND EXPANDED POSTEXPOSURE PROPHYLAXIS REGIMENS

REGIMEN CATEGORY	APPLICATION	DRUG REGIMEN
Basic	Occupation HIV exposure for which there is a recognized transmission risk[1]	4 weeks (28 days) of both zidovudine 600 mg every day in divided doses (i.e., 300 mg twice a day, 200 mg three times a day, **or** 100 mg every 4 hours) **and** lamivudine 150 mg twice a day
Expanded	Occupational HIV exposures that pose an increased risk for transmission (e.g. larger volume of blood and/or higher virus titer in blood)[1]	Basic regimen plus **either** indinavir 800 mg every 8 hours **or** nelfinavir 750 mg three times a day[2]

[1] See Figure 1 for further delineation of transmission risks

[2] Indinavir should be taken on an empty stomach (i.e., without food or with a light meal) and with increased fluid consumption (i.e., drinking six 8 oz glasses of water throughout the day); nelfinavir can be taken with or without meals.

Source: CDC. Public Health Service Guidelines for the Management of Health-Care Worker Exposures to HIV and Recommendations for Postexposure Prophylaxis. *MMWR* 47(RR-7):1-33, 1998

XIII

Figure 13-1: Determining the Need for HIV Postexposure Prophylaxis (PEP) After an Occupational Exposure[1]

STEP ONE: DETERMINE THE EXPOSURE CODE (EC)

Is the source material blood, bloody fluid, other potentially infectious material (OPIM),[2] or an instrument contaminated with one of these substances?

Yes → OPIM[3] / Blood or bloody fluid

No → No PEP needed

What type of exposure has occurred?

- Mucous membrane or skin, integrity compromised[4] → Volume
- Intact skin only[5] → No PEP needed
- Percutaneous exposure → Severity

Volume:

- **Small** (e.g., few drops, short duration) → **EC 1**
- **Large** (e.g., several drops, major blood splash and/or longer duration [i.e., several minutes or more]) → **EC 2**

Severity:

- **Less severe** (e.g., solid needle, superficial scratch) → **EC 2**
- **More severe** (e.g., large-bore hollow needle, deep puncture, visible blood on device, or needle used in source patient's artery or vein)[6] → **EC 3**

STEP TWO: DETERMINE THE HIV STATUS CODE (HIV SC)

What is the HIV status of the exposure source?

- HIV negative[7] → No PEP needed
- HIV positive[8]
  - **Lower titer exposure** (e.g., asymptomatic and high CD4 count[9]) → **HIV SC1**
  - **Higher titer exposure** (e.g., advanced AIDS, primary HIV infection, high or increasing viral load or low CD4 count[9]) → **HIV SC2**
- Status unknown / Source unknown → **HIV SC Unknown**

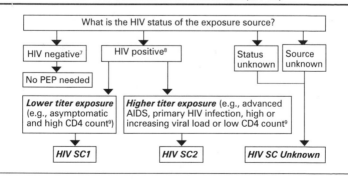

FIGURE 13-1: DETERMINING THE NEED FOR HIV POSTEXPOSURE PROPHYLAXIS (PEP) AFTER AN OCCUPATIONAL EXPOSURE *(continued)*

STEP THREE: DETERMINE THE PEP RECOMMENDATION

EC	HIV SC	PEP RECOMMENDATION
1	1	**PEP may not be warranted.** Exposure type does not pose a known risk for HIV transmission. Whether the risk for drug toxicity outweighs the benefit of PEP should be decided by the exposed HCW and treating clinician.
1	2	**Consider basic regimen.**[10] Exposure type poses a negligible risk for HIV transmission. A high HIV titer in the source may justify consideration of PEP. Whether the risk for drug toxicity outweighs the benefit of PEP should be decided by the exposed HCW and treating clinician.
2	1	**Recommend basic regimen.** Most HIV exposures are in this category; no increased risk for HIV transmission has been observed but use of PEP is appropriate.
2	2	**Recommend expanded regimen.**[11] Exposure type represents an increased HIV transmission risk.
3	1 or 2	**Recommend expanded regimen.** Exposure type represents an increased HIV transmission risk.
Unknown		If the source or, in the case of an unknown source, the setting where the exposure occurred suggests a possible risk for HIV exposure and the EC is 2 or 3, consider PEP basic regimen.

[1] This algorithm is intended to guide initial decisions about PEP and should be used in conjunction with other guidance provided in this report.

[2] Semen or vaginal secretions; cerebrospinal, synovial, pleural, peritoneal, pericardial, or amniotic fluids; or tissue.

[3] Exposures to OPIM must be evaluated on a case-by-case basis. In general, these body substances are considered a low risk for transmission in health-care settings. Any unprotected contact to concentrated HIV in a research laboratory or production facility is considered an occupational exposure that requires clinical evaluation to determine the need for PEP.

[4] Skin integrity is considered compromised if there is evidence of chapped skin, dermatitis, abrasion, or open wound.

[5] Contact with intact skin is not normally considered a risk fore HIV transmission. HOwever, if the exposure was to blood, and the circumstance suggests a higher volume exposure (e.g., and extensive area of skin was exposed or there was prolonged contact with blood), the risk for HIV transmission should be considered.

[6] The combination of these severity factors (e.g., large-bore hollow needle and deep puncture) contribute to an elevated risk for transmission if the source person is HIV-positive.

[7] A source is considered negative for HIV infection if there is laboratory documentation of a negative HIV antibody, HIV polymerase chain reaction (PCR), or HIV p24 antigen test result from a specimen collected at or near the time of exposure and there is no clinical evidence of recent retroviral-like illness.

[8] A source is considered infected with HIV (HIV-positive) is there has been a positive laboratory result fore HIV antibody, HIV PCR, or HIV p24 antigen or physician-diagnosed AIDS.

[9] Examples are used as surrogates to estimate the HIV titer in an exposure source for purposes of considering PEP regimens and do not reflect all clinical situations that may be observed. Although a high HIV titer (HIV SC 2) in an exposure source has been associated with an increased risk for transmission, the possibility of transmission from a source with a low HIV titer also must be considered.

[10] Basic regimen is four weeks of zidovudine, 600 mg per day in two or three divided doses, and lamivudine, 150 mg twice daily.

[11] Expanded regimen is the basic regimen plus either indinavir, 800 mg every 8 hours, or nelfinavir, 750 mg three times a day.

Source: CDC. Public Health Service Guidelines for the Management of Health-Care Worker Exposures to HIV and Recommendations for Postexposure Prophylaxis. *MMWR* 47(RR-7):2-3, 1998.

XIII

II. MAGNITUDE OF RISK

Correct estimation of the likelihood of transmission following occupational exposure is limited by the relative infrequency with which HIV transmission to HCWs is reported. In addition, the retrospective nature of this reporting leads to an increased potential for invalid analysis of the risks. There have been prospective and retrospective reviews of all published cases that implicate occupational exposure. The most complete prospective study performed on data from the United States estimates that the risk of HIV transmission following occupational exposure via single needle stick injury is 0.03%. (Bell, 1997) This is compared to a risk of approximately 30% for hepatitis B transmission after percutaneous exposure to HbeAg-positive blood (Alter, 1976; Grady, 1978) and 1.8%–10% infection with hepatitis C after accidental percutaneous exposure to an HCV-positive source. (Alter, 94; Puro, 1995; Mitsui, 1992) Ippolito, et al, reviewed the world literature on occupational exposure from an HIV seropositive source, and determined risk to be approximately 0.09% following a mucocutaneous exposure. (Ippolito, 1993) As noted in Table 13-2, the risk from skin exposure or exposure to body fluids/tissues other than blood has not been clearly defined. Risk of HIV transmission increases with multiple exposures and with presence of risk factors listed below.

III. RISK FACTORS FOR OCCUPATIONAL HIV TRANSMISSION

The likelihood of HIV infection following exposure is affected by the presence of certain risk factors. Cardo, et al, performed a case-control study of internationally gathered cases of percutaneous exposure of HCW in an attempt to determine factors that increased or decreased the risk of transmission. (Cardo, 1997) (See Tables 11-5 and 11-6) Their data indicate that HCW's who took AZT after potential exposure had an 81% lower risk of becoming infected (95% CI 48–94 %) not take this medication.

In general risk factors include:

- **type of contact or exposure** — Exposure has been classified into several risk categories (Table 13-1), including percutaneous, mucocutaneous, and intact skin contact, with different risks of transmission.

- **quantity of blood** — Exposure to larger quantities of blood from an HIV source, as indicated by a deep needlestick, exposure to needle placed directly into a vessel, or visible blood on the injuring device is associated with an increased risk of transmission. While the rates of transmission have been best studied regarding the use of large bore needles (< 18 gauge), suture needles appear to have a comparable rate of transmission (P=0.08). (Alter, 1976)

- **disease status of source patient** — Exposure to blood from patients with terminal illness increases risk. This likely reflects risk associated with exposure to higher levels of virus in blood (higher viral loads). HIV-RNA level has been shown to be a significant factor in the risk of perinatal transmission. Individuals with acute HIV infection also have very high HIV-RNA levels and probably represent an increased risk of transmission if occupational exposure occurs. HCW seroconversion has been reported after exposure to an HIV-infected patient with undetectable viral load. (CDC, 1998b) Other factors often present in late-stage disease, such as more virulent syncytia-inducing HIV strains, may also increased risk.

■ **host defenses** — There is some limited evidence that the immune response of the HCW may effect the risk of transmission. (Pinto, 1997) Pinto, et al, demonstrated an HIV-specific cytotoxic T-lymphocyte (CTL) response among HIV exposed but uninfected HCWs, when the peripheral blood mononuclear cells were stimulated in vitro by HIV mitogens. Along with similar responses seen in other groups with repeated exposure without infection, this suggests the possibility that the host immune response may be able to prevent establishment of HIV infection after exposure.

■ **post-exposure prophylaxis** — The data of Cardo, et al, confirm the efficacy of PEP in limiting the risk of HIV transmission to HCW's. Several cases reports of transmission in the setting of prompt initiation of PEP, however, indicates that this therapy is not 100% effective. There are greater than 14 known cases of zidovudine PEP failure following HCW exposure around the world. (Jochimsen, 1997) HIV resistance to zidovudine or delay in initiation of medication has been hypothesized to play a role in these (and other, non-HCW) prophylaxis failures.

TABLE 13-5: LOGISTIC -REGRESSION ANALYSIS OF RISK FACTORS FOR HIV TRANSMISSION AFTER PERCUTANEOUS EXPOSURE TO HIV-INFECTED BLOOD

	U.S. CASES[1]	ALL CASES[2]
RISK FACTOR	ADJUSTED ODDS RATIO (95% CI)[3]	
Deep injury	13.0 (4.4–42)	15.0 (6/0–41)
Visible blood on device	4.5 (1.4–16)	6.2 (2.2–21)
Procedure involving needle in artery or vein	3.6 (1.3–11)	4.3 (1.7–12)
Terminal illness in source patient[4]	8.5 (2.8–28)	5.6 (2.0–16)
Postexposure use of zidovudine	0.14 (0.03–0.47)	0.19 (0.06–0.52)

[1] All risk factors were significant (P < 0.02)

[2] All risk factors were significant (P < 0.01)

[3] CI denotes confidence interval. Odds ratios are for the odds of seroconversion after exposure in workers with the risk factor as compared with those without it.

[4] Terminal illness was defined as disease leading to death of the source patient from AIDS within two months after the health care worker's exposure.

Source: Cardo DM, Culver DH, Ciesielski CA, et al. *N Engl J Med* 337:1485-90, 1997.

XIII

TABLE 13-6: CHARACTERISTICS OF INJURIES SUSTAINED BY CASE PATIENTS AND CONTROLS

RISK FACTOR	CASE PATIENTS		CONTROLS		CRUDE OR (95% CI)[2]	P[3]
	NUMBER OF PATIENTS	PERCENT WITH RISK FACTOR	NUMBER OF PATIENTS[1]	PERCENT WITH RISK FACTOR		
Large-gauge (< 18) hollow-bore needle	27	15	488	1.2	14.0 (4.9-39)	0.001
Deep Injury	33	52	675	6.8	15.0 (8.0-26)	< 0.001
Visible blood on device	32	84	632	35	10.0 (4.6-23)	< 0.001
Procedure involving needle in artery or vein	33	73	669	31	5.9 (2.9-12)	< 0.001
Emergency procedure	33	12	661	2.4	5.6 (2.0-16)	0.012
Use of gloves	32	78	679	78	1.0 (0.4-2.4)	1.0
AIDS in source patient	33	82	676	70	1.9 (0.8-4.6)	0.18
Terminal illness in source patient[4]	27	48	349	16	4.8 (2.3-10)	< 0.001
Postexposure use of zidovudine	33	27	679	36	0.7 (0.3-1.4)	0.35

[1] The numbers are the number of subjects for whom data were available

[2] CI denotes confidence interval. Odds ratios are for the odds of seroconversion after exposure in workers with the risk factor as compared with those without it

[3] P values were determined by the two-tailed Fisher's exact test.

[4] Terminal illness was defined as disease leading to the death of the source patient from AIDS within two months after the health care worker's exposure.

Source: Cardo DM, Culver DH, Ciesielski CA et al. N Engl J Med 337:1485-90, 1997.

IV. PREVENTION OF OCCUPATIONAL EXPOSURE

Limiting the exposure that a health-care worker has to materials that are potentially infectious is the key to reducing the risks of occupational exposure. Universal precautions, as recommended by the Occupational Safety and Health Act (OSHA), reflects the concept that all blood and body fluids are potentially infectious and must be handled accordingly. Personal protective equipment (Table 13-7) should be used to prevent blood and other potentially infectious material from reaching a HCWs clothing, skin, eyes, mouth, or mucous membranes. (CDC, 1987)

TABLE 13-7: PERSONAL PROTECTIVE EQUIPMENT
■ Gloves
■ Gowns
■ Laboratory coats
■ Face shields
■ Eye protection
■ Mouthpieces
■ Resuscitation bags

Handwashing should be done after touching blood, body fluids or secretions, or contaminated items, whether or not gloves are worn. Hands should also be washed after removing gloves and between patient contacts. Gloves should be worn when in contact with blood or body fluids (including blood drawing), mucous membranes or nonintact skin, or items contaminated with possibly infectious material; it is strongly recommended that gloves should be worn when performing any invasive procedure. Clinicians performing surgery, deliveries, or other invasive procedures likely to generate splashes of blood or other body fluids should wear a mask and eye protection or face shield. The use of double-gloving in surgical procedures has been shown to reduce the risk of direct blood contact for operating room personnel. (Greco, 1995; Konig, 1992) Needles and other sharp instruments should be handled with great care and disposed of in approved sharps containers. As a rule, do not recap, bend or break used needles. During surgery hand-to-hand passage of sharp instruments (e.g. needles, scalpels) should be minimized-give consideration to passing these instruments first onto a surgical tray or pan.

Risk of occupational exposure and need for universal precautions applies not only to physicians, nurses and laboratory workers, but also to medical, nursing, or dental students, and to dentists. Since reports of patient-to-dentist and dentist-to-patient HIV transmission seen in the late 1980's (CDC, 1991a), both the CDC and the American Dental Association have included recommendations regarding the use of barrier precautions in dental settings and sterile technique in the preparation of dental equipment. (American Dental Association, 1988)

Another group at increased but less well-defined risk are emergency medical technicians, paramedics and law enforcement agents. These individuals are frequently in contact with patients of unknown or noncommunicated HIV status, in emergency situations. While 6 of the 133 well documented cases

XIII

occurring in the United States, (.045%) of possible transmission were among dental workers, twice that many transmissions have been reported among emergency workers (12/133, 0.09%), placing this group behind only laboratory technicians and nurses/phlebotomists in risk for occupational transmission. OSHA regulations requiring the availability of face masks, mouth shields and ventilation masks are designed to reduce the risk to emergency technicians and other public safety workers. Given the highly unpredictable nature of their risk for exposure, general infection control measures are recommended, even when the risk appears low. (International Association of Fire Fighters, 1988) Given the prevalence of HIV infection within prison populations, correctional officers are also at increased risk for occupational exposure and should use universal precautions. (Hammett, 1991) Intentional human bites and exposure to saliva are more common in correctional facilities, and may present a risk of infection transmission and should be evaluated appropriately. While Hepatitis B has been transmitted via saliva in cases involving human bites (MacQuarrie, 1974; Cancio-Bello, 1982); in the absence of visible blood in the saliva, exposure to saliva is not considered a risk for HIV transmission. (CDC, 1998b)

V. HIV INFECTION FOLLOWING OCCUPATIONAL EXPOSURE

While limited, there is some information regarding the symptomatology seen in HCW experiencing seroconversion from occupational exposure. Approximately four-fifths of cases were associated with symptoms consistent with primary HIV infection a median of 25 days after exposure . (CDC, 1998b) The average time to seroconversion is 65 days and 95% of infected HCWs have seroconverted within 6 months after exposure. (Busch, 1997) There are rare reported cases of HCW who remain negative for HIV antibody at 6 months, but seroconvert by 12 months after exposure. (Konig, 1992; Ciesielski, 1997) Delayed seroconversion has been associated with simultaneous exposure to hepatitis C in two cases, one of which resulted in fulminant and fatal HCV.(Ridzon, 1997) Further information regarding the effect of coinfection with other viral illnesses remains to be determined.

HCW's presenting for HIV exposure PEP need to be counseled regarding risks of other viral illnesses to which they may have been exposed. Occupational exposure to both Hepatitis B and Hepatitis C virus has been reported. While all three of these viruses have similar routes and modes of exposure, the risk of transmission differs due to the differing prevalence of infection. The probability of a source patient from the general population being HBsAg positive ranges from 5–15%; 6–30% on non-immunized HCW's will become infected following a needlestick injury. (CDC, 1989) HCW's at risk for occupational exposure to hepatitis B should therefore assure appropriate vaccination against this virus. PEP for HBV is available.

Hepatitis C virus is the most common chronic blood borne infection in the United States. The Third National Health and Nutrition Examination Survey (NHANES III) data estimates 3.9 million Americans have been infected with HCV, with 36,000 new infections reported per year. (CDC, 1998c) The average incidence of HCV seroconversion following a single needlestick exposure from an HCV seropositive source is 1.8%. Exposure via mucous membranes, while extremely rare, has been reported. (Sartori, 1993) Of note, there is no vaccine or immunoglobulin available for HCV PEP.

VI. POST-EXPOSURE MANAGEMENT

Health care organizations are required to have exposure-control plans, including postexposure management and follow-up for employees at risk. The Occupational Safety and Health Administration mandates reporting of exposure incidents.

A. MANAGEMENT OF THE SITE OF EXPOSURE

Wounds/puncture sites should be washed with soap and water; mucous membranes exposed should be flushed with water. The application of bleach to skin or mucosal surfaces is not recommended.

B. EVALUATION OF THE EXPOSURE

The type of body fluid involved, type of exposure (e.g., percuaneous, mucosal, intact skin, etc), and the severity of the exposure (quantity of blood, duration of contact, etc) should be evaluated and will affect decisions about PEP. (See Table 13-1)

C. EVALUATION OF SOURCE PATIENT

The source individual of the exposure should be evaluated for possible HIV infection and , if status is unknown, should be tested, after appropriate consent. Past medical information, such as past HIV test results, clinical signs, symptoms, or diagnoses, and history of risk exposures (e.g., injection drug use, etc) may be relevant in making initial decisions regarding PEP. The use of rapid HIV testing , if available, may be particularly useful in the setting of occupational exposure. Initiation of PEP, if indicate, should not be delayed while awaiting test results. If the source is known to be HIV infected, information about clinical stage of infection, recent CD4 counts, viral load testing, and antiretroviral treatment history are important in choosing an appropriate PEP regimen; however, initiation of PEP should not be delayed if this information is not immediately available.

XIII

The source patient should also be tested for anti-HCV and HbsAg to assess risk to the HCW for hepatitis B and C.

D. BASELINE AND FOLLOW-UP TESTING

Baseline testing for HIV antibody should be performed to establish serostatus at the time of exposure and should be repeated at 6 weeks, 12 weeks, and 6 months postexposure, regardless of the use of PEP. An extended duration of follow-up may be considered with simultaneous exposure to HCV or use of HAART regimens for PEP because of theoretical concerns about delay in HIV seroconversion in this situations. Pregnancy testing should be offered to HCWs of reproductive age if pregnancy status is unknown.

In addition to HIV, hepatitis B and C are significant concerns from occupational exposures. For the HCW exposed to an HCV-positive source, baseline and follow-up testing (at 4–6 months) for anti-HCV and serum alanine aminotransferase is recommended. Confirmation by a supplemental assay (such as recombinant immunoblot assay) is recommended for all positive anti-HCV results by enzyme immunoassay. (CDC, 1998b)

If the HCW has previously received HBV vaccine and anti-HBsAg level, which reflects vaccine-induced protection, is unknown, this should be tested ; if inadequate, HBIG is recommended, as well as a booster dose of vaccine.

E. COUNSELING OF THE HCW

■ Decisions regarding appropriate post-exposure management should be individualized; the HCW should be counseled about their personal risk based on considerations outlined above, and recommendations made re: initiation of PEP

■ The HCW should be informed that knowledge about the effectiveness and the toxicity of the antiretroviral drugs used for PEP is limited; only ZDV has been shown to reduce the risk of HIV transmission in occupational settings to date and failures of ZDV prophylaxis have been reported. (Jochimsen, 1997) The addition of other antiretroviral drugs to a PEP regimen is based on the superiority of combination antiretroviral regimens over monotherapy in the treatment of HIV-infected individuals and the theoretical considerations regarding possible resistance concerns and the utility of using drugs having activity at different stages in the viral replication cycle.

■ The medical history of the HCW , including medications, presence or possibility of pregnancy, or other medical conditions should be obtained and may influence decisions/recommendations about PEP, including choice of regimen

■ A specific PEP regimen should be recommended, when indicated, and the rationale for its selection should be discussed. (See Table 13-4) Information should be given about how to take the medications; potential side effects and measures to minimize these; possible drug-drug interactions with recommended regimen and any medications that should not be taken while taking PEP; clinical monitoring for toxicity; and symptoms that should prompt immediate evaluation (such as back or abdominal pain or blood in the urine, possibly suggesting renal stones in those on indinavir). The importance of adherence should be emphasized.

■ PEP may be declined by the HCW.

■ The HCW should be urged to seek medical evaluation with the development of any acute illness during the follow-up period. The differential diagnosis in this situation must include acute HIV infection, drug reaction, toxicity from the PEP regimen, or other medical illness.

■ Measures to reduce the risk of possible secondary transmission during follow-up (especially in the 6–12 weeks after exposure) should be discussed and recommended. These include use of condoms or abstinence to prevent sexual transmission and pregnancy; refrain from donation of blood, plasma, tissue or organs ; and , in lactating mothers, consideration of discontinuation of breastfeeding.

■ There is no need to modify clinical responsibilities based on HIV exposure.

■ Each HCW should be given a contact name and/or number to call with concerns or questions.

■ HBV prophylaxis: If the patient source of exposure is HbsAg positive and the HCW has not been vaccinated, hepatitis B vaccination should be initiated and a single dose of hepatitis B immune globulin (HBIG) should be administered as soon as possible after exposure and within 24 hours if possible. If the source patient is HbsAg negative and the HCW has not been vaccinated against HBV, vaccination should be initiated. (CDC, 1991b)

F. POST-EXPOSURE PROPHYLAXIS

The decision regarding which and how many antiretroviral agents to use is largely empiric. Current recommendations are to use a two- or three-drug regimen based on level of HIV transmission risk and possibility of drug resistance (See Table 13-4) . PEP should be initiated as soon as possible following exposure, and continued for 4 weeks. The HIV Postexposure Prophylaxis (PEP) Registry demonstrated no specific adverse events associated with HIV PEP in HCW's; The registry was closed in December, 1998. Information regarding this program can be obtained through the CDC's Hospital Infections Program (404-639-6425) or on the internet.(URLaddress: **http://www.cdc.gov/ncidod/hip/Blood/PEPRegistry**)

Fifty to ninety percent of HCW receiving PEP (ZDV or combination of agents) report subjective side effects and these have led to discontinuation of therapy in 24–36% of cases. (CDC, 1998b) Common side effects in those on ZDV include nausea, vomiting, fatigue, headache, and insomnia. Serious side effects, including renal stones and pancytopenia have been reported with combination PEP regimens. For more details about side effects with different antiretroviral agents, see Chapter XIV on Pharmocology. Laboratory monitoring

XIII

should include a complete blood count , renal and hepatic function tests at baseline and 2 weeks after initiation of PEP; more in-depth testing may be indicated based on underlying medical conditions or specific toxicity associated with drugs in PEP regimen (e.g., glucose testing if on a protease inhibitor).

VII. SPECIAL CONSIDERATIONS

A. ANTIRETROVIRAL RESISTANCE

It is unclear whether or how antiretroviral resistance influences risk of HIV transmission. Transmission of drug-resistant strains has been reported, (Imrie, 1997) and therefore is a possible concern in PEP situations. If resistance of the source patient's virus to one or more of the drugs in the PEP regimen is known or suspected, drugs should be selected to include agents to which the virus is likely to be sensitive. Clinical consultation with an expert in HIV treatment should be obtained for guidance in this situation. However, it is important to avoid delay in starting PEP because of resistance concerns; if resistance is known or suspected a third or fourth drug may be included in the regimen until consultation is obtained.

B. PREGNANT HCW

In addition to the counseling issues noted above, the pregnant HCW should be informed about what is known and not known about potential risks, benefits, and side effects for the fetus and herself related to the antiretroviral agents used in PEP. (Issues relating to the use of antiretroviral drugs in pregnancy are discussed in Chapter VII on HIV and Reproduction, and in Chapter XIV on Pharmacology.) PEP should not be denied on the basis of pregnancy and pregnancy should not prevent the use of an optimal PEP regimen. For breastfeeding HCWs, temporary discontinuation of breastfeeding should be considered while on PEP to avoid infant exposure to these drugs.

VIII. THE HIV SEROPOSITIVE HCW

There has been great controversy about HCWs who are infected with HIV and continue to work. The infection of several patients by an HIV seropositive dentist is well known although poorly understood. However, in four separate studies involving a total of 896 surgical and dental patients exposed to HIV infected providers, only one patient was found to be HIV seropositive and this individual had other risk factors for HIV. (CDC, 1991c) Health care workers with HIV may also themselves be at risk for contracting a communicable disease; appropriate precautions should be taken and appropriate immunizations given.

All clinicians with exudative or transudative skin lesions should refrain from direct patient care until these lesions have healed. It is believed that

HIV-positive HCWs who follow universal precautions and do not perform invasive procedures pose no risk to their patients. Furthermore, there are no current data suggesting that HIV-positive HCWs performing non-exposure-prone invasive procedures should have their practice restricted, assuming they use universal precautions, appropriate technique, and adequate sterilization and disinfection of instruments.

"Exposure-prone" procedures require more consideration. Exposure-prone characteristics include digital palpation of a needle point in a body cavity or the simultaneous presence of the HCWs fingers and a needle or sharp instrument in a poorly visualized or highly confined anatomic space. These procedures are associated with increased risk for percutaneous injury to the HCW and potential increased risk to the patient. It is recommended that all HCWs who perform these procedures know their HIV status. HIV-positive HCWs performing exposure-prone procedures should seek counsel from an expert review panel on a case-by-case basis. Mandatory testing of HCWs in not recommended. The ethics of patient notification of exposure to an HIV-infected HCW continues to be argued. (Blatchford, 2000; Donnelly, 1999)

It is imperative that institutions have a standard policy on the management of HIV-infected HCWs, as well as policies on the management of a HCW potentially infected by a patient. (CDC, 1991c)

REFERENCES

Alter MJ. Occupational exposure to hepatitis C virus: a dilemma. *Infect Control Hosp Epidemiol* 15:742–4, 1994

Alter HJ, Seef LB, Kaplan PM et al. Type B hepatitis: the infectivity of blood positive for re antigen and DNA polymerase after accidental needlestick exposure. *NEJM* 295: 909–913, 1976

American Dental Association. Infection control recommendations for the dental office and the dental laboratory. *J Am Dent Assoc* 116:241–8, 1988

Anonymous. Needlestick transmission of HTLV-III from a patient infected in Africa. *Lancet* 2:1376–7, 1984

Bell DM. Occupational risk of human immunodeficiency virus infection in healthcare workers: an overview. *Am J Med* 102(suppl 5B):9–15, 1997

Blatchford O, O'Brien SJ, Blatchford M, Taylor A. Infectious health care workers: should patients be told? *J Med Ethics.* 26(1):27–33, 2000

Busch MP, Satten GA. Time course of viremia and antibody seroconversion following human immunodeficiency virus exposure. *Am J Med* 102(suppl 5B):117–124, 1997

Cancio-Bello TP, de Medina M, Shorey J, Valledor MD, Schiff ER. An institutional outbreak of hepatits B related to a human biting carrier. *J Infect Dis* 146:652–6, 1982

Cardo DM, Culver DH, Ciesielski CA Srivastava PU, Marcus R, Abiteboul D, Heptonstall J, Ippolito G, Lot F, McKibber PS, Bell DM, and the Centers for Disease Control and Prevention Needlestick Surveillance Group. *N Engl J Med* 337:1485–90, 1997

XIII

Ciesielski CA, Metler RP. Duration of time between exposure and seroconversion in healthcare workers with occupationally acquired infection with human immunodeficiency virus. *Am J Med* 102(suppl 5B):115–6, 1997

CDC. Recommendations for Prevention of HIV Transmission in Health-Care Settings. *MMWR* 36(suppl 2S):1–16, Aug 21, 1987

CDC. Guidlines for Prevention of Transmission of Human Immunodeficiency Virus and Hepatitis B Virus to Health-Care and Public Safety Workers. *MMWR* 38(suppl 6):1–37, June 23, 1989

CDC. Epidemiologic Notes and Reports Update: Transmission of HIV Infection during an Invasive Dental Procedure — Florida.. *MMWR* 40(2):21–27, Jan 18, 1991a

CDC. Hepatitis B virus: A comprehensive strategy for eliminatng transmission in the United States through universal childhood vaccination: recommendations of the ACIP. Appendix A: Postexposure prophylaxis for hepatitis B. *MMWR* 40 (RR-13):21–25, 1991b

CDC, Recommendations for Preventing Transmission of Human Immunodeficiency Virus and Hepatitis B Virus to Patients During Exposure-prone Procedures. *MMWR* 40(RR-08); 1–9, 1991c)

CDC. Case-control study of HIV seroconversion in health-care workers after percutaneous exposure to HIV-infected blood France, United Kingdom, and United States, January 1988–August 1994. *MMWR* 44:929–33, 1995

CDC. Update: Provisional Public Health Service recommendations for chemoprophylaxis after occupational exposure to HIV. *MMWR* 45(22):468–72, 1996

CDC/National Center for HIV, STD and TB Prevention, *Fact Sheet*, October 1998a

CDC. Public Health Service guidelines for the management of health-care worker exposures to HIV and recommendations for postexposure prophylaxis. *MMWR* 47(RR-7):1–34, 1998b

CDC. Recommendations for prevention and control of hepatitis C virus (HCV) infection and HCV-related chronic disease. *MMWR* 47 (RR-19):1–39, Oct 16,1998c

Diaz RS, De Oliveira CF, Pardini R, Operskalski E, Mayer AJ, Busch MP. HIV type 1 tat gene heteroduplex mobility assay as a tool to establish epidemiologic relationships among HIV type 1-infected individuals. *AIDS Res and Hum Retroviruses* 15(13): 1151–6, 1999

Donnelly M, Duckworth G, Nelson S, Wehner H, Gill N, Nazareth B, Cummins A. Are HIV lookbacks worthwhile? Outcome of an exercise to notify patients treated by an HIV infected health care worker. *Commun Dis Public Health.* 2(2):126–9, 1999

Grady GF, Lee VÁ, Prince AM et al. Hepatitis B immune globulin for accidental exposures among medical personnel: final report of a multicenter controlled trial. *J Infect Dis* 138:625–38), 1978

Greco RJ, Garza JR. Use of double gloves to protect the surgeon from blood contact during aesthetic procedures. *Aesthetic Plast Surg* 19:265–267, 1995

Hammett TM. 1990 update: AIDS in correctional facilities. Washington; U.S. Department of Justice, 1991.

Imrie A, Beveridge A, Genn W, Vizzard J, Cooper DA, the Sydney Primary HIV Infection Study Group. Transmission of human immunodeficiency virus type 1 resistant to nevirapine and zidovudine. *J Infect Dis* 175: 1502–6, 1997

International Association of Fire Fighters. *Guidelines to prevent transmission of communicable disease during emergency care for firefighters, paramedics, and emergency medical technicians.* International Association of Fire Fighters, New York City, New York, 1988.

Ippolito G, Puro V., De Carli G, the Italian Study Group on Occupational Risk of HIV Infection. The risk of occupational human immunodeficiency virus infection in health care workers: Italian multicenter study. *Arch Intern Med* 153:1451–8, 1993

Ippolito G, Puro V, Heptonstall J, Jagger J, De Carli G, Petrosillo N. Occupational Human Immunodeficiency Virus Infection in Health Care Workers: Worldwide Cases Through September 1997. *Clin Infectious Dis* 28:365–83, 1999

Jochimsen EM. Failures of zidovudine postexposure prophylaxis. *Am J Med* 102(suppl 5B):52–55, 1997

Konig M, Bruha M, Hirsch HA. Perforation of surgical gloves in gynecologic operations and abdominal Cesarean section. *Geburtshilfe Frauenheilkd* 52:109–112, 1992

MacQuarrie MD, Forghani B, Wolochow DA. Hepatitis B transmitted by a human bite. *JAMA* 230:723–4, 1974

Mitsui T, Iwano K, Masuko K et al. Hepatitis C virus infection in medical personnel after needlestick accident. *Hepatology* 16:1109–14, 1992

Pinto LA, Landay AL, Berzofsky JA, Kessler HA, Shearer GM. Immune response to human immunodeficiency virus (HIV) in healthcare workers occupationally exposed to HIV-contaminated blood. *Am J Med* 102(suppl 5B):21–4, 1997

Puro V, Petrosillo N, Ippolito G. Italian Study Group on Occupational Risk of HIV and Other Bllodborne Infections. Risk of hepatitis C seroconversion after occupational exposures in health care workers. *Am J Infect Control* 23:273–7, 1995

Ridzon R, Gallager K, Ciesielski C, Mast EE, Ginsberg MB, Robertson BJ, Luo CC, DeMaria A. Simultaneous Transmission of Human Immunodeficiency Virus and Hepatitis C Virus from a Needle-Stick Injury. *N Engl J Med* 336:919–22, 1997

Sartori M, La Terra G, Aglietta M, Manzin A, Navino C, Verzetti G. Transmission of hepatitis C via blood splash into conjunctiva [letter]. *JAMA* 25:270–1, 1993

XIII

This *Guide* is a PRELIMINARY EDITION.

We need YOUR HELP to make the NEXT EDITION as useful as possible!

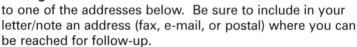

Please send your
comments
criticisms
corrections
suggested changes, and
other guidance
to one of the addresses below. Be sure to include in your letter/note an address (fax, e-mail, or postal) where you can be reached for follow-up.

Translation Partners Needed

Write to us if you can help us find partners to help us have this *Guide* translated into your native language. For instance, provide us with a contact who works with translation in your country's Ministry of Health, or tell us about a group at a medical school that translates medical texts.

Send Us Your Comments

E-mail: womencare@hrsa.gov

Fax to the attention of "Womencare": 301-443-0791 (USA)

Postal address: Womencare
Parklawn Building, Room 11A-33
5600 Fishers Lane
Rockville, Maryland 20857
USA

Note that this and subsequent editions of
A Guide to the Clinical Care of Women with HIV
will be available online.

Go to the HIV/AIDS Bureau Web site
and click on the publication *Women's Guide*:
http://www.hrsa.gov/hab

XIV: PHARMACOLOGIC CONSIDERATIONS IN HIV-INFECTED PREGNANT PATIENTS

Paul Pham, PharmD and Patricia Barditch-Crovo, MD

I. LIST OF TABLES

II. INTRODUCTION

The decision to administer drugs to a pregnant woman is largely based on the therapeutic benefit to the mother and/or fetus versus the perceived risk to the developing fetus. Clinicians are usually advised to avoid prescribing drugs for pregnant patients since human safety data in pregnancy are lacking for many medications. However in some clinical situations the benefits far outweigh the risks. These are important considerations when selecting agents to treat patients with human immunodeficiency virus (HIV), to prevent its transmission, and to prevent associated opportunistic infections.

There is limited information concerning the safety of many antiretrovirals in pregnancy. Mutagenicity and teratogenicity studies in animals are the basis for most safety in pregnancy data. Animals are administered doses 5- to 20-times higher that those given to humans; clinical applicability is not always evident.

It is now standard care to treat for HIV-infected patients with an "antiretroviral cocktail" making it increasingly difficult to assess the safety of a single antiretroviral agent. More prospective clinical data are needed. Clinicians are

XIV

encouraged to report all in utero exposures to The Antiretroviral Pregnancy Registry (1-800-258-4263), a collaborative effort between the National Institutes of Health, Centers for Disease Control and pharmaceutical companies: Outcome data compiled from the Registry are used to monitor birth defects.

The Food and Drug Administration (FDA) has developed a classification system to help clinicians choose agents safe for use in pregnancy. (Tables 14-1, 14-2, 14-3, and 14-6)

III. RISKS OF ANTIRETROVIRAL DRUGS IN PREGNANCY

Certain antiretroviral agents should be avoided during pregnancy, either because of effects inherent to the drug itself, or the potential for dangerous interactions. Administration of efavirenz to pregnant cynomolgus monkeys is associated with anenecephaly, unilateral anophthalmia, microopthalmia and cleft palate in newborns[1]. Hydroxyurea produces mutagenesis and teratogenesis in many animal species; it should not be given during pregnancy[2].

Antiretroviral therapy is often complicated by side effects in relatively healthy HIV-infected nonpregnant adults which could be exacerbated in pregnancy or put the fetus at risk. Protease inhibitors, for example, have been associated with the development of glucose intolerance and even diabetes mellitus. Hyperglycemia in pregnancy leads to increased risk of macrosomia, fetal distress, pre-eclampsia and stillbirth[3]. In patients taking indinavir, 10% develop indirect bilirubinemia (i.e., > 2.5%) and nephrolithiasis has been reported in 5-15%[4]. Any of these adverse effects will complicate a pregnancy.

Because many patients turn to so-called complimentary or alternative therapies, it is important to take a complete medication history, including over-the-counter drugs and nutritional supplements . St John's wort lowers trough indinavir drug concentrations (Cmin) by 81% when administered concurrently [Lancet 2000; 355(9203): 547-8]. Because St John's wort induces cytochrome P450 3A enzymes, it will likely decrease levels of other protease inhibitors and non-nucleoside reverse transcriptase inhibitors. Therefore, St John's wort should not be taken with antiretroviral medications. Since safety data for herbal alternative therapies are scarce, these agents should be avoided during pregnancy. Table 14-6 summarizes data on alternative therapies to avoid during pregnancy.

IV. BENEFITS OF ANTIRETROVIRAL DRUGS IN PREGNANCY: DRUGS TO CONSIDER

One example in which the benefit far outweighs the risk of drug administration during pregnancy is evident in the use of zidovudine (AZT) in preventing perinatal HIV transmission (ACTG study 076)[5]. Administration of AZT to the pregnant HIV-infected mother after the first trimester, during labor, after labor and to the newborn reduced the perinatal acquisition of HIV. In addition, uninfected infants exposed to AZT in this study and followed to a median age of 3.9 years, have not shown a significant difference in growth, neurological development or immune status when compared to uninfected infants exposed to placebo[6]. The use of AZT during pregnancy and delivery has become the standard of care in the United States; however due to its high cost, its administration during pregnancy is not feasible in developing countries.

The HIVNET 012 trial compared the administration of one dose of nevirapine given orally to the mother during labor followed by one dose of nevirapine to the infant within 72 hours after birth to the administration of AZT during labor followed by AZT to the infant for 7 days. The 14-16 week post delivery data showed that while both regimens were well tolerated, 25.1% of infants in the AZT arm and 13.1% of infants in the nevirapine arm were infected with HIV (p=0.0006)[7]. Although long-term safety data are not currently available for nevirapine, this regimen may provide a simple and inexpensive regimen to prevent perinatal transmission of HIV in less developed countries. The current guidelines state that pregnancy per se should not preclude use of optimal therapeutic regimens. Therefore pregnant women should be treated according to standard guidelines for antiretroviral therapy in adults, with sustained reduction of viral load as the primary objective. (*MMWR* 1998; 47[RR-2])

V. PHARMACOKINETICS OF ANTIRETROVIRAL DRUGS IN PREGNANCY

Although many physiologic changes occur during pregnancy, few trials have been conducted to evaluate their clinical significance on the pharmacokinetics of commonly used drugs. Physiologic changes that may affect drug pharmacokinetics include: delayed gastric emptying, decreased intestinal motility, increased volume of distribution (an average increase of 8L), increased renal blood flow (by 25-50%) and glomerular filtration rate (by 50%)[8, 9, 10]. The serum half-life of nevirapine is reduced from 66 hours in non-pregnant women to 45 hours in pregnant women; this decrease is not likely to be clinically significant[11]. Pregnancy does not change the pharmacokinetics of AZT, 3TC and ddI.[12, 13, 14]

The absorption and pharmacokinetics of many of the anti-HIV drugs are affected by food. Table 14-5 lists pertinent food-drug interactions that are probably as valid for pregnant women as for a non-gravid population.

Table 14-1, on the following pages, provides a quick reference on dosing recommendations, FDA Pregnancy Risk Classification, animal teratogenicity and human experience in pregnancy for the most commonly prescribed drugs in the treatment of HIV infection.

XIV

Table 14-1: Antiretrovirals

Drug Name	Dosing	Adverse Effects	FDA Class	Animal Data	Human Experience in Pregnancy	Comments
Nucleoside Reverse Transcriptase Inhibitor (NRTIs)						
Abacavir (Ziagen®)	300 mg bid	Hypersensitivity reaction-fever, rash, fatigue, malaise, GI symptoms and arthralgias (noted in 2-3% of patients). **Mandatory discontinuation with hypersensitivity reaction. Do not rechallenge (2 deaths reported upon rechallenge);** rare cases of lactic acidosis and severe hepatomegaly with steatosis.	C	Rodent studies demonstrated placental passage, anasarca, skeletal malformation at 1000 mg/kg dose (35 times human therapeutic levels) during organogenesis. However rabbits receiving 8.5 times human therapeutic levels did not have fetal malformation.	Based on ex vivo data, placental transfer was 32-66% (Infect Dis Obstet Gynecol, 1998 6 (6): 244-6).	Inadequate data to recommend routine use during pregnancy.
Zidovudine (Retrovir®, AZT)	300 mg po bid, or 200 mg po tid. PACTG protocol dosing: Prenatal: 100 mg 5x per day (alternatively 300 mg twice a day) beginning at weeks 14-34; Intrapartum 2mg/kg IV for first hour then 1mg/kg IV until birth. Infant received 2mg/kg po q6h for the first 6 weeks of life beginning 8-12 hrs after birth	GI intolerance, malaise; headache (in 5-10%); bone marrow suppression (anemia and neutropenia seen more commonly with late stage AIDS); myalgia; myopathy; transaminase elevation; fingernail discoloration; rare cases of lactic acidosis and severe hepatomegaly with steatosis.	C	Rodent studies of doses that resulted in serum levels 350 times higher than levels in humans demonstrated maternal toxicity and fetal malformations. Vaginal squamous tumors seen in 13% of rodents exposed to high dose AZT.	Human studies demonstrated 85% placental passage. No maternal toxicities or fetal defects noted with AZT during pregnancy. Long-term toxicity data (up to 3.9 years) for infants exposed to AZT in utero and post partum did not show an increased risk of adverse effects or developmental abnormalities.	The only nucleoside analog with extensive clinical data on safety and efficacy during pregnancy. When feasible all antiretroviral regimens for the prevention of perinatal transmission should include AZT.

Table continues . . .

TABLE 14-1: ANTIRETROVIRALS (continued)

DRUG NAME	DOSING	ADVERSE EFFECTS	FDA CLASS	ANIMAL DATA	HUMAN EXPERIENCE IN PREGNANCY	COMMENTS
Stavudine (Zerit®, D4T)	Wt > 60kg dose: 40 mg po bid. Wt < 60kg dose: 30 mg po bid	Peripheral neuropathy (in 5-15% of patients); transaminase elevation (in 8% of patients); rare cases of lactic acidosis and severe hepatomegaly with steatosis.	C	Studies in rhesus monkeys demonstrated 76% placental passage. Not teratogenic in rodent, but decreased sternal bone calcium developed. Carcinogenic studies not completed.	Insufficient information to provide reliable and definitive conclusions regarding the risk to pregnant women and their developing fetuses.	Use as an alternative for patients unable to tolerate AZT-containing regimens. *Note*: Due to the antagonism between AZT and d4T, they should never be used together as a part of a HAART regimen.
Didanosine (Videx, DDI)	Wt > 60kg dose: 400 mg po qd (tabs) or 500 mg po qd (powder). Wt < 60kg dose: 250 mg po qd (tabs) or 334 mg po qd (powder). Total daily dose may also be taken in two divided doses	GI intolerance (diarrhea, mouth sores), peripheral neuropathy in (5-12% of patients); pancreatitis (in 1-9% of patients with 6% cases fatal); transaminase elevation; rare cases of lactic acidosis and severe hepatomegaly with steatosis.	B	Not teratogenic or carcinogenic in rodent studies.	Human studies demonstrated 35% (range 23-59%) placental passage. In 8 patients studied, no toxicities were observed in mothers, infants. (5th Conference Retroviral Oppor Infect 1998 Feb 1-5: 121 (Abst. No 226). Due to the small number of patients no firm conclusion can be made. PACTG 249 Phase I study showed that ddI was well tolerated by mother and fetus when started at weeks 26-36.	GI side effects may limit use. The pediatric powder formulation is better tolerated (for every 4Gm of ddI, mix with 200 cc of Maalox®).

Table continues . . .

XIV

TABLE 14-1: ANTIRETROVIRALS

DRUG NAME	DOSING	ADVERSE EFFECTS	FDA CLASS	ANIMAL DATA	HUMAN EXPERIENCE IN PREGNANCY	COMMENTS
Lamivudine, (Epivir, 3TC)	150 mg po bid	Generally very well tolerated; occasional headache; nausea; diarrhea; abdominal pain; and insomnia; rare cases of lactic acidosis and severe hepatomegaly with steatosis.	C	Not teratogenic or carcinogenic in rodent studies.	Human studies demonstrated 100% placental passage. In a multicenter trial 39 pregnant patients received AZT and 3TC; mild anemia and aspartate aminotransferase elevations were noted in 60% of the neonates. Long term outcome is not known (Infect Dis Obstet Gynecol 1998; 6(6):237-43). PETRA Safety Data.	PETRA trial demonstrated that AZT+3TC starting at 36 wks plus 1week of AZT+3TC postpartum to mother and infant or AZT+3TC during labor plus 1 week AZT+3TC postpartum to mother and infant resulted in a 42% and 37% reduction of transmission rates, respectively. AZT and 3TC given during labor only was not effective.(1999; 6th COROI Abst.S-7)

Table continues . . .

TABLE 14-1: ANTIRETROVIRALS *(continued)*

DRUG NAME	DOSING	ADVERSE EFFECTS	FDA CLASS	ANIMAL DATA	HUMAN EXPERIENCE IN PREGNANCY	COMMENTS
Zalcitabine, (Hivid®; Dideoxycytidine, ddC)	0.75 mg po tid	High incidence of peripheral neuropathy (17-31% of patients); stomatitis, apthous ulcers; hepatitis; rare cases of pancreatitis reported; rare cases of lactic acidosis and severe hepatomegaly with steatosis.	C	Studies in rhesus monkey demonstrated 30-50% placental passage. Carcinogenic in rodent studies resulting in thymic lymphoma. Teratogenic in rodent studies resulting in hydrocephalus.	Insufficient information to provide reliable and definitive conclusions regarding the risk to pregnant women and their developing fetuses.	ddC is not recommended as part of any HAART regimen due to sub-optimal virologic response and toxicity, therefore use in the prevention of perinatal transmission is not recommended.
NON-NUCLEOSIDE REVERSE TRANSCRIPTASE INHIBITOR (NNRITs)						
Efavirenz (Sustiva®)	600 mg po q hs	Morbilliform rash in 15-27% of patients with 1-2% requiring discontinuation; one case of Steven Johnson Syndrome reported; CNS effects (confusion, depersonalization, abnormal dreams) usually seen on day 1 in up to 52% of patients and resolves in 2-4 weeks; transaminase elevation in 2-3% of patients, hyperlipidemia	C	Placental passage of 100% seen in cynomalgus monkeys, rats and rabbits. Teratogenicity demonstrated in cynomalgus monkeys resulting in anencephaly, anophthalmia, microphthalmia. No data on carcinogenicity.	No data	Due to the teratogenicity data in the cynomalgus monkeys most experts agree that **Efavirenz should be avoided during pregnancy.**

Table continues . . .

XIV

Table 14-1: Antiretrovirals

Drug Name	Dosing	Adverse Effects	FDA Class	Animal Data	Human Experience in Pregnancy	Comments
Nevirapine (Viramune)	200 mg po qd for 14 days then 200 mg po bid	Rash in 17% of patients (7% discontinued due to rash, many patient require hospitalization) Stevens Johnson Syndrome reported; transaminase elevation; severe hepatitis; fever; nausea; headache	C	Not teratogenic in rodent studies. No data on carcinogenicity.	Placental passage of 100% in humans. In HIVNET 006 trial (nevirapine 200 mg given to 21 HIV-infected pregnant patients) nevirapine was well tolerated and no fetal defects were noted (AIDS 1999 March 11; 13(4): 479-86.).	In HIVNET 012 administration of single-dose nevirapine given to mother during labor and to infants within 72 hours of delivery was compared with administration of AZT during labor and AZT for 7 days to infants. The 14-16 week data showed that 25.1% of infants in the AZT and 13.1% of infants in the nevirapine arm were infected (p=0.0006)(Lancet 1999 Sep 4; 354 (9181): 795-802.) The nevirapine regimen represents a simple and inexpensive therapy for the prevention of perinatal transmission.

Table continues . . .

TABLE 14-1: ANTIRETROVIRALS (continued)

DRUG NAME	DOSING	ADVERSE EFFECTS	FDA CLASS	ANIMAL DATA	HUMAN EXPERIENCE IN PREGNANCY	COMMENTS
Delavirdine (Rescriptor®)	400 mg po tid	Rash in 18% of patients (4.3% discontinued due to rash, usually does not require discontinuation unless mucous membrane involvement); rare erythema multiforme or Stevens-Johnson syndrome; headache	C	Placental passage of 4-15% in late-term rodent studies. Teratogenic in rodent studies resulting in ventricular septal defects. Maternal toxicity, embryotoxicity and decrease pup survival seen with doses five times the human dose. No data on carcinogenicity.	Insufficient information to provide reliable and definitive conclusions regarding the risk to pregnant women and their developing fetuses.	Due to the availability of more potent NNRTIs (e.g., nevirapine) use of delavirdine is generally not recommended.
PROTEASE INHIBITORS (PIS)						
Ritonavir (Norvir®)	600 mg po bid	Severe GI intolerance (N/V/D; abdominal pain, common with 600 mg bid dosing); taste perversion; asthenia; circumoral and peripheral paresthesias; lipodystrophy syndrome; hyperglycemia; increased triglycerides and/or cholesterol; transaminase elevation; (increased incidence seen with Hep B and C co-infection); elevated CPK and uric acid.	B	Placental passage of 115% mid-term and 15-64% late-term demonstrated in rodent studies. In human placental perfusion model, ritonavir showed little accumulation in the fetal compartment and no accumulation in placental tissue. Not teratogenic but cryptochidism reported in rodents studies. No data on carcinogenicity.	Insufficient information to provide reliable and definitive conclusions regarding the risk to pregnant women and their developing fetuses.	Use may be limited by GI intolerance. Dose of ritonavir may be lowered if used with another protease inhibitor (e.g., ritonavir 400 mg /saquinavir 400 mg BID)

Table continues . . . .

XIV

TABLE 14-1: ANTIRETROVIRALS

DRUG NAME	DOSING	ADVERSE EFFECTS	FDA CLASS	ANIMAL DATA	HUMAN EXPERIENCE IN PREGNANCY	COMMENTS
Saquinavir (Invirase® Fortovase®)	Invirase® 600 mg po tid (not recommended as sole PI); Fortovase® 1200 mg po tid	GI intolerance (nausea, diarrhea, abdominal pain); lipodystrophy syndrome; hyperglycemia; increased triglycerides and/or cholesterol; transaminase elevation	B	Placental passage in humans unknown. Placental passage in rat and rabbit is minimal. No teratogenicity reported in rodent studies. No data on carcinogenicity.	Insufficient information to provide reliable and definitive conclusions regarding the risk to pregnant women and their developing fetuses.	Fortovase® 1200 mg tid is not a practical regimen due to the high pill burden and resulting marginal drug levels. Used in combination with ritonavir, allows for an acceptable alternative PI regimen (see above for dosing).
Indinavir (Crixivan®)	800 mg tid	Nephrolithiasis +/- hematuria in 5-15% of patients (48oz of fluid recommended to decrease incident); indirect hyperbilirubinemia (> or = 2.5 mg/dl in 10-15% of patients); lipodystrophy syndrome; hyperglycemia; increased triglycerides and/or cholesterol; transaminase elevation	C	Placental passage is significant in rats, but low in rabbits. Not teratogenic in rodent studies (but extra ribs have been reported). Incidence of hyperbilirubinemia in neonatal Rhesus monkeys approximately 4-fold above controls. No data on carcinogenicity.	Insufficient information to provide reliable and definitive conclusions regarding the risk to pregnant women and their developing fetuses.	Due to theoretical concerns of hyperbilirubinemia and nephrolithiasis, **Indinavir should be avoided during pregnancy.**

Table continues . . . .

TABLE 14-1: ANTIRETROVIRALS *(continued)*

DRUG NAME	DOSING	ADVERSE EFFECTS	FDA CLASS	ANIMAL DATA	HUMAN EXPERIENCE IN PREGNANCY	COMMENTS
Nelfinavir (Viracept®)	**750 mg po tid or 1250 mg po bid**	Diarrhea (treatable with imodium or pancrealipase); lipodystrophy syndrome; hyperglycemia; increased triglycerides and/or cholesterol; transaminase elevation	B	Placental passage unknown. Not teratogenic in rodent studies. No data on carcinogenicity.	Insufficient information to provide reliable and definitive conclusions regarding the risk to pregnant women and their developing fetuses.	The combination of AZT, 3TC and nelfinavir has been well tolerated during pregnancy [personal communication with Jean Anderson, MD].
Amprenavir (Agenerase®)	**1200 mg po bid**	GI intolerance most common (N/V/D); oral paresthesias; headache; rash (in 11% of patients); lipodystrophy syndrome; hyperglycemia; increased triglycerides and/or cholesterol; transaminase elevation	C	Placental passage unknown. Rat studies, using half the human dose, resulted in thymic elongation and incomplete ossification of bones. Rabbit studies using one-twentieth of human therapeutic doses were associated with abortions and skeletal abnormalities.	No data	There is not sufficient data to date to support use of amprenavir in pregnancy.

XIV

TABLE 14-2: COMMONLY USED ANTIMICROBIALS FOR THE TREATMENT AND PREVENTION OF OPPORTUNISTIC INFECTIONS IN HIV-INFECTED PATIENTS

DRUG NAME	DOSING	ADVERSE EFFECTS	FDA CLASS	ANIMAL DATA	HUMAN EXPERIENCE IN PREGNANCY	COMMENTS
Trimethoprim-Sulfamethoxazole (Bactrim, Septra, Cotrim, Sulfatrim)	**PCP prophylaxis:** 1 DS po qd, 1SS po qd, 1 DS po TIW **PCP treatment:** 5mg/kg (based on the trimethoprim component) po or IV q 8h	Fever; leukopenia; rash and/or GI intolerance (in 25-50% of HIV-infected persons, most patients tolerate readministration of lower dose after 2 weeks of discontinuation); megaloblastic anemia; neutropenia; thrombocytopenia. Hematologic toxicity increased with folate depletion and high doses-treat with leucovorin 3-15 mg qd x 3 days. Reversible hyperkalemia (with high doses); photosensitivity; renal failure; hemolytic anemia with G6PD deficiency; hepatitis including cholestatic jaundice; thrush; erythema multiforme; Stevens Johnson syndrome	C	Cleft palate has been observed in some animals.	In a surveillance study of Michigan Medicaid recipients, 2,296 exposures to sulfamethoxazole/trimethoprim in the first trimester resulted in a 5.5% incidence of birth defects. This incidence suggests an association between the drug and congenital defects (cardiovascular), however other factors such as mother's disease, concurrent drug use, and chance, may be involved[15].	Most authorities consider sulfonamides safe in pregnancy. **Sulfonamides may cause kernicterus in neonates, therefore should be avoided in pregnant women at term.**

Table continues . . . .

TABLE 14-2: COMMONLY USED ANTIMICROBIALS FOR THE TREATMENT AND PREVENTION OF OPPORTUNISTIC INFECTIONS IN HIV-INFECTED PATIENTS *(continued)*

DRUG NAME	DOSING	ADVERSE EFFECTS	FDA CLASS	ANIMAL DATA	HUMAN EXPERIENCE IN PREGNANCY	COMMENTS
Azithromycin (Zithromax®)	**MAI prophylaxis:** 1200 mg po q week; **MAI treatment: 500 mg po qd (in combination with ethambutol and/or rifabutin)**	GI intolerance (4%); diarrhea; nausea; abdominal pain; vaginitis; reversible hearing loss (more common with 500 mg x 30-90 days); increased transaminases	B	Animal studies show no harm to the fetus.	Azithromycin and erythromycin were compared for the treatment of chlamydia in pregnancy. The authors recommended using azithromycin due to efficacy and better tolerability. Effect on the fetus was not evaluated. (Obstet Gyn 1998 Feb; 91 (2): 165-8.)	The benefit of azithromycin administration for MAI prophylaxis or treatment outweighs the risks of congenital malformations.

Table continues . . .

XIV

TABLE 14-2: COMMONLY USED ANTIMICROBIALS FOR THE TREATMENT AND PREVENTION OF OPPORTUNISTIC INFECTIONS IN HIV-INFECTED PATIENTS *(continued)*

DRUG NAME	DOSING	ADVERSE EFFECTS	FDA CLASS	ANIMAL DATA	HUMAN EXPERIENCE IN PREGNANCY	COMMENTS
Clarithromycin (Biaxin®)	**MAI prophylaxis: 500 mg po bid** **MAI treatment: 500 mg po bid (in combination with ethambutol and/or rifabutin.)**	GI intolerance (4%); diarrhea; headache; reversible dose-related hearing loss; taste disturbances	C	Studies in monkeys show growth retardation, cleft palate and embryonic loss	The Teratogen Information Service in Philadelphia reported that the outcome of 34 first or second trimester exposures were similar to those expected in the non-exposed population. The 122 pregnancies exposed to clarithromycin in the 1st trimester did not have increased major or minor malformations when compared to matched controls. Incidence of spontaneous abortion was higher in clarithromycin-exposed group compared to controls (14% vs 7%) (p=0.04)(Schick B et al. Reprod Toxicology 1996; 10:162)	The benefit from clarithromycin administration for MAI prophylaxis or treatment outweighs the risks of congenital malformations.

Table continues . . .

TABLE 14-2: COMMONLY USED ANTIMICROBIALS FOR THE TREATMENT AND PREVENTION OF OPPORTUNISTIC INFECTIONS IN HIV-INFECTED PATIENTS *(continued)*

DRUG NAME	DOSING	ADVERSE EFFECTS	FDA CLASS	ANIMAL DATA	HUMAN EXPERIENCE IN PREGNANCY	COMMENTS
Pyrazinamide	15-30 mg/kg/day in 2-4 divided doses; usually 500 mg po tid	Non-gouty polyarthralgia; asymptomatic hyper-uricemia; hepatitis (dose related, frequency not increased when given with INH or rifampin, rarely serious); GI intolerance; gout	C	No animal data available.	No human data available.	**Due to insufficient data pyrazinamide should be avoided.** INH, rifampin and ethambutol are recommended as first line agents.
Isoniazid (INH, Tubizid®, Nydrazid®)	300 mg po qd	Age-related hepatitis- < 20 years old-nil/35 yrs old-6%/45 yrs old-11%/ 55 yrs old-18%; drug should be discontinued if transaminase levels are greater or equal to 3-5 x normal limits; allergic reactions; fever; peripheral neuropathy (especially with pre-existing alcoholism, diabetes, pregnancy, malnutrition); glossitis	C	C-Animal studies show embryocidal effect, but not teratogenic.	Retrospective analysis of more than 4900 exposures to INH did not show increased fetal malformations. (Snider DE et al. Am Rev Respir Dis 1980; 122:65-79)	The American Academy of Pediatrics and the American Thoracic Society recommend that pregnant women with a positive PPD should receive INH if HIV-positive, have had recent TB contact, or have an X-ray showing old TB; start after 1st trimester if possible.

Table continues . . .

XIV

TABLE 14-2: COMMONLY USED ANTIMICROBIALS FOR THE TREATMENT AND PREVENTION OF OPPORTUNISTIC INFECTIONS IN HIV-INFECTED PATIENTS *(continued)*

DRUG NAME	DOSING	ADVERSE EFFECTS	FDA CLASS	ANIMAL DATA	HUMAN EXPERIENCE IN PREGNANCY	COMMENTS
Rifampin (Rifadin)	**600 mg po qd**	Orange discoloration of urine, tears, sweat; hepatitis-usually cholestatic changes during first month (frequency not increased when given with INH); jaundice (usually reversible with dose reduction and/or continued use); GI intolerance; hypersensitivity reactions; flu-like syndrome with intermittent use characterized by dyspnea, wheezing	C	Animal data show congenital malformations-cleft palate, spina bifida, and embryotoxicity. Isolated cases of fetal abnormalities reported. Administration in last weeks of pregnancy may cause postnatal hemorrhage.	Several reviews have evaluated treatment of TB in pregnancy. All concluded that rifampin was not teratogenic and recommended use of the drug with INH and ethambutol if necessary (Am Rev Respir Dis 1986; 134:355-63).	The American Thoracic Society recommends rifampin in combination with INH and ethambutol if treatment for TB is needed during pregnancy.
Rifabutin (Mycobutin®)	**300 mg po qd (dose is decreased to 150 mg when used with protease inhibitor e.g., indinavir or nelfinavir)**	Orange discoloration of urine, tears, sweat; uveitis with eye pain, photophobia, redness and blurred vision-usually seen with high doses (600mg/day or concurrent use of fluconazole or clarithromycin); hepatitis; GI intolerance; allergic reactions	B	Animal data showed skeletal abnormalities.	No human data available.	For MAI prophylaxis azithromycin is preferred; for MAI treatment clarithromycin + ethambutol is recommended in pregnancy. Rifabutin cannot be routinely recommended in pregnancy due to the lack of data.

Table continues . . .

TABLE 14-2: COMMONLY USED ANTIMICROBIALS FOR THE TREATMENT AND PREVENTION OF OPPORTUNISTIC INFECTIONS IN HIV-INFECTED PATIENTS *(continued)*

DRUG NAME	DOSING	ADVERSE EFFECTS	FDA CLASS	ANIMAL DATA	HUMAN EXPERIENCE IN PREGNANCY	COMMENTS
Ethambutol (Myambutol®)	**15-25 mg/kg po qd**	Optic neuritis (decreased acuity, reduced color discrimination, constricted fields, scotomata-dose related and infrequent with 15mg/kg); GI intolerance; confusion, precipitation of acute gout	B	Teratogenic in animal studies	No congenital defects have been reported. In 38 patients exposed to ethambutol during pregnancy, no increased risk of birth defects observed (including embryonic optic nerve). (Chest 1974; 66:20-4)	The CDC considers ethambutol safe in pregnancy
Atovaquone (Mepron®)	**750 mg po bid**	GI intolerance (nausea, vomiting and diarrhea); headache; rash. 7-9% required discontinuation due to side effects	C	Not teratogenic in rat studies. Maternal and fetal toxicities (decreased fetal weight, early fetal resorption and post-implantation fetal loss) reported in rabbits	No human data available	Not recommended for PCP treatment due to poor clinical efficacy. Not recommended for PCP prophylaxis due to high cost, poor GI tolerance and lack of safety data in pregnancy. Preferred regimens for PCP prophylaxis include trimethoprim/sulfamethoxazole and dapsone.

Table continues . . .

TABLE 14-2: COMMONLY USED ANTIMICROBIALS FOR THE TREATMENT AND PREVENTION OF OPPORTUNISTIC INFECTIONS IN HIV-INFECTED PATIENTS *(continued)*

DRUG NAME	DOSING	ADVERSE EFFECTS	FDA CLASS	ANIMAL DATA	HUMAN EXPERIENCE IN PREGNANCY	COMMENTS
Hydroxyurea (Hydrea®, Droxia®)	**500 mg po bid**	Dose-dependent leukopenia, anemia and thrombocytopenia; GI intolerance (N/V/D, constipation), stomatitis; rash; alopecia	D	Hydroxyurea is teratogenic in several animal studies; anomalies include nervous system, palate, skeleton, neural tube and cardiac defects.	Eight case reports of hydroxyurea exposure during pregnancy did not demonstrate teratogenicity, however the data are too limited to draw any conclusions[15].	**Contraindicated due to high incidence of teratogenicity in animal studies and limited human experience.**
Amphotericin B (Fungizone®)	**0.5-1.2 mg/kg IV qd**	40-50% incidence of fever and chills; 30-40% incidence of renal tubular acidosis-dose dependent and reversible in absence of prior renal damage and dose < 3 Gm (reduced with hydration and sodium loading); 20% incidence of hypokalemia; hypomagnesemia; anemia; phlebitis and pain at infusion site; hypotension; nausea; vomiting; metallic taste; headache	B	Animal studies demonstrated amphotericin to be harmless in pregnancy	The Collaborative Perinatal Project identified 9 1st trimester exposures to amphotericin and found no adverse fetal effect[15].	Many authorities feel that amphotericin can be used in pregnancy for the treatment of serious fungal infections.

Table continues . . .

TABLE 14-2: COMMONLY USED ANTIMICROBIALS FOR THE TREATMENT AND PREVENTION OF OPPORTUNISTIC INFECTIONS IN HIV-INFECTED PATIENTS (continued)

DRUG NAME	DOSING	ADVERSE EFFECTS	FDA CLASS	ANIMAL DATA	HUMAN EXPERIENCE IN PREGNANCY	COMMENTS
Flucytosine (Ancobon®)	25 mg/kg q6h (monitor levels)	GI intolerance (N/V/D); marrow suppression with leukopenia or thrombocytopenia (dose related with renal failure, serum concentration > 100mcg/ml or concurrent amphotericin); confusion; rash; hepatitis (dose related); enterocolitis; headache; photosensitivity reaction	C	Teratogenicity reported in animal studies.	Three case reports of second and third trimester exposure resulted in no defects in the newborns, however no conclusion can be drawn[15].	4% of administered dose converts to 5FU in the fungal organism. 5FU has been associated with congenital malformations. Its use with amphotericin for the treatment of cryptococcal meningitis did not result in added efficacy (ACTG 159. NEJM 1997; 337:15) **Avoid in pregnancy.**
Nystatin	500,000 units 5x/day	GI intolerance (N/V/D)	B	No animal data	489 first trimester exposures to nystatin were observed in a Michigan Medicaid recipients surveillance study. No association between nystatin and congenital defects was observed[15].	Due to low systemic absorption nystatin may be used in the management of thrush during pregnancy

Table continues . . .

XIV

TABLE 14-2: COMMONLY USED ANTIMICROBIALS FOR THE TREATMENT AND PREVENTION OF OPPORTUNISTIC INFECTIONS IN HIV-INFECTED PATIENTS *(continued)*

DRUG NAME	DOSING	ADVERSE EFFECTS	FDA CLASS	ANIMAL DATA	HUMAN EXPERIENCE IN PREGNANCY	COMMENTS
Clotrimazole	10 mg troches 5x/day	GI intolerance (N/V); transaminase elevation	C	Embryotoxic in rats and mice. Not teratogenic in mice, rabbits and rats.	2,624 exposures to clotrimazole were observed in the first trimester in a Michigan Medicaid recipients surveillance study. No association between clotrimazole and congenital defects were observed[15].	Due to low systemic absorption nystatin is preferred over clotrimazole in the management of thrush during pregnancy.
Fluconazole (Diflucan®)	100-800 mg po qd	Dose-related GI intolerance including bloating, nausea, vomiting, pain, anorexia, weight loss (8-11% with dose < 400mg/day, 30% with dose > 400mg/day); reversible alopecia in 10-20% of receiving >/= 400mg/day for 3 months; transaminase elevation to > 8 x normal, rare cases of fatal hepatitis and Stevens Johnson Syndrome.	C	Teratogenic in animal studies.	Craniofacial, limb and cardiac defects have been reported in 3 infants with 1st trimester exposure to high dose fluconazole (CID 1996; 22:336-40). The risk of low dose intermittent use has not been fully evaluated but appears to be low. In a prospective follow up of 226 patients exposed to low dose fluconazole, teratogenicity was not reported. (Am J Obstet Gyn 1996; 175:1645-50)	**Contraindicated in the 1st trimester due to potential for teratogenicity.**

Table continues . . .

TABLE 14-2: COMMONLY USED ANTIMICROBIALS FOR THE TREATMENT AND PREVENTION OF OPPORTUNISTIC INFECTIONS IN HIV-INFECTED PATIENTS *(continued)*

DRUG NAME	DOSING	ADVERSE EFFECTS	FDA CLASS	ANIMAL DATA	HUMAN EXPERIENCE IN PREGNANCY	COMMENTS
Itraconazole (Sporanox®)	**200-400 mg po qd**	Headache; GI intolerance-nausea (10%) and vomiting; rash (8%); hypokalemia reported with high doses (600mg per day); adrenal insufficiency; impotence; gynecomastia; leg edema; transaminase elevation, rare cases of fatal hepatitis	C	Teratogenic in rats and mice (encephaloceles, macroglossia and skeletal malformation).	FDA has received 14 case reports of malformations following use of itraconazole, 4 were limb defects. However in another report of 80 exposures to single-dose itraconazole or fluconazole no malformations were reported (Rosa F et al. Presented at the Ninth International Conference of the Organization of Teratology Information Services, May 2-4, 1996, Salt Lake City, Utah).	Contraindicated in the 1st trimester due to potential for teratogenicity.

Table continues . . .

XIV

TABLE 14-2: COMMONLY USED ANTIMICROBIALS FOR THE TREATMENT AND PREVENTION OF OPPORTUNISTIC INFECTIONS IN HIV-INFECTED PATIENTS *(continued)*

DRUG NAME	DOSING	ADVERSE EFFECTS	FDA CLASS	ANIMAL DATA	HUMAN EXPERIENCE IN PREGNANCY	COMMENTS
Pyrimethamine (Daraprim®)	**Acute treatment of Toxoplasmosis** Pyrimethamine 50-100 mg po qd (in combination with Sulfadiazine 4-8 Gm po qd in four divided doses for 6 weeks); **Toxoplasmosis maintenance dose:** Sulfadiazine 2-4 Gm po qd in four divided dose (plus pyrimethamine 25-75 mg po qd after acute treatment). **Toxoplasmosis prophylaxis:** 50-75 mg po q week (in combination with dapsone 100 po qd) / administer with leucovorin	Folic acid deficiency with megaloblastic anemia and pancytopenia (dose-related and reversed with leucovorin); allergic reactions; GI intolerance (nausea, anorexia, vomiting)	C	Teratogenic in animal studies.	No adverse fetal effects were reported in two reviews of treatment of toxoplasmosis in pregnancy (CID 1994; 18:853-62; Clin Peritonol 1994;21:675-88). If pyrimethamine is used during pregnancy, concomitant leucovorin (folinic acid) supplementation (25 mg/day) is recommended, especially during the 1st trimester.	When use in pregnancy is indicated, leucovorin 25mg pc qd should be administered concomitantly to prevent hematologic toxicity.

Table continues . . .

Table 14-2: Commonly Used Antimicrobials for the Treatment and Prevention of Opportunistic Infections in HIV-Infected Patients (continued)

Drug Name	Dosing	Adverse Effects	FDA Class	Animal Data	Human Experience in Pregnancy	Comments
Sulfadiazine	**Acute treatment of Toxoplasmosis:** Sulfadiazine 4-8 Gm po qd in four divided doses (in combination with Pyrimethamine 50-100 mg po qd for 6 weeks); **Toxoplasmosis maintenance dose:** Pyrimethamine 25-75 mg po qd (plus Sulfadiazine 2-4 Gm po qd in four divided dose after acute treatment)	Allergic reactions-rash, pruritus; crystalluria with renal damage, urolithiasis and oliguria; GI intolerance; photosensitivity; hepatitis; fever; periarteritis nodosum, Stevens-Johnson Syndrome; serum sickness	C	At high doses, animals developed cleft palate and bone abnormalities.	Extensive use in humans without complication except one case of agranulocytosis that was possibly associated[15].	**Due to the potential of kernicterus in the newborn, sulfa drugs should be avoided near term.** May be used in the 2nd and 3rd trimester without complications.

Table continues . . .

XIV

TABLE 14-2: COMMONLY USED ANTIMICROBIALS FOR THE TREATMENT AND PREVENTION OF OPPORTUNISTIC INFECTIONS IN HIV-INFECTED PATIENTS *(continued)*

DRUG NAME	DOSING	ADVERSE EFFECTS	FDA CLASS	ANIMAL DATA	HUMAN EXPERIENCE IN PREGNANCY	COMMENTS
Aerosolized pentamidine	**PCP prophylaxis- 300 mg nebulized q month**	Asthma reaction reported in 2-5% of patients; cough seen in 30% of patients			Aerosolized pentamidine given to 15 women during the 2nd and 3rd trimesters did not alter pregnancy outcome or cause fetal harm (Am J Obstet Gyn 1992; 166:387).	CDC and manufacturer advise against the use of pentamidine during pregnancy due to the lack of data, however some feel that aerosolized pentamidine may be considered safe due to minimal systemic absorption (CID 1995; 21 suppl 1:S24)

Table continues . . .

TABLE 14-2: COMMONLY USED ANTIMICROBIALS FOR THE TREATMENT AND PREVENTION OF OPPORTUNISTIC INFECTIONS IN HIV-INFECTED PATIENTS *(continued)*

DRUG NAME	DOSING	ADVERSE EFFECTS	FDA CLASS	ANIMAL DATA	HUMAN EXPERIENCE IN PREGNANCY	COMMENTS
Intravenous pentamidine	PCP treatment- 3-4 mg/kg IV qd	Nephrotoxicity-seen in 25% (usually reversible with discontinuation); hypotension (administer IV over 60 min to decrease risk); hypoglycemia-seen in 5-10% (usually occurs after 5 days of treatment including past treatment, may last days or weeks) may lead to insulin dependent diabetes; marrow suppression (leukopenia; thrombocytopenia); GI intolerance with nausea, vomiting, abdominal pain, anorexia and bad taste; transaminase elevation; pancreatitis; toxic epidermal necrolysis; fever	C	Not teratogenic in rat studies, however has been shown to be embryocidal	Spontaneous abortion reported, but causal relationship has not been established.	**Both manufacturer and CDC advise against the use of intravenous pentamidine in pregnancy.**
Primaquine	15-30 mg (base) po qd (in combination with Clindamycin for the treatment of PCP)	Hemolytic anemia (G6PD deficiency); methemoglobinemia; GI intolerance; neutropenia	C	No animal studies available.	No human data available	Theoretical concern is hemolytic anemia in G6PD deficient fetus. Should screen for G6PD deficiency in mother prior to use

Table continues . . .

TABLE 14-2: COMMONLY USED ANTIMICROBIALS FOR THE TREATMENT AND PREVENTION OF OPPORTUNISTIC INFECTIONS IN HIV-INFECTED PATIENTS *(continued)*

DRUG NAME	DOSING	ADVERSE EFFECTS	FDA CLASS	ANIMAL DATA	HUMAN EXPERIENCE IN PREGNANCY	COMMENTS
Albendazole (Albenza®)	400-800 mg bid x 3 weeks	Diarrhea; abdominal pain; transaminase elevation; hepatotoxicity; reversible pancytopenia and neutropenia	C	Teratogenic and embryotoxic in rodent and rabbit studies.	No human data available	**Contraindicated in pregnancy.**
Dapsone	100 mg po qd (PCP prophylaxis)	Rash; blood dyscrasias including methemoglobinemia and sulfhemoglobinemia and hemolytic anemia (with or without G6PD deficiency); nephrotic syndrome; fever, nausea, anorexia; blurred vision; photosensitivity; tinnitis; insomnia; irritability; headache (transient); rare "sulfone syndrome"-fever, exfoliative dermatitis, jaundice, adenopathy; methemoglobinemia and anemia	C	No animal teratogenicity studies conducted. Carcinogenic risk in rats.	No adverse effects reported. (Drug Saf 1993;8:295-311).	Dapsone has been used extensively in the treatment of malaria and for chemoprophylaxis of leprosy without producing major fetotoxicity or causing birth defects. Recommend screening for G6PD deficiency in mother prior to use.

Table continues . . .

TABLE 14-2: COMMONLY USED ANTIMICROBIALS FOR THE TREATMENT AND PREVENTION OF OPPORTUNISTIC INFECTIONS IN HIV-INFECTED PATIENTS (continued)

DRUG NAME	DOSING	ADVERSE EFFECTS	FDA CLASS	ANIMAL DATA	HUMAN EXPERIENCE IN PREGNANCY	COMMENTS
Acyclovir (Zovirax®)	5-10 mg/kg IV q8h; 200-800 mg po x3-5 times per day	GI intolerance (nausea and vomiting; diarrhea); renal toxicity (esp with rapid IV infusion); dizziness; transaminase elevation; itching, headache. Toxicities are infrequent.	C	Not teratogenic but potential to cause chromosomal damage at high doses.	Birth defects reported in 23 out of 1002 exposures however this was not statistically different from the expected rate. (Glaxo Wellcome, Acyclovir Pregnancy Registry, 1996)	CDC recommends use of acyclovir for life threatening disease but does NOT advocate use for treatment or prophylaxis of genital herpes.
Valacyclovir (Valtrex®)	1000 mg po tid (for Zoster); 500 mg po bid (for recurrent HSV)	GI intolerance-nausea, vomiting, diarrhea; headache; constipation	B	Not teratogenic in animal studies	No human data available but likely to be similar to acyclovir.	Recommendation is likely to be similar to acyclovir since valacyclovir is converted to acyclovir. However it may be more prudent to use acyclovir in pregnancy due to more extensive pregnancy data.

Table continues . . .

XIV

TABLE 14-2: COMMONLY USED ANTIMICROBIALS FOR THE TREATMENT AND PREVENTION OF OPPORTUNISTIC INFECTIONS IN HIV-INFECTED PATIENTS *(continued)*

DRUG NAME	DOSING	ADVERSE EFFECTS	FDA CLASS	ANIMAL DATA	HUMAN EXPERIENCE IN PREGNANCY	COMMENTS
Famciclovir (Famvir®)	500 mg po q8h (for zoster); 125 mg q12h (HSV)	Headache; nausea; fatigue	B	Carcinogenic, but not embryotoxic or teratogenic in animal studies.	No human data	Until more data are available, it may be prudent to use acyclovir in pregnancy.
Ganciclovir (Cytovene®)	CMV retinitis- Induction: 5mg/kg IV q12h x 2 weeks then Maintenance: 5 mg/kg IV qd	Neutropenia (ANC < 500 in 15-20%; usually early in treatment and responds within 3-7 days to drug holiday or to G-CSF); thrombocytopenia (platelet count < 20,000 in 10%, reversible). Monitor CBC 2-3/week and discontinue if ANC < 500-750 or platelet count < 25,000; anemia; fever; rash; CNS-headache, seizures, confusion, changes in mental status; abnormal liver function tests (2-3%)	C	Teratogenic and embryogenic; growth retardation; aplastic organ in animal studies.	No human data	Most authorities recommend the use of foscarnet for treatment of CMV infection during pregnancy due to the potential teratogenic effect of ganciclovir.

Table continues . . .

A Guide to the Clinical Care of Women with HIV

Pharmacologic Considerations of ARV Therapy in HIV-Infected Pregnant Patients

Table 14-2: Commonly Used Antimicrobials for the Treatment and Prevention of Opportunistic Infections in HIV-Infected Patients (continued)

Drug Name	Dosing	Adverse Effects	FDA Class	Animal Data	Human Experience in Pregnancy	Comments
Cidofovir (Vistide®)	**CMV retinitis** **Induction: 5mg/kg q week x 2 weeks then q2 weeks (give concurrently with probenecid and hydration)**	Nephropathy-dose dependent, reduced with hydration and probenecid. (Side effect of probenecid includes chills, fever, headache, rash and nausea in 30-50% of patients); uveitis; ocular hypotony; GI intolerance; neutropenia; metabolic acidosis	C	Carcinogenic in animal studies	No human data available.	Due to lack of data on cidofovir during pregnancy, most authorities recommend the use of foscarnet for the treatment of CMV infection in pregnancy.
Foscarnet (Foscavir®)	**CMV retinitis** **Induction: 90 mg/kg IV q12h;** **Maintenance: 90-120 mg/kg IV qd.**	Renal failure (usually reversible; 30% get serum creatine (Cr) > 2mg/dl; (Monitor Cr 1-3 times per week and discontinue if Cr > 2.9 mg/dl); Mineral and electrolyte changes-reduced magnesium, phosphorus, ionized calcium, potassium (monitor serum electrolytes 1-2 times per week and monitor for symptoms of paresthesias); seizures (10%); fever; GI intolerance; anemia; genital ulceration; neuropathy	C	Skeletal malformation or variation in animal studies.	No human data available	Some experts recommend that foscarnet should be used as first line treatment for sight-threatening CMV retinitis in pregnant women. Due to high incidence of nephrotoxicity, antepartum testing of the fetus and close monitoring of the aminiotic fluid to observe for fetal nephrotoxicity is recommended.

Table continues . . .

U.S. Department of Health and Human Services, Health Resources and Services Administration, HIV/AIDS Bureau   423

Table 14-2: Commonly Used Antimicrobials for the Treatment and Prevention of Opportunistic Infections in HIV-Infected Patients *(continued)*

Drug Name	Dosing	Adverse Effects	FDA Class	Animal Data	Human Experience in Pregnancy	Comments
Ribavirin (Rebetrol®)	**Treatment of Hepatitis C (in combination with interferon):** < 75kg-400 mg q am and 600 mg q pm. > 75kg-600 mg bid	Hemolytic anemia (mean hgb decrease is 3 gm/dl); leukopenia; hyperbilirubinemia; increased uric acid.	X	Ribavirin has been demonstrated teratogenic in rodents (and in all animals data tested), but not in primates when given during the first trimester	No data available	**Both the CDC and the manufacturer consider the use of ribavirin contraindicated during pregnancy.**
Interferon (Roferon®, Intron®)	**Treatment of Hepatitis C (in combination with ribavirin): 3 million units 3x/week.**	Flu-like syndrome; GI intolerance (N/V/D, anorexia); CNS toxicity (delirium; obtundation and depression); neutropenia, anemia, thrombocytopenia, increased transaminase; rash; alopecia; proteinuria	C	Abortifacient in Rhesus monkeys when given 20-500 times the human dose.	Limited case reports of interferon exposure during pregnancy do not suggest an association with birth defects, however data are too limited to draw a conclusion.	Due to the anti-proliferative properties of interferon, it should be used cautiously in pregnancy.

Table 14-3: Safety of Commonly Used Antimicrobials

Drug Name	FDA Class	Animal Data	Human Experience in Pregnancy	Comments
Metronidazole	B	Animal (rodents) data show risk of carcinogenicity.	The use of metronidazole in pregnancy is controversial; most studies show no risk).	The manufacturer and CDC consider use of metronidazole **contraindicated** during 1st trimester. However most authorities feel metronidazole is safe in the 2nd and 3rd trimester.
Clindamycin	B	No fetal harm demonstrated in rat studies. Cleft palate observed in one mouse strain.	In a surveillance study of Michigan Medicaid recipients, 647 exposures to clindamycin during the first trimester resulted in a 4.8% incidence of birth defects. These data do not support an association between clindamycin and congenital effects[15].	Clindamycin is considered to be safe in the 2nd and 3rd trimesters of pregnancy.
Penicillins	B	Carcinogenicity demonstrated in rats after prolonged subcutaneous administration of penicillin in peanut oil.	Several collaborative perinatal project reports involving over 12,000 exposures to penicillin derivatives during the 1st trimester indicated no association between penicillin derivative drugs and birth defects[15].	Penicillins are usually considered safe to use during pregnancy.
Cephalosporins	B	Not teratogenic or fetotoxic.	Extensive pregnancy exposure was not associated with birth defects.	Cephalosporins are usually considered safe to use during pregnancy.
Erythromycin	B	No teratogenic effect in rat studies.	In a surveillance study of Michigan Medicaid recipients, 6,972 patients exposed to erythromycin during the first trimester resulted in a 4.6% incidence of birth defects. These data do not support an association erythromycin and congenital malformations.	**Avoid estolate salt** (due to hepatotoxicity in 10% of patients). The CDC recommends the use of erythromycin for the treatment of chlamydia during pregnancy.

Table continues . . .

XIV

TABLE 14-3: SAFETY OF COMMONLY USED ANTIMICROBIALS *(continued)*

DRUG NAME	FDA CLASS	ANIMAL DATA	HUMAN EXPERIENCE IN PREGNANCY	COMMENTS
Tetracyclines	D	Teratogenic in animal studies resulting retardation of skeletal development and embryotoxicity.	Tetracyclines are contraindicated in pregnancy due to retardation of skeletal development and bone growth, enamel hypoplasia, and discoloration of teeth of fetus. Maternal liver toxicity has also been reported.	**Contraindicated**
Fluoroquinolones	C	Animal data demonstrated arthropathy in immature animals resulting in erosions in joint cartilage.	In a prospective follow-up study conducted by the European Network of Teratology Information Services (ENTIS), 666 cases of fluoroquinolone exposure (the majority during the 1st trimester) showed a congenital malformation rate of 4.8%. From previous epidemiologic data, this rate did not exceed the background rate.(Eur J Obstet Gyn Reprod Bio 1996; 69:83-9)	Based on animal data and the availability of alternative antimicrobial agents, **the use of fluoroquinolones during pregnancy is contraindicated.**
Aminoglycoside	D	Fetotoxicity reported in rodent studies	Eighth cranial nerve toxicity in the fetus is well documented with exposure to kanamycin and streptomycin and can potentially occur with other aminoglycosides.	**Consider use only in life-threatening infections when no alternative is available.** Gentamicin is classified by the FDA as "C" (although it has the same potential adverse effects.)
Imipenem	C	Animal studies (monkeys) show increased embryogenic loss.	No data in humans.	Due to the lack of human data, use only in life-threatening infections
Meropenem	B	No risk	No data in humans	Due to the lack of human data, use only in life-threatening infections

Table continues . . .

TABLE 14-3: SAFETY OF COMMONLY USED ANTIMICROBIALS (continued)

Drug Name	FDA Class	Animal Data	Human Experience in Pregnancy	Comments
Chloramphenicol	C	No animal data	A collaborative perinatal project monitored 98 exposures during the first trimester and 348 exposures anytime during pregnancy. No relationship between chloramphenicol and malformations were found[15]	**Although apparently non-toxic to the fetus, chloramphenicol should not be used near term due to the potential of cardiovascular collapse (Gray Baby Syndrome).**
Aztreonam	B	Animal studies show no harm to the fetus.	No human data available	Likely to be safe in pregnancy, but due to the lack of data, use only if absolutely needed.
Methenamine	C	No animal data	In a surveillance study of Michigan Medicaid recipients, 209 exposures to methenamine during the first trimester resulted in a 3.8% incidence of birth defects. This data did not support an association between methenamine and congenital defects.	The benefit of methenamine therapy is not likely to be worth the risk of use during pregnancy.
Nitrofurantoin	B	Not teratogenic or fetotoxic in rat and rabbit studies	In a surveillance study of Michigan Medicaid recipients, 1,292 exposures to nitrofurantoin resulted in a 4.0% incidence of birth defects. These data did not support an association between nitrofurantoin and congenital defects[15].	Most authorities feel that use of nitrofurantoin is safe during pregnancy.
Vancomycin	C	No animal data	The manufacturer has received reports of vancomycin use during pregnancy without adverse fetal effects.	Consider use only when the benefit outweighs the risk of drug administration.

Table continues . . .

TABLE 14-3: SAFETY OF COMMONLY USED ANTIMICROBIALS *(continued)*

CATEGORY	PREGNANCY RISK FACTOR
A	Controlled studies in women fail to demonstrate a risk to the fetus in the 1st trimester (and there is no evidence of a risk in later trimesters), and the possibility of fetal harm appears remote.
B	Either animal-reproduction studies have not demonstrated a fetal risk but there are no controlled studies in pregnant women *or* animal-reproduction studies have shown an adverse effect (other than a decrease in fertility) that was not confirmed in controlled studies in women in the 1st trimester (and there is no evidence of a risk in later trimesters).
C	Either studies in animals have revealed adverse effects on the fetus (teratogenic or embryocidal or other) and there are no controlled studies in women *or* studies in women and animals are not available. Drugs should be given only if the potential benefit justifies the potential risk to the fetus.
D	There is positive evidence of human fetal risk, but the benefits from use in pregnant women may be acceptable despite the risk (e.g., if the drug is needed in a life-threatening situation or for a serious disease for which safer drugs cannot be used or are ineffective).
X	Studies in animals or human beings have demonstrated fetal abnormalities *or* there is evidence of fetal risk based on human experience *or* both, *and* the risk of the use of the drug in pregnant women clearly outweighs any possible benefit. The drug is contraindicated in women who are *or* may become pregnant.

TABLE 14-4: DRUG INTERACTIONS OF ANTIMICROBIALS

PRIMARY DRUG	INTERACTING DRUG	MECHANISM OF INTERACTION	EFFECT	TIME COURSE	SEVERITY	COMMENTS/RECOMMENDATION
NUCLEOSIDE REVERSE TRANSCRIPTASE INHIBITORS						
AZT (Zidovudine) (Retrovir®)	Ganciclovir	Pharmacodynamic interaction/Additive toxicity.	Enhanced bone marrow toxicity.	Delayed	Moderate	May require decreased dose of AZT: Switch to alternative antiretroviral or use concomitant G-CSF. Monitor CBC frequently.
	Acetaminophen	Competitive inhibition of glucuronidation	May rarely result in granulocytopenia and hepatotoxicity	Delayed	Minor	Intermittent use of acetaminophen is considered safe. Adverse effects not consistently reported.
	Stavudine	In vitro and in vivo antagonism	Decreased antiviral efficacy	Immediate	Major	Concomitant administration not recommended
	Rifampin	Enzymatic induction resulting in increased glucuronidation of AZT	Increased clearance of AZT	Delayed	Moderate	Monitor for antiretroviral failure (e.g., increased viral load). May require increasing the dose of AZT.
ddl (Didanosine) (Videx®)	Oral Ganciclovir	Unknown	ddl AUC increased by 70% with concomitant dosing	Delayed	Moderate	Monitor for ddl toxicity (e.g., peripheral neuropathy, pancreatitis). Dose reduction may be required.
	Indinavir Ritonavir Delavirdine	Increase in gastric pH due to the buffer in ddl formulation	Decreased absorption of indinavir, ritonavir and delavirdine	Immediate	Moderate	Separate administration time by at least 2 hours

Table continues . . .

XIV

Table 14-4: Drug Interactions of Antimicrobials (continued)

Primary Drug	Interacting Drug	Mechanism of Interaction	Effect	Time Course	Severity	Comments
ddl (Didanosine) (Videx®) (continued)	Dapsone	Increase in gastric pH due to the buffer in ddl formulation	Decreased absorption of dapsone	Immediate	Moderate	Separate administration time by at least 2 hours.
	Itraconazole Ketoconazole	Increase in gastric pH due to the buffer in ddl formulation	Decreased absorption of antifungal agent	Immediate	Major	Separate administration time by at least 2 hours. Fluconazole may be preferred as an alternative azole antifungal.
	Ciprofloxacin (Fluoroquinolone) Tetracyclines	Chelation of fluoroquinolones and tetracyclines by the divalent cation in ddl	Significant decrease in antibiotic absorption results in sub therapeutic levels	Immediate	Major	Administer quinolones or tetracyclines 2 hours before or 6 hours after ddl administration.
	Pentamidine Ethambutol	Pharmacodynamic interaction / additive toxicity	May increase the risk of pancreatitis	Delayed	Moderate	Avoid in patients with current alcohol use. Use caution when administering to patients with a history of alcoholism.
	DDC,D4T,INH, Cisplatin, Disulfiram Vincristine, Gold	Pharmacodynamic interaction/Additive toxicity	May increase the risk of peripheral neuropathy.	Delayed	Moderate	Avoid co-administration or give with careful monitoring for symptoms of peripheral neuropathy. Incidence of peripheral neuropathy increases with low CD4 count.
	Methadone	Unknown	ddl levels decreased by 41%, methadone levels remains unchanged.	Delayed	Moderate	Consider ddl dose increase.

Table continues . . .

TABLE 14-4: DRUG INTERACTIONS OF ANTIMICROBIALS *(continued)*

PRIMARY DRUG	INTERACTING DRUG	MECHANISM OF INTERACTION	EFFECT	TIME COURSE	SEVERITY	COMMENTS
DDC (Zalcitabine) (Hivid®)	DDI,D4T,INH Cisplatin, Disulfiram, Vincristine, Gold-	Pharmacodynamic interaction/ Additive toxicity	May increase the risk of peripheral neuropathy.	Delayed	Moderate	Avoid or give with careful monitoring of symptoms of peripheral neuropathy. Peripheral neuropathy increases with low CD4 count.
D4T (Stavudine) (Zerit®)	DDC,DDI,INH Cisplatin, Disulfiram, Vincristine, Gold	Pharmacodynamic interaction/Additive toxicity	May increase the risk of peripheral neuropathy	Delayed	Moderate	Avoid or give with careful monitoring of symptoms of peripheral neuropathy. Peripheral neuropathy increases with low CD4 count.
	Methadone	Unknown	D4T drug levels decreased by 27%. Methadone levels unchanged	Delayed	Mild	Clinical significance unknown, no dose adjustment needed.
	Zidovudine	In vitro and in vivo antagonism	Decreased efficacy of the combination therapy	Immediate	Major	Concomitant administration not recommended due to antagonism.
3TC (Lamivudine) (Epivir®)	Bactrim	Trimethoprim competitively inhibits renal tubular secretion.	Lamivudine AUC increased by 44%	Immediate	Minor	No dosage adjustment required due to the safety profile of 3TC.
Abacavir (Ziagen®)						No known drug interactions

Table continues . . .

XIV

TABLE 14-4: DRUG INTERACTIONS OF ANTIMICROBIALS *(continued)*

PRIMARY DRUG	INTERACTING DRUG	MECHANISM OF INTERACTION	EFFECT	TIME COURSE	SEVERITY	COMMENTS
Nevirapine (Viramune®) (NVP)	*NON-NUCLEOSIDE REVERSE TRANSCRIPTASE INHIBITORS*					
	Ethinyl estradiol (Oral contraceptive)	Induction of hepatic metabolism	May decrease ethinyl estradiol AUC	Delayed	Major	Although there are no data on this interaction, patients should be aware of the potential interaction. Alternative birth control method **recommended**.
	Methadone	Induction of hepatic metabolism	May substantially decrease methadone AUC	Delayed	Moderate	**Opiate withdrawl** may occur. May need increased dose of methadone (some patients may required doses of greater than 150 mg per day)
	Ketoconazole	Induction of hepatic metabolism by nevirapine. Inhibition of hepatic metabolism by Ketoconazole	Ketoconazole levels decreased by 63%. Nevirapine levels increased by 15-30%.	Delayed	Moderate	**Co-administration not recommended.** Ketoconazole dose may need to be increased.
	Rifampin/ Rifabutin	Induction of hepatic metabolism	Nevirapine levels decreased by 37% with rifampin and 16% with rifabutin	Delayed	Major	Co-administration not recommended with rifampin. Rifabutin may be a preferred alternative agent.
	Clarithromycin	Induction of hepatic metabolism by nevirapine	Clarithromycin AUC decreased by 30%, but active hydroxy-metabolite is increased.	Delayed	Minor	No dose modification needed. Use standard dose of nevirapine and clarithromycin
		Inhibition of hepatic metabolism by clarithromycin.	Nevirapine AUC increased by 26%	Immediate	Minor	

Table continues . . .

TABLE 14-4: DRUG INTERACTIONS OF ANTIMICROBIALS *(continued)*

PRIMARY DRUG	INTERACTING DRUG	MECHANISM OF INTERACTION	EFFECT	TIME COURSE	SEVERITY	COMMENTS
Nevirapine (Viramune®) (NVP) *(continued)*	Saquinavir	Induction of hepatic metabolism	Saquinavir AUC decreased by 25%	Delayed	Moderate	Avoid concurrent use.
	Ritonavir	Induction of hepatic metabolism	Ritonavir AUC decreased by 11%.	Delayed	Minor	Use standard doses.
	Indinavir	Induction of hepatic metabolism	Indinavir AUC decreased by 28%	Delayed	Minor	Clinical trials demonstrated efficacy with standard dose. Some experts recommend increasing the indinavir dose to 1000 mg q8h.
	Nelfinavir	Induction of hepatic metabolism	Nelfinavir levels increase by 10%.	Delayed	Minor	Use standard doses.
Delavirdine (Rescriptor®) (DLV)	Indinavir	Inhibition of hepatic metabolism	Indinavir AUC increased by 40%	Immediate	Moderate	May reduce indinavir dose to 600 mg q8h
	Nelfinavir	Inhibition of hepatic metabolism by delavirdine	Nelfinavir AUC increased by 2 fold	Immediate	Moderate	Monitor for neutropenia and complication for the first few months. Insufficient data for dosing recommendation.
		Induction of hepatic metabolism by nelfinavir.	Delavirdine AUC decreased by 50%	Delayed		
	Ritonavir	Inhibition of hepatic metabolism	Ritonavir AUC increased by 70%. No effect on delavirdine concentration.	Immediate	Minor	No data on dosage.

Table continues . . .

XIV

Table 14-4: Drug Interactions of Antimicrobials *(continued)*

Primary Drug	Interacting Drug	Mechanism of Interaction	Effect	Time Course	Severity	Comments
Delavirdine (Rescriptor®) (DLV) *(continued)*	Saquinavir	Inhibition of hepatic metabolism	Invirase C min increased by six-fold	Delayed	Minor	Beneficial interaction. No dosage adjustment needed. Monitor transaminases.
	ddI and antacid	Decrease delavirdine absorption due to antacid content in ddI	Delavirdine AUC decreased by 41%	Immediate	Moderate	Separate administration by at least 1 hour.
	Simvastatin/ Lovastatin	Inhibition of hepatic metabolism	Increased serum levels of simvastatin and lovastatin	Immediate	Moderate	**Avoid concurrent administration.** Consider alternatives such as atorvastatin, pravastatin, cerivastatin, fluvastatin. Monitor for adverse effects due to limited clinical data.
	H2 blockers, Proton pump inhibitors (e.g., omeprazole)	Decreased delavirdine absorption due to increased gastric pH	May decrease delavirdine concentration	Immediate	Moderate	Though not thoroughly evaluated, the **manufacturer does not recommend** long-term concurrent administration.
	Terfenadine, Astemizole, Cisapride	Inhibition of hepatic metabolism	Increased levels of terfenadine, astemizole, cisapride	Immediate	Major	**Concurrent administration contraindicated** due to potential for serious cardiac arrhythmias.
	Midazolam, Triazolam	Inhibition of hepatic metabolism	Midazolam and triazolam AUCs increased	Immediate	Major	**Concurrent administration contraindicated** due to potential for prolonged sedation. Lorazepam and Temazepam may be safe alternatives.

Table continues . . .

Table 14-4: Drug Interactions of Antimicrobials *(continued)*

Primary Drug	Interacting Drug	Mechanism of Interaction	Effect	Time Course	Severity	Comments
Delavirdine (Rescriptor®) (DLV) *(continued)*	Ergot Alkaloid	Inhibition of hepatic metabolism	Possible acute ergot toxicity characterized by peripheral vasospasm and ischemia of extremities	Immediate	Major	**Concurrent administration contraindicated.**
	Sildenafil	Inhibition of hepatic metabolism	Potential increase in sildenafil drug levels	Immediate	Moderate	**Caution** with concurrent use. Do not exceed 25 mg sildenafil in a 48-hour period.
	Clarithromycin	Inhibition of hepatic metabolism	Clarithromycin levels increased by 100%, and delavirdine levels increased by 44%.	Immediate	Minor	May require dose adjustment.
	Rifampin	Induction of hepatic metabolism	Delavirdine Cmin decreased below the level of detection.	Delayed	Major	**Concurrent administration contraindicated** due to sub-therapeutic level of delavirdine
	Rifabutin	Inhibition of hepatic metabolism by delavirdine	Rifabutin AUC increased by 100%	Immediate	Moderate	**Concurrent administration contraindicated** due to sub-therapeutic level of delavirdine
		Induction of hepatic metabolism by rifabutin	Delavirdine AUC decreased by 80%	Delayed	Major	

Table continues . . .

XIV

TABLE 14-4: DRUG INTERACTIONS OF ANTIMICROBIALS *(continued)*

PRIMARY DRUG	INTERACTING DRUG	MECHANISM OF INTERACTION	EFFECT	TIME COURSE	SEVERITY	COMMENTS
Efavirenz (Sustiva®) (EFV)	Fortovase® (Saquinavir soft gel)	Induction of hepatic metabolism	Fortovase® AUC decreased by 60%. Efavirenz AUC decreased by 12%	Delayed	Moderate	Avoid using Fortovase® monotherapy with efavirenz. If ritonavir/saquinavir/efavirenz regimen used, dose Fortovase 800 mg bic.
	Nelfinavir	Inhibition of hepatic metabolism	Nelfinavir AUC increased by 21%	Immediate	Minor	May be a beneficial pharmacokinetic interaction. No dose adjustment needed.
	Amprenavir	Induction of hepatic metabolism	Amprenavir AUC decreased by 36%	Delayed	Moderate	Clinical significance not known. Recommended empiric dose of amprenavir 1200 mg q8h + efavirenz 600 mg qhs is reasonable. Amprenavir 1200 mg q12h + ritonavir 200 mg q12h + efavirenz 600 mg qhs resulted in a 5-fold increase in amprenavir level. May consider decreasing the dose of amprenavir to 600 mg q12h when used with ritonavir and efavirenz.
	Indinavir	Induction of hepatic metabolism	Indinavir AUC decreased by 31%	Delayed	Moderate	May need to increase indinavir dose to 1000 mg q8h.
	Ritonavir	Dual Inhibition of hepatic metabolism	Efavirenz AUC increased by 21%. Ritonavir AUC increased by 17%.	Immediate	Minor	No adjustment needed. May be able to reduce dose of ritonavir to 500 mg bid if GI intolerance occurs.

Table continues . . .

TABLE 14-4: DRUG INTERACTIONS OF ANTIMICROBIALS *(continued)*

PRIMARY DRUG	INTERACTING DRUG	MECHANISM OF INTERACTION	EFFECT	TIME COURSE	SEVERITY	COMMENTS
Efavirenz (Sustiva®) (EFV) *(continued)*	Ergot Alkaloid	Inhibition of hepatic metabolism	Potential acute ergot toxicity characterized by peripheral vasospasm and ischemia of extremities	Immediate	Major	**Concurrent administration contraindicated.**
	Midazolam, Triazolam	Inhibition of hepatic metabolism	AUCs of midazolam and triazolam increased	Immediate	Major	**Concurrent administration contraindicated** due to potential for prolonged sedation. Lorazepam and Temazepam may be safe alternatives
	Terfenadine, Astemizole, Cisapride	Inhibition of hepatic metabolism	Levels of terfenadine, astemizole, cisapride increased	Immediate	Major	**Concurrent administration contraindicated** due to potential for serious cardiac arrhythmia.
	Clarithromycin	Induction of hepatic metabolism	Clarithromycin AUC decreased by 39%	Immediate	Moderate	Incidence of rash increased to 46% with concurrent administration. No interaction with azithromycin, a better alternative.
	Ethinyl estradiol (oral contraceptive)	Inhibition of hepatic metabolism	Ethinyl estradiol AUC increased by 37%	Immediate	Minor	No dose changes recommended. Clinical significance of interaction unknown. No data on progesterone component of oral contraceptive available. Alternative form of birth control recommended.
	Rifabutin	Induction of hepatic metabolism	Rifabutin AUC decreased by 35%. No effect on Efavirenz AUC	Delayed	Moderate	If concurrent administration required, increase dose of rifabutin to 450 mg or 600 mg po qd.

Table continues . . .

XIV

TABLE 14-4: DRUG INTERACTIONS OF ANTIMICROBIALS (continued)

PRIMARY DRUG	INTERACTING DRUG	MECHANISM OF INTERACTION	EFFECT	TIME COURSE	SEVERITY	COMMENTS
	Rifampin	Induction of hepatic metabolism	Efavirenz AUC decreased by 26%. No change in rifampin levels.	Delayed	Moderate	**Concurrent administration contraindicated.** Rifabutin dose adjusted to 450-600 mg qd is a better alternative to rifamycin.
PROTEASE INHIBITORS						
Indinavir (Crixivan®) (IDV)	DDI	Impairment of indinavir absorption by ddI buffer	Decreases absorption of indinavir	Immediate	Moderate	Separate indinavir and ddI doses by at least 1 hour.
	Simvastatin/ Lovastatin	Inhibition of hepatic metabolism.	Increased serum levels of simvastatin and lovastatin	Immediate	Moderate	**Avoid concurrent administration.** Possible alternatives include atorvastatin, pravastatin, cerivastatin, fluvastatin. Monitor for adverse effect due to limited clinical data with these agents
	Rifabutin	Inhibition of hepatic metabolism by indinavir	Rifabutin AUC increased by 2 fold.	Immediate	Moderate	Decrease rifabutin dose by half (150mg once a day).
		Induction of hepatic metabolism by rifabutin.	Indinavir AUC decreased by 32%	Delayed	Moderate	May need to increase indinavir dose to 1Gm po tid.
	Rifampin	Induction of hepatic metabolism	Indinavir AUC decreased by 90%	Immediate	Major	**Concurrent administration contraindicated.**
	Sildenafil	Inhibition of hepatic metabolism.	Sildenafil AUC increased by 2 to 11 fold.	Immediate	Major	**Caution** with concurrent use, Do not exceed 25 mg of sildenafil in a 48-hour period.

Table continues . . .

TABLE 14-4: DRUG INTERACTIONS OF ANTIMICROBIALS (continued)

PRIMARY DRUG	INTERACTING DRUG	MECHANISM OF INTERACTION	EFFECT	TIME COURSE	SEVERITY	COMMENTS
Indinavir (Crixivan®) (IDV) (continued)	Terfenadine Astemizole Cisapride	Inhibition of hepatic metabolism	Drug levels increased by 3-fold or greater.	Immediate	Major	**Concurrent administration contraindicated** due to potential for cardiac arrhythmias. Alternative antihistamines include loratidine, fexofenadine or cetirizine. Alternative pro-kinetic agent includes metoclopramide.
	Ergot Alkaloid	Inhibition of hepatic metabolism	Potential acute ergot toxicity characterized by peripheral vasospasm and ischemia of extremities	Immediate	Major	**Concurrent administration contraindicated.**
	Ketoconazole Itraconazole	Inhibition of hepatic metabolism	Indinavir AUC increased by 70%.	Immediate	Moderate	Dose indinavir at 600mg Q8h.
	Midazolam, Triazolam	Inhibition of hepatic metabolism	AUCs of midazolam and triazolam are increased.	Immediate	Major	**Concurrent administration contraindicated** due to potential for prolonged sedation.
	Nelfinavir	Inhibition of hepatic metabolism.	Indinavir AUC increased by 50% Nelfinavir AUC increased by 80%	Immediate	Minor	Limited dosing data using indinavir 1200 mg bid + nelfinavir 1250 mg bid.
	Amprenavir	Inhibition of hepatic metabolism	Amprenavir AUC increased by 26%. Indinavir AUC increased by 38%.	Immediate	Minor	No dose adjustment recommended.

Table continues . . .

XIV

TABLE 14-4: DRUG INTERACTIONS OF ANTIMICROBIALS *(continued)*

PRIMARY DRUG	INTERACTING DRUG	MECHANISM OF INTERACTION	EFFECT	TIME COURSE	SEVERITY	COMMENTS
Indinavir (Crixivan®) (IDV) *(continued)*	Ritonavir	Inhibition of hepatic metabolism	Indinavir AUC increased by 2 to 5-fold.	Immediate	Minor	Interaction allows indinavir to be given twice-daily (400 mg bid, 600 mg bid or 800 mg bid). Most experience has been with co-administration of 400 mg of indinavir and 400 mg of ritonavir twice-daily. Other dosing regimens studied include indinavir 600 mg bid + ritonavir 200mg bid or indinavir 800mg bid + ritonavir 100 or 200 mg bid.
	Saquinavir	Inhibition of hepatic metabolism	Saquinavir AUC increased 4- to 7-fold. No effect on Indinavir level	Immediate	Moderate	In vitro antagonism. Avoid co-administration.
Saquinavir (Invirase®) (Fortovase®) (SQV)	Ritonavir	Inhibition of hepatic metabolism	Saquinavir AUC increased by 20-fold.	Immediate	Minor	Dual protease inhibitor combination with the most clinical experience. Recommended doses: ritonavir 400 mg bid and saquinavir 400 mg bid
	Indinavir	Inhibition of hepatic metabolism	Saquinavir AUC increased 4- to7- fold No effect on indinavir	Immediate	Moderate	In vitro antagonism. Avoid co-administration
	Nelfinavir	Inhibition of hepatic metabolism	Fortovase® AUC increased by 3 to 5-fold. Nelfinavir AUC increased by 20%	Immediate	Minor	Recommended doses are nelfinavir 750mg tid and Fortovase® 800mg tid.

Table continues . . . .

TABLE 14-4: DRUG INTERACTIONS OF ANTIMICROBIALS *(continued)*

PRIMARY DRUG	INTERACTING DRUG	MECHANISM OF INTERACTION	EFFECT	TIME COURSE	SEVERITY	COMMENTS
Saquinavir (Invirase®) (Fortovase®) (SQV) *(continued)*	Amprenavir	Induction of hepatic metabolism	Saquinavir level decreased by 18%. Amprenavir level decreased by 36%.	Delayed	Minor	Insufficient data to recommend dose adjustment.
	Ketoconazole	Inhibition of hepatic metabolism	Saquinavir level increased by 3-fold.	Immediate	Minor	Beneficial pharmacokinetic interaction. Use standard doses.
	Midazolam, Triazolam	Inhibition of hepatic metabolism	Midazolam and triazolam AUCs increased	Immediate	Major	**Concurrent administration contraindicated** due to potential for prolonged sedation.
	Terfenadine Astemizole Cisapride	Inhibition of hepatic metabolism	Drug levels increased by 3-fold or greater.	Immediate	Major	**Concurrent administration Contraindicated** due to potential for cardiac arrhythmias. Alternative antihistamines include loratidine, fexofenadine or cetirizine. Alternative pro-kinetic agent includes metoclopramide.
	Ergot Alkaloid	Inhibition of hepatic metabolism	Acute ergot toxicity characterized by peripheral vasospasm and ischemia of extremities	Immediate	Major	**Concurrent administration contraindicated.**

Table continues . . .

XIV

TABLE 14-4: DRUG INTERACTIONS OF ANTIMICROBIALS *(continued)*

PRIMARY DRUG	INTERACTING DRUG	MECHANISM OF INTERACTION	EFFECT	TIME COURSE	SEVERITY	COMMENTS
Saquinavir (Invirase®) (Fortovase®) (SQV) *(continued)*	Simvastatin/ Lovastatin	Inhibition of hepatic metabolism.	Simvastatin and lovastatin serum level increased	Immediate	Moderate	**Avoid co-administration.** Recommended alternatives include atorvastatin, pravastatin, cerivastatin, fluvastatin. Monitor for adverse effects due to limited clinical data with these agents
	Rifabutin/ Rifampin	Induction of hepatic metabolism	Rifabutin and rifampin decrease AUC of saquinavir by 40% and 80% respectively.	Delayed	Major	**Concurrent administration contraindicated.**
	Sildenafil	Inhibition of hepatic metabolism.	Sildenafil AUC increased by 2- to 11-fold.	Immediate	Major	**Caution** with concurrent use. Do not exceed 25 mg of sildenafil in a 48-hour period
Ritonavir (Norvir®) (RTV)	Metronidazole	Alcohol in ritonavir liquid may precipitate a disulfiram-like reaction.	Unexpected nausea	Immediate	Moderate	Warn patient of the alcohol content in ritonavir liquid.
	Ethinyl estradiol (Oral contraceptive)	Induction and increase in glucuronosyl transferase activity.	Ethinyl estradiol level decreased by 40%	Delayed	Major	Warn patient of interaction. Recommend another method of contraception.
	Sildenafil	Inhibition of hepatic metabolism.	Sildenafil AUC increased by 2 to 11-fold.	Immediate	Major	**Caution** with concurrent use. Do not exceed 25 mg of sildenafil in a 48 hour period

Table continues . . .

TABLE 14-4: DRUG INTERACTIONS OF ANTIMICROBIALS *(continued)*

PRIMARY DRUG	INTERACTING DRUG	MECHANISM OF INTERACTION	EFFECT	TIME COURSE	SEVERITY	COMMENTS
Ritonavir (Norvir®) (RTV) *(continued)*	Theophylline	Induction of glucuronosyl transferase activity.	Theophylline AUC dcreased by 43%	Delayed	Moderate	Monitor theophylline levels; dose may need to be increased if subtherapeutic.
	Ketoconazole	Inhibition of hepatic metabolism	Ketoconazole AUC increased more than 3-fold.	Immediate	Moderate	May need to decrease ketoconazole dose.
	Rifabutin	Inhibition of hepatic metabolism	Rifabutin AUC increased 4-fold	Immediate	Moderate	Concurrent use of rifabutin and ritonavir is contraindicated by the manufacturer. Some experts recommend one-fourth the dose (150mg every other day) of rifabutin if needed, however no data support this recommendation.
	Rifampin	Induction of hepatic metabolism	Ritonavir AUC decreased by 35%	Delayed	Moderate	Monitor for therapeutic efficacy of ritonavir. May need to increase ritonavir dose. There may be an increase in liver toxicity
	Ergot Alkaloid	Inhibition of hepatic metabolism	Acute ergot toxicity characterized by peripheral vasospasm and ischemia of extremities	Immediate	Major	**Concurrent administration contraindicated.**
	Terfenadine Astemizole Cisapride	Inhibition of hepatic metabolism	Drug level increased by 3-fold or greater.	Immediate	Major	**Concurrent administration contraindicated** due to potential for cardiac arrhythmias. Alternative antihistamines include loratidine, fexofenadine or cetirizine. Alternative pro-kinetic agents include metoclopramide.

Table continues . . .

XIV

TABLE 14-4: DRUG INTERACTIONS OF ANTIMICROBIALS *(continued)*

PRIMARY DRUG	INTERACTING DRUG	MECHANISM OF INTERACTION	EFFECT	TIME COURSE	SEVERITY	COMMENTS
Ritonavir (Norvir®) (RTV) *(continued)*	Benzodiazepines	Inhibition of hepatic metabolism	Prolonged sedation due to accumulation of benzodiazepine	Delayed	Major	**Concurrent administration of zolpidem, lorazepate, midazolam, diazepam, estazolam, flurazepam and triazolam is contraindicated.** Alternative benzodiazepine that can be used : temazepam and lorazepam.
	Antiarrhythmics	Inhibition of hepatic metabolism	AUC of antiarrhythmics increased	Immediate	Major	**Concurrent administration of propafenone, quinidine, flecainide, amiodarone, bepridil, encainide is contraindicated.**
	Methadone	Induction of hepatic metabolism	Methadone levels decreased by 37%.	Delayed	Moderate	Monitor for withdraw symptoms; may require dose increase of methadone.
	Ketoconazole	Inhibition of hepatic metabolism	Ketoconazole levels increased by 3-fold.	Immediate	Moderate	Use with caution; do not exceed 200 mg ketoconazole per day.
	Antidepressant/ Antipsychotic	Inhibition of hepatic metabolism	Antidepressant and antipsychotic AUCs are increased	Immediate	Major	**Concurrent administration of buproprion, pimozide, nefazadone and clozapine is contraindicated.** Fluoxetine can be used. Desipramine may be used but dose may have to be reduced if used concurrently with ritonavir.
	Simvastatin/ Lovastatin	Inhibition of hepatic metabolism.	Increased simvastatin and lovastatin serum levels.	Immediate	Moderate	**Avoid co-administration.** Alternatives include atorvastatin, pravastatin, cerivastatin, fluvastatin. Monitor for adverse effect due to limited clinical data.

Table continues . . .

TABLE 14-4: DRUG INTERACTIONS OF ANTIMICROBIALS (continued)

PRIMARY DRUG	INTERACTING DRUG	MECHANISM OF INTERACTION	EFFECT	TIME COURSE	SEVERITY	COMMENTS
Ritonavir (Norvir®) (RTV) (continued)	Opioid analgesic	Inhibition of hepatic metabolism	Prolong sedation and possible respiratory depression	Immediate	Major	**Concurrent administration of meperidine and propoxyphene is contraindicated.** Oxycodone can be used.
	NSAID	Inhibition of hepatic metabolism	NSAID AUCs may be increased	Immediate	Major	**Concurrent administration of Piroxicam is contraindicated.** ASA can be used.
	Saquinavir	Inhibition of hepatic metabolism	Saquinavir AUC increased by 20-fold.	Immediate	Minor	Dual protease inhibitor with the most clinical experience. Recommended doses: ritonavir 400mg bid and Fortovase® or Invirase® 400 mg bid.
	Indinavir	Inhibition of hepatic metabolism	Indinavir AUC increased by 2 to 5-fold.	Immediate	Minor	Interaction allows indinavir to be dosed twice-daily (400 mg bid, 600 mg bid or 800 mg bid) which reduces renal stones caused by indinavir. Most experience has been with indinavir 400 mg bid and ritonavir 400 mg bid. Other dosing regimens include indinavir 600 mg bid + ritonavir 200mg bid or indinavir 800mg bid + ritonavir 100 or 200 mg bid.
	Nelfinavir	Inhibition of hepatic metabolism	Nelfinavir AUC increased by 1.5 fold.	Immediate	Minor	Ongoing clinical trials are using ritonavir 400mg bid and nelfinavir 500 or 750 mg bid.
	Amprenavir	Inhibition of hepatic metabolism	Amprenavir AUC increased by 2.5-fold.	Immediate	Minor	Insufficient data for dose recommendation. May be able to use a lower dose of amprenavir.

Table continues . . .

XIV

TABLE 14-4: DRUG INTERACTIONS OF ANTIMICROBIALS (continued)

PRIMARY DRUG	INTERACTING DRUG	MECHANISM OF INTERACTION	EFFECT	TIME COURSE	SEVERITY	COMMENTS
Nelfinavir (Viracept®) (NFV)	Ketoconazole	Inhibition of hepatic metabolism	Nelfinavir AUC increased by 35%	Immediate	Minor	No dose adjustment needed.
	Fluconazole	Inhibition of hepatic metabolism	Nelfinavir AUC increased by 30%	Immediate	Minor	May be beneficial. No dose adjustment needed.
	Simvastatin/ Lovastatin	Inhibition of hepatic metabolism.	Simvastatin and lovastatin serum levels increased.	Immediate	Moderate	Avoid co-administration: Alternatives include atorvastatin, pravastatin, cerivastatin, fluvastatin. Monitor for adverse effects due to limited clinical data
	Rifampin	Induction of hepatic metabolism	Nelfinavir AUC decreased by 82%	Delayed	Major	Concurrent administration contraindicated.
	Rifabutin	Induction of hepatic metabolism by rifabutin	Nelfinavir AUC decreased by 32%	Delayed	Moderate	If co-administration required, increase nelfinavir to 1000mg po tid.
		Inhibition of hepatic metabolism by nelfinavir	Rifabutin levels increased 3-fold	Immediate	Moderate	If co-administration required, decrease rifabutin to 150 mg po qd.
	Benzodiazepines	Inhibition of hepatic metabolism	Prolonged sedation due to accumulation of benzodiazepine.	Immediate	Major	Midazolam and triazolam are contraindicated. Alternative benzodiazepines include temazepam and lorazepam.

Table continues . . .

TABLE 14-4: DRUG INTERACTIONS OF ANTIMICROBIALS *(continued)*

PRIMARY DRUG	INTERACTING DRUG	MECHANISM OF INTERACTION	EFFECT	TIME COURSE	SEVERITY	COMMENTS
Nelfinavir (Viracept®) (NFV) *(continued)*	Ergot Alkaloid	Inhibition of hepatic metabolism	Acute ergot toxicity characterized by peripheral vasospasm and ischemia of extremities	Immediate	Major	**Concurrent administration contraindicated.**
	Terfenadine Astemizole Cisapride	Inhibition of hepatic metabolism	Drug levels increased by 3-fold or greater.	Immediate	Major	**Concurrent administration contraindicated** due to potential cardiac arrhythmia. Recommended alternative antihistamine: loratidine, fexofenadine or cetirizine. Alternative pro-kinetic agent: metoclopramide
	Ethinyl Estradiol (oral contraceptive)	Induction of hepatic metabolism	Ethinyl estradiol AUC decreased by 47%	Delayed	Major	Advise patient to use **alternative method of contraception.**
	Sildenafil	Inhibition of hepatic metabolism.	Sildenafil AUC increased by 2-11 fold.	Immediate	Major	**Caution** with concurrent use. Do not exceed 25 mg of sildenafil in a 48 hour period
	Indinavir	Inhibition of hepatic metabolism.	Indinavir AUC increased by 50% Nelfinavir AUC increased by 80%	Immediate	Minor	Limited data for dosing IDV 1200mg bid + NFV 1250 mg bid.
	Saquinavir	Inhibition of hepatic metabolism	Fortovase® AUC increased by 3-5 fold. Nelfinavir AUC increased by 20%	Immediate	Moderate	Dose nelfinavir 750mg tid and Fortovase 800mg tid.

Table continues . . .

XIV

TABLE 14-4: DRUG INTERACTIONS OF ANTIMICROBIALS *(continued)*

PRIMARY DRUG	INTERACTING DRUG	MECHANISM OF INTERACTION	EFFECT	TIME COURSE	SEVERITY	COMMENTS
Nelfinavir (Viracept®) (NFV) *(continued)*	Amprenavir	Inhibition of hepatic metabolism	Nelfinavir AUC increased by 15%, Amprenavir AUC increased by 50%.	Immediate	Minor	No dose adjustment. Insufficient data to recommend a dosage adjustment.
	Ritonavir	Inhibition of hepatic metabolism	Nelfinavir AUC increased by 1.5 fold. Increase in nelfinavir M8 metabolite.	Immediate	Moderate	Ongoing clinical trials are using ritonavir 400mg bid and nelfinavir 500 mg or 750 mg bid.
Amprenavir (Angenerase®) (APV)	Rifampin	Induction of hepatic metabolism	Amprenavir AUC decreased by 80%	Delayed	Major	**Concurrent administration contraindicated.**
	Rifabutin	Induction of hepatic metabolism	Amprenavir AUC decreased by 14%. Rifabutin AUC increased by 204%	Delayed	Moderate	Decrease rifabutin dose by one-half: Dose rifabutin 150mg qd. No change in amprenavir dose.
	Ketoconazole	Inhibition of hepatic metabolism	Amprenavir AUC increased by 32%. Ketoconazole AUC increased by 44%.	Immediate	Minor	May be beneficial. No dose adjustment needed.
	Clarithromycin	Inhibition of hepatic metabolism	Amprenavir AUC increased by 18%	Immediate	Minor	No dose adjustment needed.
	Ethinyl Estradiol (oral contraceptive)	Induction of hepatic metabolism	Potential decreases in ethinyl estradiol level.	Delayed	Major	Advise patient of potential risk and to use an alternative contraceptive method.

Table continues . . .

TABLE 14-4: DRUG INTERACTIONS OF ANTIMICROBIALS (continued)

PRIMARY DRUG	INTERACTING DRUG	MECHANISM OF INTERACTION	EFFECT	TIME COURSE	SEVERITY	COMMENTS
Amprenavir (Angenerase®) (APV) (continued)	Sildenafil	Inhibition of hepatic metabolism.	Sildenafil AUC increased by 2-11 fold.	Immediate	Major	**Caution** with concurrent use. Do not exceed 25 mg of sildenafil in a 48-hour period
	Simvastatin/ Lovastatin	Inhibition of hepatic metabolism.	Simvastatin and lovastatin levels increased.	Immediate	Moderate	Avoid concurrent administration. Alternative agents include atorvastatin, pravastatin, cerivastatin, fluvastatin. Monitor for adverse effects due to limited clinical data.
	Saquinavir	Induction of hepatic metabolism.	Saquinavir level decreased by 18%. Amprenavir level decreased by 36%.	Delayed	Minor	No dose adjustment. Insufficient data for dose recommendation
	Indinavir	Inhibition of hepatic metabolism.	Amprenavir AUC increased by 33%. Indinavir AUC decreased by 38%.	Immediate	Minor	No dose adjustment.
	Nelfinavir	Inhibition of hepatic metabolism.	Nelfinavir AUC increased by 15%, Amprenavir AUC increased by 50%.	Immediate	Minor	No dose adjustment. Insufficient data for dose recommendation.
	Ritonavir	Inhibition of hepatic metabolism.	Amprenavir AUC increased 2.5-fold.	Immediate	Minor	Insufficient data for dose recommendation.

Table continues . . .

XIV

TABLE 14-4: DRUG INTERACTIONS OF ANTIMICROBIALS *(continued)*

PRIMARY DRUG	INTERACTING DRUG	MECHANISM OF INTERACTION	EFFECT	TIME COURSE	SEVERITY	COMMENTS
Amprenavir (Agenerase®) (APV) *(continued)*	Efavirenz	Induction of hepatic metabolism	Amprenavir AUC decreased by 36%. Efavirenz AUC increased by 15%	Delayed	Moderate	Further studies needed for dosage recommendation.
	Bepridil	Inhibition of hepatic metabolism	Bepridil AUC Increased	Immediate	Major	**Concurrent administration contraindicated.**
	Ergot Alkaloid	Inhibition of hepatic metabolism	Acute ergot toxicity characterized by peripheral vasospasm and ischemia of extremities	Immediate	Major	**Concurrent administration contraindicated.**
	Midazolam, Triazolam	Inhibition of hepatic metabolism	AUCs of midazolam and triazolam are increased.	Immediate	Major	**Concurrent administration contraindicated** due to potential for prolonged sedation. Lorazepam and Temazepam may be safe alternatives
	Terfenadine Astemizole Cisapride	Inhibition of hepatic metabolism	Cardiotoxic drug level increased by 3-fold or greater.	Immediate	Major	**Concurrent administration contraindicated** due to potential for cardiac arrhythmias. Alternatives include loratidine, fexofenadine or cetirizine. Alternative prokinetic agent includes metoclopramide.

AUC= Area Under the Concentration Time Curve
Cmax= Peak serum concentration
Cmin= Trough serum concentration

Time course: *Delayed* = maximal interaction occurring at 14 days
Immediate = interaction occurring immediately.

Severity: *Major* = Do not co-administer; contraindicated.
Moderate = Can be co-administered with caution and possible dose adjustment.
Minor = Can be co-administered

TABLE 14-5: CLINICALLY PERTINENT FOOD-DRUG INTERACTIONS

GANCICLOVIR CAPSULE/ ITRACONAZOLE CAPSULE / NELFINAVIR / RITONAVIR:
Should be taken with food or within 2 hours of eating.

AZT :
Can be taken with food to decrease GI side effects.

SAQUINAVIR (FORTOVASE® AND INVIRASE®) / ATOVAQUONE:
Should be administered with a high fat meal

EFAVIRENZ / AMPRENAVIR:
High fat meal should be avoided

DIDANOSINE / INDINAVIR / ITRACONAZOLE SOLUTION:
Should be taken on an empty stomach (1 hour before or 2 hours after meals).

GRAPEFRUIT JUICE:
Increases saquinavir levels 40-100% but decreases indinavir AUC by 26%.

TABLE 14-6: DRUGS OF SPECIAL CONSIDERATION IN WOMEN

DRUG NAME	FDA CLASS	COMMENTS
Terbutaline	B	Terbutaline has produced significant increases in birth weights (Briggs et al, 1998). Follow-up studies did not show increased adverse fetal outcomes (Acta Obstet Gynecol Scand Suppl 1982; 108:67-70.)
Ritodrine	B	The manufacturer reports that ritodrine administration after the 20th week of gestation has not been associated with an increase in fetal abnormalities.
Methergine	C	Indicated for postpartum uterine bleeding. According to the manufacturer, oral methylergonovine 0.2 milligram 3-to 4-times daily may be administered to nursing mothers for a MAXIMUM of 1 week postpartum to control uterine bleeding
Pain Medication		
Acetaminophen	B	Acetaminophen is considered safe for short term use in all stages of pregnancy
Aspirin	C	**Avoid in pregnancy.** However if absolutely needed, doses of 80 mg per day may be used. Avoid full dose aspirin in third trimester due to potential for bleeding complication in the newborn and prolongation of gestation and labor.
Non-steroidal anti-inflammatory drugs (NSAIDs)	C	**Avoid in pregnancy.** Due to the prostaglandin synthesis inhibition, constriction of ductus arteriosus has been reported. Persistent pulmonary hypertension in the newborn has occurred when NSAIDs were used in 3rd trimester or near term. NSAIDs have been shown to inhibit labor and prolong pregnancy.
Narcotic analgesic	B	Narcotic analgesics can be used short term in . pregnancy. **Avoid the use of high doses for prolong periods near term as neonatal withdrawal can occur.**

XIV

TABLE 14-7: ALTERNATIVE/ COMPLIMENTARY MEDICATION TO AVOID IN PREGNANCY

DRUG NAME	ANIMAL DATA	HUMAN EXPERIENCE IN PREGNANCY	COMMENTS
Vitamin A	A known teratogen at high doses in animal data.	A double-blind randomized trial of low dose supplementation with Vitamin A or beta carotene (7,000 mcg retinol equivalent) in malnourished pregnant women reported a 40% decrease in newborn mortality (BMJ 1999 Feb 27; 318 (7183): 570-5). In a prospective case controlled study of 423 exposures to 10,000 IU vit A during the first 9 weeks. An increased risk of major malformations was not reported. (Teratology 1999 Jan; 59(1): 7-11)	Further research is needed to recommend Vitamin A intake. **Until more data are available it is prudent to consume only the recommended dietary allowance of 8,000 IU (which can be obtained by a balanced diet).**
Vitamin B6 *(in doses above 100 mg a day)*	None	None	**Avoid use of high doses in pregnancy.** **Possible health hazard: ataxia and peripheral neuropathy.** (FDA Statement before Senate Committee on Labor and Human Resources, Oct 21, 1993).

Table continues . . .

TABLE 14-7: ALTERNATIVE/ COMPLIMENTARY MEDICATION TO AVOID IN PREGNANCY *(continued)*

DRUG NAME	ANIMAL DATA	HUMAN EXPERIENCE IN PREGNANCY	COMMENTS
Niacin *(in doses above 500mg immediate-release or 750mg sustained-release)*	None	None	**Avoid use of high doses in pregnancy.** **Possible health hazard: GI symptoms (N/V/D, abdominal cramps); liver disease.** (FDA Statement before Senate Committee on Labor and Human Resources, Oct 21, 1993).
Selenium *(in doses of greater than 800-1000 mcg per day)*	None	None	**Avoid use of high doses in pregnancy.** **Possible health hazard: Tissue damage.** (FDA Statement before Senate Committee on Labor and Human Resources, Oct 21, 1993).
Ma-huang (Ephedra Sinica)	None	None	**Avoid use in pregnancy.** **The FDA warns against using Ma-huang (Ephedra Sinica) due to possible health hazards including: high blood pressure, irregular heartbeat, nerve damage, injury, insomnia, tremor, headache, seizure, heart attack, stroke, and death (FDA Statement before Senate Committee on Labor and Human Resources, Oct 21, 1993). Over 500 reports of adverse events including 8 fatalities have been reported to the FDA. (MMWR August 16,1996).**
St John's Wort (Hypericum perforatum)	None	None	Meta-analysis of St John's wort suggests that it was more effective than placebo and as effective as low dose tricyclic antidepressants for short-term management of mild-to-moderately severe depression. (J Nervous and Mental dis 1999; 187 (9), 532-538). **Due to the lack of data in pregnancy the routine use of St John's Wort cannot be recommended.** **Major drug interaction:** Indinavir trough concentration (Cmin) decreases by 81% when co-administered with St John's wort.

Table continues . . . .

XIV

TABLE 14-7: ALTERNATIVE/ COMPLIMENTARY MEDICATION TO AVOID IN PREGNANCY *(continued)*

DRUG NAME	ANIMAL DATA	HUMAN EXPERIENCE IN PREGNANCY	COMMENTS
Chaparral herb (traditional American Indian medicine)	None	None	**Avoid use in pregnancy.** **Possible health hazard: liver disease, possibly irreversible.** (FDA Statement before Senate Committee on Labor and Human Resources, Oct 21, 1993).
Comfrey herb	None	None	**Avoid in pregnancy.** **Possible health hazard: obstruction of blood flow to liver, possibly leading to death.** (FDA Statement before Senate Committee on Labor and Human Resources, Oct 21, 1993).
Slimming/ dieter's tea	None	None	**Avoid in pregnancy.** **Possible health hazard: nausea, diarrhea, vomiting, stomach cramps, chronic constipation, fainting, possibly death.** (FDA Statement before Senate Committee on Labor and Human Resources, Oct 21, 1993).
Germander herb	None	None	**Avoid in pregnancy.** **Possible health hazard: liver disease, possibly leading to death.** (FDA Statement before Senate Committee on Labor and Human Resources, Oct 21, 1993).
Lobelia herb (Indian tobacco)	None	None	**Avoid in pregnancy.** **Possible health hazard: respiratory distress, tachycardia, hypotension, and possibly coma and death at higher doses.** (FDA Statement before Senate Committee on Labor and Human Resources, Oct 21, 1993).
Magnolia-Stephania herb	None	None	**Avoid in pregnancy.** **Possible health hazard: renal failure which may be irreversible.** (FDA Statement before Senate Committee on Labor and Human Resources, Oct 21, 1993).

Table continues . . .

TABLE 14-7: ALTERNATIVE/ COMPLIMENTARY MEDICATION TO AVOID IN PREGNANCY *(continued)*

DRUG NAME	ANIMAL DATA	HUMAN EXPERIENCE IN PREGNANCY	COMMENTS
Willow bark herb	None	None	**Avoid in pregnancy.** **Possible health hazard: allergic reaction (marketed as aspirin-free product, although it actually contains a precursor of aspirin with subsequent conversion to aspirin.)** (FDA Statement before Senate Committee on Labor and Human Resources, Oct 21, 1993).
Wormwood herb	None	None	**Avoid in pregnancy.** **Possible health hazard: neurological symptoms, paresthesia, delirium and paralysis.** (FDA Statement before Senate Committee on Labor and Human Resources, Oct 21, 1993).
Germanium mineral	None	None	**Avoid in pregnancy.** **Possible health hazard: kidney damage, possibly death.** (FDA Statement before Senate Committee on Labor and Human Resources, Oct 21, 1993).
L-tryptophan amino acid	None	None	**Avoid in pregnancy.** **Possible heath hazard: eosinophilic myalgia syndrome, a potentially fatal blood dyscrasia. (FDA has limited its import into the US).** (FDA Statement before Senate Committee on Labor and Human Resources, Oct 21, 1993).

XIV

REFERENCES

[1] Sustiva (Efavirenz) Capsules Product Monograph. Wilmington: DE: DuPont Pharmaceutical; 1998.

[2] Shepard TH, Catalog of Teratogenic *Agents. 7th ed. Baltimore, MD: JHU, Press. 1992:* 206-7.

[3] Ndiaye O, Gbaguidi A, Ba M et al. Newborn infant with macrosomia: etiologic factors and perinatal complications. *Dakar Med* 1997: 42(2): 159-61.

[4] Crixivan (Indinavir) Capsules Product Monograph. West Point; Pa: Merck & Co; 1998.

[5] Connor E and Mofenson L. Zidovudine for the reduction of perinatal human immunodeficiency virus transmission: Pediatric AIDS Clinical Trials Group Protocol 076-results and treatment recommendations. *Pediatric Infect. Dis J*, 1995; 14:536-41.

[6] Hanson C, Antonelli TA; Sperling RS et al. Lack of tumors in infants with perinatal HIV exposure and fetal neonatal exposure to zidovudine. *J Acquir Immune Defic Syndr Hum Retrovirol* 1999 Apr 15;20(5):463-7

[7] Guay LA, Musoke P; Fleming T et al. Intrapartum and neonatal single-dose nevirapine compared with zidovudine for prevention of mother-to-child transmission of HIV-1 in Kampala, Uganda: HIVNET 012 randomized trial. *Lancet* 1999 Sep 4; 354(9181): 795-802.

[8] Dunihoo DR. Maternal physiology. In: Dunihoo DR, editor. *Fundamentals of Gynecology and Obstetrics.* Philadelphia: J.B. Lippincott Co. 1992: 280-4

[9] Parry E, Shields R, Turnbull A. Transit time in the small intestine in pregnancy. *J Obstet Gynaecol Br Commonw* 1970; 77:900-1.

[10] Davidson JM, Hytten FE. Glomerular filtration during and after pregnancy. *J Obstet Gynaecol* 1974; 81: 588-95.

[11] Mirochnick M; Fenton T; Gagnier P et al. Pharmacokinetics of nevirapine in human immunodeficiency virus type 1- infected pregnant women and their neonates. Pediatric AIDS Clinical Trials Group Protocol 250 Team. *J Infect Dis* 1998 Aug;178(2):368-74.

[12] Pharmacokinetic and antiretroviral acitivity of lamivudine alone or when coadministered with zidovudine in human immunodeficiency virus type 1-infected pregnant women and their offspring.

[13] Schuman P; Kauffman R; Crane LR et al. Pharmacokinetics of zidovudine during pregnancy. Int Conf AIDS. 1990 Jun 20-23; 6 (2): 94 (abstract no. F.B.17)

[14] Wang Y; Liningston E; Patil S et al. Pharmacokinetics of didanosine in antepartum and postpartum human immunodeficiency virus-infected pregnant women and their neonates: an AIDS clinical trial group study. *JID* 1999 Nov; 180(5): 1536-41.

[15] Briggs, Freeman and Yaffe; *Drugs in Pregnancy and Lactation: A Reference Guide to Fetal and Neonatal Risks,* Williams and Wilkins.

XV: RESOURCES
ARRANGED ACCORDING TO TOPIC

Topics included in this section are:

I. Clinical care

II. Clinical trials/research

III. Consumer resources

IV. Adherence

V. Adolescents

VI. Psychosocial care

VII. Substance abuse

VIII. Palliative care

IX. Prevention

X. Occupational exposure

XI. Professional associations

XII. International resources

If a resource is listed once, it is not listed under subsequent topics.

I. CLINICAL CARE/PRIMARY CARE

■ **AIDS Treatment Information Service (ATIS):** Provides all the PHS Treatment guidelines, updated as new data become available. ATIS also provides documents on general treatment information, anergy skin testing, nutrition and food safety, hepatitis C co-infection, and other relevant clinical topics.

- **http://www.hivatis.org**
- Public Health Service Treatment guidelines: **http://www.hivatis.org/trtgdlns.html**
  - ▶ Click on *Adult and Adolescent Treatment Guidelines**
  - ▶ Click on *Pediatric Treatment Guidelines**
  - ▶ Click on *Perinatal Guidelines*
  - ▶ Click on *Health Care Worker Exposure Guidelines*
  - ▶ Click on *Nonoccupational Exposure Considerations*

XV

> ▶ Click on *Opportunistic Infection Guidelines*
>
> ▶ Click on *Tuberculosis Guidelines*

*This document is periodically updated as new data become available.

- Other ATIS documents:
  - ▶ Click on *General Treatment Information*
  - ▶ Or click on *Drug Treatment*
  - ▶ Or click on *Hepatitis C Co-infection*
  - ▶ Or click on *Nutrition and Food Safety*
  - ▶ Or click on *ATIS Publication List*
  - ▶ Or click on *Anergy Skin Testing*
- ATIS by phone: 1-800-HIV-0440 (Monday-Friday 9am-7pm ET, and in Spanish); Fax: 301-519-6616; TTY: 800-480-3739

■ **AIDS Education and Training Centers Warmline:** Medical and health care professionals can call with questions on any topic related to HIV care.
- 1-800-933-3413
- Monday – Friday from 7:30 am to 5 pm, western standard time.

■ **Johns Hopkins University AIDS Service:** A comprehensive Web site of HIV information and resources, including publications, medical education, provider and consumer interactive forums for seeking answers to questions, and resources and information on managed care, epidemiology, prevention and treatment.
- http://www.hopkins-aids.edu.
- http://www.hopkins-aids.edu/publications/index_pub.html:
  - ▶ Click on *1999 Medical Management of HIV Infection*, John G. Bartlett, M.D (a comprehensive manual of HIV/AIDS treatment) To order a copy of this manual, call 1-800-787-1254.
  - ▶ Or click on *Hopkins HIV Report*, a bimonthly newsletter for practitioners. A range of topics, such as: *Update on STDs from IDSA*. To receive this newsletter free, write to *The Hopkins HIV Report*, P.O. Box 5252, Baltimore MD 21224, Attn: Distribution.

■ **University of California at San Francisco:** A comprehensive Web site of HIV information and resources.
- http://www.HIVInSite/ucsf.edu
  - ▶ Click on *The AIDS Knowledge Base* for the text of this comprehensive manual of HIV/AIDS treatment (**http://www.HIVInSite/ucsf.edu/akb/1997/**)

■ **The Body:** A comprehensive Web site of HIV information and resources, including complete library on AIDS Basics and Prevention, Treatment, Conferences, Quality of Life, and Government.
- http://www.thebody.com

■ **Aegis:** A comprehensive Web site of HIV information and resources. Clinical and treatment information as well as information on women and children. A very good source of up-to-date information from the mainstream press, professional journals, and legal and legislative sources.

- http://www.aegis.com
- Publications such as: *Guidelines for the education and foster care of children infected with HIV.*

■ **American Foundation for AIDS Research (AMFAR) Treatment Directory:** A list of treatments and treatment protocols, updated biannually (On-line and book form)

- http://www.amfar.org/td
- Or order from National AIDS Clearinghouse (listed under Prevention).

■ **Centers for Disease Control National Prevention Information Network:** Offers up-to-date epidemiological information, including downloadable slides, daily updates on HIV/AIDS, and patient-oriented information.

- http://www.cdcnpin.org/
- Daily news updates in both general media and professional journals
- Numerous resources: distance learning, description of and contact information for model centers, linkages to many other sites

■ **NIAID Database for Anti-HIV Compounds:** Computerized databases containing chemical structures and biological data have been established at the Division of AIDS (DAIDS) NIAID to monitor developments in the chemotherapy of HIV and opportunistic infections (OI's) and to serve as an information source. A portion of the HIV database is presented, and there are plans to make the entire database, consisting of more than 20,000 compounds, available on the Internet.

- http://www.niaid.nih.gov/daids/dtpdb

■ **FDA Background on Protease Inhibitors:** Profiles of the similarities and differences of each approved protease inhibitor, and provide useful information about dosing, storage, potential drug interactions, and therapeutic options.

- http://www.fda.gov/oashi/aids/piindex.html

■ **HIV Medication Guide:** A Web site providing drug information as well as software to assess for potential drug interactions.

- http://www.jag.on.ca/asp_bin/Main.asp
- Click on *HIV Medication Guide* 2.05 to download PC software with which to store information about patients (schedules, laboratory values including CD4+ and viral load, weight, etc. (in English and French)
- Or click on *pamphlets* for patient information pamphlets on antiretroviral agents.

xv

- CD-ROM version for $20 USD call (705) 523-1782 or write: JAG enterprises, 2408 South Shore Road, Sudbury, Ontario P3G 1M3

- This site is made possible by an unrestricted educational grant from Glaxo Wellcome and BioChem Pharma

■ **Resistance mutations:** Web sites that deal with viral resistance to anti-retrovirals.

- http://www.viral-resistance.com

- http://www.hiv-web.lanl.gov

■ **New York Online Access to Health (NOAH):** The NY State Web site on health provides a range of topics relevant to HIV/AIDS and women.

- http://www.noah.cuny.edu/about.html

  ➤ Click on *Health topics*, then click on *HIV/AIDS*

  ➤ Then click on *Gender, age and race* for numerous topics (such as menstrual problems) and resources

■ **AIDS Alliance for Children, Youth & Families** (formerly the AIDS Policy Center for Children, Youth & Families): The national association providing advocacy, education and support for children and families affected by HIV/AIDS.

- http://www.aids-alliance.org

■ **Health Care Financing Administration (HCFA):** The federal agency that administers the Medicare, Medicaid and Child Health Insurance Programs.

- http://www.hcfa.gov

- Preventing HIV transmission:
  http://www.hcfa.gov/hiv/babies.htm

- The Maternal AIDS Project:
  http://www.hcfa.gov/hiv/subpg6.htm

■ **National Pediatric & Family HIV Resource Center (NPHRC):** A comprehensive Web site of HIV information and resources for professionals who care for children, adolescents and families with HIV infection and AIDS.

- http://www.pedHIVAIDS.org

- To order the *Pediatric Treatment Guidelines* and other documents:

  ➤ http://www.pedHIVAIDS.org/catalog

  ➤ Or call: 1-800-448-0440 or (800) 362-0071

  ➤ Or write to: University of Medicine and Dentistry, 30 Bergen Street, ADMC #4, Newark, NJ 07107

  ➤ Fax: (973) 972-0399

- Publications (in English and Spanish) include:

  ➤ *HIV and AIDS in Children: Questions and Answers*

  ➤ *The Family Information Guide*

> ➤ *What Women Need to Know: The HIV Treatment Guidelines for Pregnant Women*
>
> ➤ *Women's Initiative for HIV Care and Reduction of Perinatal Transmission (WIN): Program Findings*
>
> ➤ *Medication Adherence for Children and Families: Guidelines for Assessment and Support*

■ **National Library of Medicine (NLM):** Literature searches of the professional medical and HIV/AIDS-related literature including abstracts from relevant conferences.

● **http://www.nlm.nih.gov**

➤ Then click on *Medline*;

➤ Then click on *Internet Grateful Med.*

■ **HIV Dent:** Information on the dental manifestations of HIV and AIDS, including information for persons living with HIV/AIDS and their dental care providers.

● **http://www.hivdent.org**

■ **The Journal of the American Medical Association:** HIV/AIDS site with an extensive array of information for providing clinical care to people living with HIV and AIDS.

● **http://www.ama-assn.org/special/hiv/hivhome.htm**

■ **The Kaiser Family Foundation (KFF):** Provides numerous publications about HIV/AIDS policy and the healthcare system, such as *Medicaid and HIV/AIDS Policy: A Basic Primer*

● **http://www.kff.org**

■ **The HRSA HIV/AIDS Bureau (HAB):** The Web site of the Federal agency that administers the Ryan White CARE Act funding (Health Resources and Services Administration – HRSA). Numerous types of information related to models of care for women:

● **http://www.hrsa.gov/HAB**

➤ Click on *Title IV-Women, Infants, Children, and Youth*

➤ Click on *SPNS-Special Projects of National Significance*

♦ Then click on *SPNS Snapshots* for model programs for women, youth, and homeless youth;

♦ Or click on *New SPNS Initiatives*:

■ Then click on *adherence to anti-retroviral therapies,*

■ Or *palliative care/end-of-life treatment for HIV positive individuals.*

■ Or *HIV care for incarcerated populations,*

■ Or *care for HIV positive substance abusers*

XV

- Publications: Numerous publications such as the ones listed below can be obtained by calling (301) 443-6652 or writing HIV/AIDS Bureau Office of Communications, 5600 Fishers Lane, Room 7-46, Rockville, Maryland 20857 or faxing (301) 443-0791

    ➤ *Helping Adolescents with HIV Adhere to HAART*— 1999

    ➤ *HIV Disease in Women of Color* — May 1999

    ➤ *Hispanics Living with HIV Disease: Barriers to Care* — April 1999

    ➤ *HIV/AIDS in Racial and Ethnic Minorities* — February 1999

    ➤ *Women and HIV/AIDS* — December 1998

■ **National Maternal and Child Health Clearinghouse:** Provides publications on topics related to maternal and child health, including HIV/AIDS.

- Write: 2070 Chain Bridge Road, Suite 450,Vienna, VA 22182-2536
- Phone: (703) 356-1964

II. CLINICAL TRIALS/RESEARCH

■ **AIDS Clinical Trials and Women:** The ATIS Web site provides women-specific information.

- **http://www.hivatis.org/womninfo.html**
    ➤ Click on *NIAID Resources for Studying HIV/AIDS in Women*

■ **AIDS Clinical Trials Information Service (ACTIS):** Nationwide access to NIH-funded clinical trials at this Web site and phone number.

- **http://www.actis.org**
- 1-800-874-2572, TDD 1-800-243-7012

■ **Pediatric AIDS Clinical Trials:** Nationwide access to Pediatric AIDS Clinical Trials.

- **http://www.pactg.s-3.com**

■ **AIDS Clinical Trials Group:** The Web site for the NIH-funded AIDS Clinical Trials Groups. No.

- **http://www.actg.s-3.com**

■ **Terry Beirn Community Programs for Clinical Research on AIDS(CPCRA):** A network of research units composed of community-based health care providers who offer their patients the opportunity to participate in research where they get their health care.

- **http://www.cpcra.org**

■ **The Bulletin of Experimental Treatments for AIDS (BETA),** is published four times a year by the San Francisco AIDS Foundation:

- **http://www.sfaf.org/treatment**

- Or Contact *BETA*, 10 U.S. Plaza No. 660, San Francisco, CA 94102.
- 1-800-959-1059 or 415-487-8060.

III. CONSUMER RESOURCES

■ **Project Inform:** A national project targeting consumers with up-to-date treatment information, strategies for adherence, and other tools for people living with HIV.
- **http://www.Projectinform.org**
  - ➤ Click on *Wise Women* for the newsletter *WISE Words*
  - ➤ Or click on *Fact Sheets* for topics such as gynecological problems
  - ➤ Or click on other categories of information, such as treatment information and an extensive list of consumer organizations around the country.
- Phone: 1-800-822-7422
- Project WISE EMail Address: WISE@projinf.org

■ **Women Alive:** An organization by and for women living with HIV
- **http://www.women-alive.org**
- National treatment hot line: 1-800-554-4876
- Phone: 323-965-1564
- e-mail: info@women-alive.org
- Now available free: "Knowledge, Action, Health A woman's guide to HIV treatments" (Tambien en espanol)

■ **The Community AIDS Treatment Information Exchange (CATIE):** A Canadian network that provides information on the treatment options available to people living with HIV/AIDS, including drugs, other medical treatments and complementary therapies, in English and French
- **http://www.catie.ca**

■ **New Jersey Women and AIDS Network:** A hotline staffed by women with HIV. Also provides information and advocacy for women with HIV/AIDS.
- 1-800-747-1108 M-F 9-5 ET
- Publications include *NJWAN Newsletter; Pregnancy and You; Me First; Medical Manifestations of HIV in Women.*

■ **Women Organized to Respond to Life-threatening Disease (WORLD):** Organization for women with HIV that provides peer advocacy, treatment education training and retreats for HIV positive women (HIV University).
- **http://www.womenhiv.org**
- 1-510-986-0340 M-F 10-6 PST
- Newsletter: *WORLD.*

■ **Seattle Treatment Education Project (STEP):** Agency that provides treatment information for people with HIV/AIDS, healthcare providers, and ASOs, including a peer-staffed Treatment TalkLine.

- http://www.thebody.com/step/steppage.html
- 1-206-329-4857 M-F 1-5 PST
- Or call (877) 597-STEP [7837] toll-free, from the Pacific Northwest: Washington, Oregon, Idaho, Alaska, and Montana.
- Publications include *Step Perspective; Babes Perspective* (for women)

■ **PWA Health Group:** Organization that provides treatment education and support, advocacy, policy and early treatment programs, and information about alternative treatments. It started as an AIDS buyers' when there were no approved drugs for AIDS, to import promising therapies from other countries. The PWA Health Group was founded in 1987 by Thomas Hannan and Michael Callen, both people with AIDS, and their doctor, Joseph Sonnabend, as a not-for-profit organization.

- http://www.aidsinfonyc.org/pwahg
- 1-212-255-0520 M-F 10-6, Sa 12-4 ET
- Publications include *Notes from the Underground; Smart Women*

■ **Critical Path AIDS Project:** Comprehensive HIV/AIDS Web site. Founded by Persons With AIDS (PWAs) to provide treatment, resource, and prevention information in wide-ranging levels of detail — for researchers, service providers, treatment activists, but first and foremost, for other PWAs who often find themselves in urgent need of information quickly and painlessly. Hosts other HIV/AIDS organizations..

- http://www.critpath.org

■ **HIV/AIDS Phone resources:**

- National AIDS Hotline: 1-800-342-2437, Spanish 1-800-344-7432, TDD 1-800-243-7889
- AIDS Clinical Trials Information Service (ACTIS) : 1-800-874-2572, TDD 1-800-243-7012
- HIV/AIDS Treatment Information Service (ATIS): 1-800-448-0440, TDD 1-800-243-7012, 1-888-480-3739
- CDC National Prevention Information Network: 1-800-458-5231, TDD 1-800-243-7012
- AIDS Treatment Data Network: 1-800-734-7104
- National AIDS Treatment Advocacy Project (NATAP): 212-219-0106
- 1-888-26 NATAP
- Treatment Action Group: 212-260-0300
- National Minority AIDS Council: 202-483-6622

- National Association of People with AIDS: 202-898-0414
- Latino Commission on AIDS (CIEST): 212-675-3288
- The Mother's Initiative: 1-800-828-3280 (Mothers available to talk)
- Community Prescription Service: 1-800-842-0502
- Direct AIDS Alternative Information Resources: 1-888-951-5433

■ **Other Phone resources:**
  - STD Hotline: 1-800-227-8922, TDD 1-800-243-7889
  - National Institute on Drug Abuse Hotline: 1-800-662-HELP (4357), 1-800-66-AYUDA (662-9832)
  - National Drug and Alcohol Treatment Referral Service: 1-800-662-4357
  - Cocaine Treatment: 1-800-COCAINE
  - Al-A-Teen: 1-800-344-2666
  - Marijuana treatment: 1-800-766-6779
  - Domestic violence local phone numbers of domestic violence hotlines: 1-800-SAFE, TDD 1-800-787-3224

IV. ADHERENCE

■ **The HIV/AIDS Project Development and Evaluation Unit (HAPDEU)** Online and downloadable guide for the development of HIV antiretroviral treatment adherence programs
  - http://www.hapdeu.org/adherence
  - HIV/AIDS Client Services and Early Intervention Program, P.O. Box 47841, Olympia, WA 98504
  - Or call: Audie Lemke at (206) 685-1679.

■ **University of San Francisco HIVInSite Adherence Resources:**
  - http://www.HIVInSite.ucsf.edu/topics/adherence/2098. 4504.html
  - Resources include:
    - ➤ AIDS Education and Training Center Adherence Curriculum by Helen Miramontes and Linda Frank, 1999.
    - ➤ ACTG Adherence Baseline Questionnaire
    - ➤ ACTG Adherence Follow Up Questionnaire

■ **The Body: Treatment Strategies for HIV/AIDS**
  - http://www.thebody.com/treat/adherence.html

XV

V. ADOLESCENTS

■ **Health Initiatives for Youth (HIFY):** Adolescent health information, and youth education and advocacy.
   ● **http://www.hify.com**
   ● 1-415-487-5777

■ Publications:

   ► Chabon, B and Futterman, D. Adolescents and HIV. *AIDS Clinical Care* 11(2):9-16.

   ► DiClemente, Ralph J. *Adolescents and AIDS: A Generation in Jeopardy.* Newbury Park, CA: SAGE Publications, 1992.

   ► Hoffman ND, Futterman D, Myerson A. Treatment Issues for HIV+ Adolescents. *AIDS Clinical Care* 11(3):17-24.

   ► Ryan, C. and Futterman, D. *Lesbian and Gay Youth: Care and Counseling.* New York: Columbia University Press, 1998.

■ Also see Substance Abuse Resources related to adolescents.

VI. PSYCHOSOCIAL CARE

■ **National directory of state and local hotlines** for rape crisis centers and other services for women in distress:
   ● **http://www.feminist.org/911/harass_af.html**

■ **National Domestic Violence Hotline**
   ● **http://www.feminist.org/911/crisis.html**
   ● Telephone: 1-800-799-SAFE (7233), or 1-800-787-3224 (TDD)
   ● Staffed 24 hours a day by trained counselors who can provide crisis assistance and information about shelters, legal advocacy, health care centers, and counseling.

■ **National Clearinghouse on Child Abuse and Neglect Information**
   ● **http://www.calib.com/nccanch**
   ● Telephone: (800) 394-3366 or (703) 385-7565
   ● A national resource for professionals seeking information on the prevention, identification, and treatment of child abuse and neglect and related child welfare issues.

■ **The American Psychological Association Office on AIDS:** Information, training, and technical assistance on a wide range of HIV/AIDS-related topics associated with coping, mental health services, prevention, technology transfer, community collaboration, public policy, and ethics.
   ● **http://www.apa.org/pi/aids/activities.html**
   ● Provides the APA HOPE Program: Federally funded program for

training mental health providers about working with people with
HIV\AIDS.

- Also publications such as the Psychology and AIDS Exchange
  Newsletter.

■ *The Invisible Epidemic: The Story of Women and AIDS.* By Gena Corea.
NY: HarperCollins, 1992.

VII. SUBSTANCE ABUSE

■ **National Clearinghouse for Alcohol and Drug Information (NCADI):**
Numerous documents on diagnosis and treatment of substance abuse,
including specific to people living with HIV and vulnerable populations,
including youth.

- http://www.health.org/pubs/hivaids.htm
- http://www.health.org/pubs/catalog/intr.htm or call 1-800-729-
  6686
- 1-800-729-6686, TDD 1-800-487-4889

VIII. PALLIATIVE CARE

■ *A Handbook for Palliative Care* By Linda Wrede-Seaman, MD

- Published by Intellicard 2nd Edition: 1999, ISBN: 188841107-4
- Decision algorithms for assessment and management of pain and
  common symptoms in terminal illness.

■ *Recovering from the Loss of a Loved One to AIDS Help for Surviving Family, Friends, and Lovers Who Grieve* By Katherine Fair Donnelly. Fawcett
Books,1995

■ **Growth House Search Engine:** Comprehensive database for end of life
issues, including death with dignity, hospice, palliative care, grief, bereavement, and related topics.

- http://www.growthhouse.org/search.htm

■ *The Oxford Textbook of Palliative Medicine*, 2nd edition.

IX. PREVENTION

■ **The National AIDS Clearinghouse**

- 1-800-458-5231
- Provides numerous free prevention documents on specific topics such
  as: *What are adolescents' prevention needs? And How do HIV, STD and
  unintended pregnancy prevention work together?*

XV

■ **Nonoccupational HIV Exposure Guidelines:**

- http://www.hivatis.org/trtgdlns.html
  - ➤ Click on *Non-occupational exposure*

■ **Perinatal HIV prevention:**

- http://www.hivatis.org/trtgdlns.html
  - ➤ Click on *Perinatal Guidelines*
- http://www.hivatis.org/womninfo.html
  - ➤ Click on *National Pediatric and Family HIV Resource Center*
  - ➤ Then click on *Perinatal prevention*
  - ➤ Then click on *Research Literature Updates:*
    - ♦ *What Women Need to Know: The HIV Treatment Guidelines for Pregnant Women*
    - ♦ *Reduction of Perinatal HIV Transmission: Guide for Providers* (May 1997)

■ *Reducing the Odds: Preventing Perinatal Transmission of HIV in the United States:* National Academy of Science Report on perinatal transmission.

- http://www.nap.edu/readingroom/books/rto

X. OCCUPATIONAL EXPOSURE

■ **HRSA/CDC National Clinicians' Post-Exposure Prophylaxis Hotline (PEPline)**

- National toll-free hotline to help counsel and treat health care workers with job-related exposure to blood-borne diseases and infections, including hepatitis and HIV infection.
- 1-888-448-4911

■ *PHS Guidelines for the Management of Health Care Worker Exposures to HIV and Recommendations for Post Exposure Prophylaxis.*

- http://www.cdc.gov/epo/mmwr/preview/mmwrhtml/ 00052722.htm
- Guidelines published 15 May 1998

XI. PROFESSIONAL ASSOCIATIONS

■ **International Association of Physicians in AIDS Care (IAPAC)** This organization provides on its Web site policy information about ongoing efforts to expand access to healthcare services and life-saving drugs and technologies.

- http://www.iapac.org
- Phone: 312 795-4930

- Publications include the monthly *Journal of the International Association of Physicians in AIDS Care*

■ **Association of Nurses in AIDS Care (ANAC)** Professional association that provides information and advises members about clinical and policy issues related to nursing and HIV care.

- http://www.anacnet.org
- 1-800-260-6780
- Publications include the monthly *Journal of Nurses in AIDS Care.*
- ANAC is responsible for development of the HIV/AIDS Nursing Certification Board, which provides nationally recognized HIV/AIDS Certification (ACRN), based on eligibility requirements and successful completion of the certification exam.
- http://www.ptcny.com
- Call 202-356-0660

■ **American College of Obstetricians and Gynecologists (ACOG)** Professional association that provides resources to and advises members about a range of issues such as domestic violence and cultural competency.

- http://www.acog.org
- Resource center: 1-800-762-2264
- Publications include a newsletter and an annual compendium of selected publications, including educational and technical bulletins.

XII. INTERNATIONAL RESOURCES

■ **The Panos Institute:**

- http://www.oneworld.org/panos
  - ► Click on *HIV/AIDS*
  - ► Or click on *Women and Health*

■ **Integrated Regional Information Network**

- ► Click on *Publications*
- ► Then click on *Non-U.S. Groups*
- ► Then click on *IRIN* for publications such as:
  - ♦ "UN says violence against women linked to HIV/AIDS"
  - ♦ "New research links high HIV rates in teenage girls"

■ *Women's Experiences: An International Perspective.* Long, Lynellyn D and Ankrah, E Maxine, Eds. NY: Columbia University Press, 1996.

■ **The Joint UN Programme on AIDS (UNAIDS):** Offers up-to-date epidemiological and other data that can be downloaded.

- http://www.unaids.org

XV

This *Guide* is a PRELIMINARY EDITION.

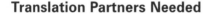

We need YOUR HELP to make the NEXT EDITION as useful as possible!

Please send your
comments
criticisms
corrections
suggested changes, and
other guidance
to one of the addresses below. Be sure to include in your letter/note an address (fax, e-mail, or postal) where you can be reached for follow-up.

Translation Partners Needed

Write to us if you can help us find partners to help us have this *Guide* translated into your native language. For instance, provide us with a contact who works with translation in your country's Ministry of Health, or tell us about a group at a medical school that translates medical texts.

Send Us Your Comments

E-mail: womencare@hrsa.gov

Fax to the attention of "Womencare": 301-443-0791 (USA)

Postal address: Womencare
Parklawn Building, Room 11A-33
5600 Fishers Lane
Rockville, Maryland 20857
USA

Note that this and subsequent editions of
A Guide to the Clinical Care of Women with HIV
will be available online.

Go to the HIV/AIDS Bureau Web site
and click on the publication *Women's Guide*:
http://www.hrsa.gov/hab

INDEX

> *Note:* Because this is a preliminary editon, this Index is also preliminary. It's future development depends on you, and we welcome your input.
>
> ### Send Us Your Comments
> *E-mail:* womencare@hrsa.gov
> *Fax to the attention of* "Womencare": 301-443-0791 (USA)
> *Postal address:* Womencare
> Parklawn Building, Room 11A-33
> 5600 Fishers Lane
> Rockville, Maryland 20857
> USA

INDEX

INDEX

INDEX